namaslay

ROCK YOUR YOGA PRACTICE,
TAP INTO YOUR GREATNESS, AND DEFY YOUR LIMITS

by **candace moore**

Victory Belt Publishing

Las Vegas

First Published in 2016 by Victory Belt Publishing Inc.

ISBN-13: 978-1-628601-12-1

The information included in this book is for educational purposes only. It is not intended or implied to be a substitute for professional medical advice. The reader should always consult his or her healthcare provider to determine the appropriateness of the information for his or her own situation or if he or she has any questions regarding a medical condition or treatment plan. Reading the information in this book does not create a physician-patient relationship.

Book design by Yordan Terziev and Boryana Yordanova

Printed in Canada
TC 0116

"You've been criticizing yourself for too long.
Try approving of yourself and see what happens."

—LOUISE HAY

For my Sittee, Mary Palmer, who
always said, "You can have any. thing.
you want." (She was referring to food
in her house, but I've come to realize
that my grandmother's little mantra is
applicable to life in general.)

TABLE OF CONTENTS

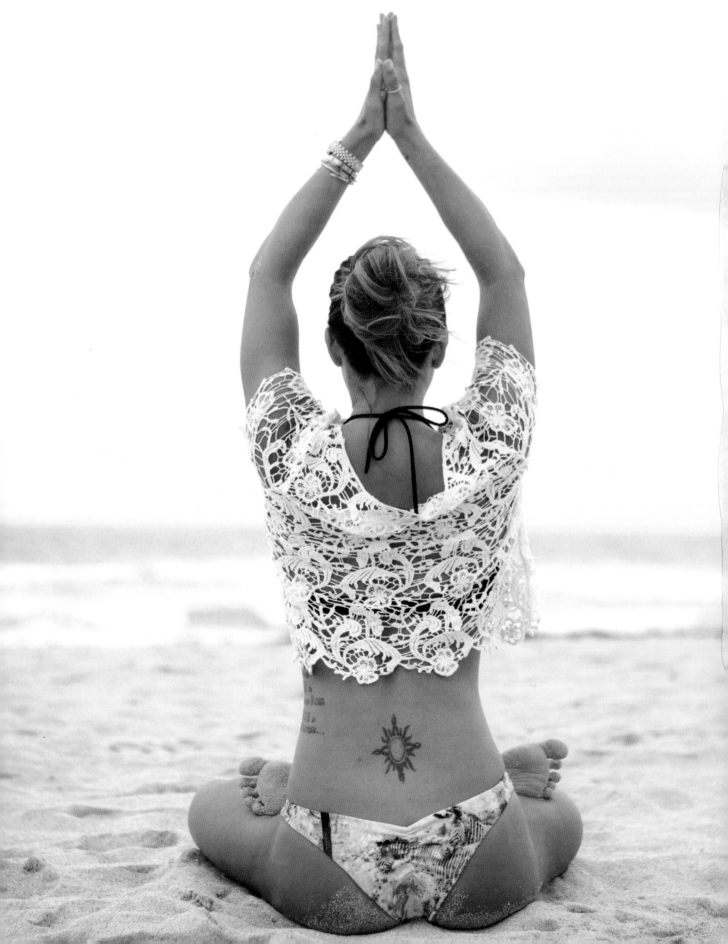

introduction

I don't know about you, but when I look back on years past, I shake my head at all the time I wasted. I wasted a lot of time being angry, irritable, and way too hard on myself. I made decisions based on fear, and my life was dominated by stress. Approaching life with a victim mentality, I wore a permanent scowl. It felt like life was always out to get me. I was anxious and depressed, and I constantly felt like I was on the defensive.

And then one day, everything changed. I was bitten by a dog, and I subsequently fell ill. Really, really ill. The dog bite was the beginning of the most horrific chapter of my life. The mystery illness shook me to my core. It took away my ability to walk, and about eight months in, it invaded my brain to the point that I couldn't quite comprehend the words of those around me.

The disease stole years of my life. My friends were getting married, buying houses, and having babies; their lives were moving forward, evolving, filled with light and laughter. And there I was, laid up in bed in a dark, stale room, with my physical and emotional health declining day by day. I had no answers as to why my health continued to deteriorate, despite having consulted with doctor after doctor.

When I tell my story, people sometimes look at me with eyes like saucers and exclaim, "Oh, you poor thing!"

I used enjoy this. I used to revel in the Poor Me's. It was a comfortable spot.

But then I realized that the Poor Me's aren't the place to be. Nothing good happens there. So I turned the Poor Me's into an attitude of gratitude.

Yeah, you read that right. I am grateful for that mystery illness. For the lost time. For all the doctor consults and the coming up empty. For the thousands of dollars in medical bills. For the uncertainty. For the depression. For finally getting a diagnosis. For the struggle of not knowing whether I'd ever get better.

If your brow is furrowed and you're wondering how in the world someone can be grateful for the absolute worst time of her life, I get it. But when you are brought to your knees and dragged through your darkest hour, you are left with a decision.

One option is to lie down and give in to the Poor Me's. Now, I've been using "the Poor Me's" as a cutesy way to describe absolute misery. So let's get rid of the cute. What I'm really talking about here is lying down and giving in to the darkness, the emptiness, the despair that you feel when you are going through what seems like hell on earth. Lying down, admitting that you don't have the strength to fight anymore, and letting yourself burn.

Or you can get back up and find your way out, arms outstretched like Frankenstein's as you feel your way through the smoke, danger, and confusion. Rely on your blind faith in your own strength.

I chose to get back up.

Not literally, because I physically could not get up. But figuratively, I got back up. I listened to the little voice within that said, "Actually, I can," and opened my arms, surrendering to something bigger than me and trusting that my strength, courage, and innate wisdom would get me through.

Perhaps at this point you're flipping to the cover to make sure that you picked up the right book. You might be thinking, *It's a yoga book, right? What does this have to do with anything?*

Yeah, this is a yoga book. But yoga is not just the pretzel poses that you see on social media. Yoga is not just inspirational quotes and playful transitions and creative sequences. Sure, those are cool and sometimes inspiring, and I'm not going to lie to you—I will double-tap those pics faster than you can say "one-handed handstand on your fingertips," but really, that's not all there is to yoga.

Yoga is a state of being. The word *yoga* means "union." As in, we're in this together. As in, you are not alone. And that's ultimately what I want you to take away from this book. We're not separate. I'm not special because I got through the worst time of my life. I don't have any more talent or wisdom than you do. We *all* bring significant value to the table. I'm just showing up (Sheryl Sandberg would be so proud) and sharing what I know to be true based on my experiences.

Yes, one of the components of yoga is a physical practice. The downward dogs, the child's poses, and even the one-handed handstands on your fingertips. But through the physical practice, something pretty incredible happens. When you look closely, the practice is reflective of your life, your thoughts, and your spirit.

If you're new to yoga and you're rolling your eyes at this woo-woo mumbo jumbo, I totally get you. There is little that irritates me more than taking a trip down flowery language lane, circling 'round and 'round and not getting to the point. But please hear me out: I am a dreamer, but I take my brain with me.

This book that you're holding in your hands? It's about yoga—the way of life *and* the poses. It's about struggle. It's about digging deep and tapping into your inherent greatness. It's about going through the worst of the worst, being brought to your knees, taking a cold, hard look at the person you are, and making a decision about what you will *do*.

This decision about what you will do? You make it every single day. You don't have to be sick with a mystery illness. You make this choice every morning before your feet hit the floor.

So I implore you to ask yourself: *How am I doing?*

It sounds so simple, but our lives are fast-paced. We have jobs to work, groceries to shop for, and bills to pay. We have kids to chauffeur around, laundry to do, dinners to make, and lawns to mow. Ain't nobody got time to stop and check in with how we're doing!

But chances are, if you're reading this book, you do have a minute to spare. So take a second and do it right now. On a scale of 1 to 10, with 1 being as miserable as a bride with food poisoning on her wedding day and 10 being as happy as an audience member on an episode of Oprah's "Favorite Things," how are you *doing?*

If you're below an 8, keep reading. This book will help inspire you both on and off the yoga mat. It'll help you find your way to a 9 or even a 10.

If you're at 8 or above, put the book down; you don't need it.

Just kidding! Keep reading, then reach out to me on social media with your tips for living a fulfilling life. Because above all, this book is about sharing insights, experiences, and knowledge. Remember, we're in this together. Yoga. Union. One-handed handstand on your fingertips.

So what, exactly, is Namaslay?

Namaslay is a life philosophy that mixes old-world yogic principles with a modern can-do attitude. It marries *Namaste,* the ancient yogic greeting that means "the light in me acknowledges the light in you," and *slay,* which means "to slaughter." But for our purposes, *slay* is not meant literally. I am not encouraging you to go out and kill anyone. Rather, it's meant figuratively, as in, go out there and kill it at whatever it is you're working at—your job, your relationship, your *life.*

Are you scratching your head and wondering, *How can two polar opposites come together like this? Isn't* slay *a little, um, violent for a yogic life philosophy?*

Nah. It's the yin and yang coming together and working as one. Yoga. Union. Let me explain.

In yogic philosophy, *niyamas* are guidelines for self-discipline. The five niyamas are as follows:

- SAUCHA means "cleanliness," and yeah, while we want to be physically clean (pro tip: it's a good idea to bathe regularly; you're welcome), it's also important to evaluate the cleanliness of everything around you. How is the energy that you're bringing onto your yoga mat? With what kind of attitude do you approach your work, your relationships, and even your daily errands? How clean is your diet? Tune in to each facet of your life and see where you can do a little tidying up.

- SANTOSA is about manifesting contentment with whatever it is you're going through. This doesn't mean that you have to keep a giant smile plastered to your face. You don't have to be happy 100 percent of the time. Rather, it's about seeing the bigger picture and letting go of singular events. So I got a mystery illness and lost the ability to walk for a while. Am I supposed to just laugh it off in the name of santosa? No. It's fine (and normal!) to fear the unknown. It's fine (and normal!) to feel angry, sad, and frustrated. Feel it. Feel it *fully.* Cry it out, kick it out, or dance it out, but then? Move on. Move *forward.* Decide what you will do and *go do it.*

- TAPAS is about discipline and passion. It's about developing the determination to live your life without getting in your own way. And man, we *really* get in our own way. Take the yoga practice, for instance. Maybe you're in class and the teacher has you holding what feels like eight hundred breaths in warrior 2. Your arms are shaking, you have sweat dripping out of places that shouldn't be sweating, and you aren't sure whether you want to cry, scream, storm out of the room, or at least get out of the pose. But instead, you take a deep breath. You let go of your thoughts and trust that you can do anything you put your mind to and work toward. This is honing the tapas. So you flick the switch in your mind and continue to hold the pose for the rest of the eight hundred breaths. Because you, my friend, are Namaslayin' it.

- SVADHYAYA means "self-study," and it is my favorite of the niyamas. It wasn't until I came down with the mystery illness that I truly started to get to know myself. And when you know who you are, things just fall into place in your life. That was one of the most valuable lessons I learned from my illness. But, if I'm being honest, what was maddening to me was that I'd lived in my body for twenty-five years before getting sick. I mean, how do you know someone for twenty-five years and *still* not really know who she is? Kind of a waste of time, right? So take every opportunity to get to know yourself. Think about what your actions, words, and choices say about you—even in seemingly meaningless situations (although, full disclosure, there is no such thing), like what you say to the barista at your local coffee haunt. If you're not doing, saying, and being what you want to do, say, and be, adjust accordingly. You are in charge of your own life.

- ISHVARAPRANIDHANA is about surrendering and trusting that everything is happening exactly as it should. This is a tough one, especially if you've gone through some really difficult times. But Ishvarapranidhana is a big-picture thing, just like santosa. Essentially, it's about letting go and accepting that it is what it is. It's not an easy thing to do, I acknowledge that. So I understand if you're skeptical. And we've all gone through some awful stuff, so I can appreciate the tendency to want to shake your fist to the sky and say, "Really? My dad is diagnosed with cancer and I'm just supposed to *accept* it, no questions asked? It is what it *is*?!? No!"

On the other hand, acceptance makes life easier. When I had been bedridden for days, I reached a breaking point and felt like I was going crazy. I had been in mental and physical agony for so long, and there were no promises that I was going to get better. There came a time when I had to decide—either keep jamming out to the woe-is-me violin or throw the violin out the window, let it all go, and trust that everything would be okay in the end. Something magical happens when you surrender and choose to trust. Your world softens when you soften. Your world reflects love when you choose to love. And nothing feels as good as being able to walk through your world wrapped up in a soft love blanket. Okay, that sounds weird, but you get what I'm trying to say, right?

So how does all of that relate to Namaslay? Namaslay is a life philosophy that's based on these niyamas. Here are the Namaslay "commandments," if you will:

1. BELIEVE IN YOURSELF.

Know that deep within each and every one of us lies a strength and courage bigger than any obstacle we could ever encounter. Lead your life with confidence. And remember that confidence and ego are not the same thing. Confidence serves those around you; ego is self-serving and self-destructive. Be quietly secure, led by an undercurrent of determination, knowing how truly powerful you are.

2. GET OUT OF YOUR OWN WAY.

Both on the yoga mat and off, we are often filled with self-doubt. We put unnecessary pressure on ourselves, and we have these ideas about what we *should* be able to do or what we *should* have accomplished by now. This negative self-talk is no good. It holds us back from our inherent greatness. Whether it's a yoga pose that you've been working toward or a life goal that you've been striving to meet, make a conscious effort to get out of your own way. Stop clinging to limiting ideas about your abilities. Be kind and generous to yourself and to others. Start speaking to yourself like you would speak to someone you love. Get out of your own way.

3. CONTINUE TO LEARN.

Read everything. Take classes. Engage in conversation. Ask lots of questions. Befriend people who are not your age, who come from different backgrounds, who listen to different music, and who are in completely different lines of work. Even as you grow and become an expert in your own field, always maintain a beginner's mindset. Remember that everyone knows something you don't, and therefore we all have things to teach each other. We are all teachers. And the best teachers are the ones who know that there is always more to learn.

4. GET COMFORTABLE BEING UNCOMFORTABLE.

Comfort is a safe place, and it's a fine place to hang around. I'd even argue that it's a necessary place to be at certain times of your life, like when you're dealing with health issues or after you go through a rough breakup. But discomfort is where growth happens. So when you find yourself in a particularly challenging situation, see if you can set aside your worries and fears. Then take a deep breath and be fully present. Settle into your little nook carved out within the discomfort, pull out your imaginary notebook, and sit in on the lesson at hand. Continue to challenge yourself not just to endure uncomfortable situations, but to learn and prosper from them.

5.
DO THE
LITTLE THINGS.

Return your grocery cart. Call your grandma. Floss your teeth. Ask how the cashier is and listen to the response. Make eye contact and smile. Practice random acts of kindness. These are the things that bring us together, that connect us. Remember: Yoga. Union. Do the little things so often that they become habit, and watch how they add richness to your life.

6.
MANIFEST
GRATITUDE.

Look for ways to feel gratitude throughout your day, from the moment you wake up until the moment you go to sleep. Make "thank you" a daily mantra. While brushing your teeth—thank you for another day! While eating a bomb breakfast—thank you for this delicious food! I'm grateful for the sweet car I'm driving to work. Sure, it's a rust bucket, but it gets me from point A to point B, and the speakers work great! Look around you and count your blessings. Not only does it make life more enjoyable, but it physically transforms you internally. No joke! Feeling gratitude may lower your stress level, which alters what's going on chemically within you. As Janice Kaplan explains in her book *The Gratitude Diaries*, it also decreases cortisol, which may help reduce inflammation, improve your ability to sleep, and boost your metabolism. So say "thank you." It's like a verbal happy pill that you can't overdose on. Say it more.

7.
BE A
HELL YEAH
PERSON.

My favorite people are the ones who have a can-do attitude. I love these types of people because they bring good energy into every situation and pretty much march to an upbeat rhythm of "Hell Yeah!" What's better and more powerful than that? What's more *uplifting* than that? There's only one thing better than seeing a group of Hell Yeah people from afar, and that's *being* one of the Hell Yeah people.

So how do you do it? It's easy. You just do the opposite of what the No I Can't people do.

Do you know them? I do. I see them everywhere.

Sometimes they're in my yoga classes. I'll demonstrate a fun arm balance, and they will side-eye the people next to them and groan. "Ugh, I can't do that," they'll mutter. "Not with that attitude," I'll cheerfully respond. (I know, I know, I've turned into *that* yoga teacher!)

Ironically, since I used to be a No I Can't person, it blows my mind that people automatically assume they can't do something. They come from a boring little town called NoICan't. People there walk around all downcast and miserable. Worst town ever; don't go there.

Here's the annoyingly chipper truth: if you believe you can, you're halfway there. And that applies to anything from yoga poses to landing your dream job. However crazy your dreams may be, you've got to be a Hell Yeah person. A Hell Yeah person gets. shit. done.

If you want to be a Hell Yeah person but can't fully commit to saying "Hell Yeah" because you were raised not to say "Hell," try saying, "Why *not* me?" Say it often enough, and you'll be a Hell Yeah (or Heck Yeah) person before you know it. I believe in you because I am a Hell Yeah person, and I know you can do it.

8.
TAP INTO YOUR GREATNESS.

When you're doing all of the above, you're dialed in. You're tapping into your greatness—the greatness that we all have deep within us. And, oh man, when you're tapping into your greatness? There's really no better feeling. It's like being plugged into this buzzing electrical current of goodness. When you're plugged in, you are *on*. You are shining and vibrant and honoring all your gifts and talents. You're giving and receiving good things, and everything is in perfect harmony. Life just doesn't get any better than that.

9.
DEFY YOUR LIMITS.

When you're totally dialed in and tapping into your greatness, you'll discover that your limits were perceived. They weren't real. None of them.

All the things that you've picked on yourself for, all the lies that you've told yourself as you stared into the mirror, all the reasons you came up with for not being good enough over the years? None of that is the truth. Your imperfections are what make you the incredible person you are. Own who you are and watch how your so-called limits fizzle away.

10.
TAKE NO SHIT.

Think of your life as your great masterpiece—something you're constantly working on, with the goal of creating the most breathtaking, inspiring work of art you've ever seen. It's your piece; you're the artist. So edit, erase, and re-create as much as you need to in order to make your masterpiece.

So what does that mean in a real-world situation?

As you probably know, I run a popular yoga blog, YogaByCandace (you can find it at yogabycandace.com). I created this little space on the Internet, and somehow it attracted my kind of people. The people who comment on the posts and participate on our forum (forum.yogabycandace.com) are knowledgeable, funny, and inclusive. And because the Internet is pretty much Big Brother, I know that they log in everywhere from Brussels to Berlin to Brunei to Boston. They are students and doctors and fitness enthusiasts. They are stay-at-home moms and soldiers stationed overseas. They are professional dancers and people living with HIV. They are wine drinkers, vegans, and meat eaters. They are *kind*. And therefore, they are my kind of people. This didn't happen by accident. I attracted these people by being myself. Had I pretended to be someone else, I would've attracted people who were *not* my kind of people. Over the years, through our interactions online and in person at workshops and retreats, I've gotten to know some of these people well, and I absolutely adore them. Ah, the beauty of the Internet.

But, as you know, the Internet also has a dark side. A while back, I shared a snippet of my personal yoga practice on Instagram. I'd just started lifting weights more seriously, and I'd put on a little muscle. Someone commented that I was getting "too big" for yoga and implied that I should stop my workouts if I wanted to continue practicing yoga.

Immediately, I was hurt. I thought, A) *Eff you for your unsolicited opinion about my body composition,* and B) *Your comment implies that yoga is for some elite group.*

The latter point has always been a *thing* for me. We all have our things, you know? You've probably heard of this elitist yoga thing. This holier-than-thou thing. This you-can-only-practice-yoga-if-you're-rich-and-white-and-wear-lululemon thing. This you-can-only-practice-yoga-if-you-don't-drink-coffee-and-are-a-vegan thing. This you're-only-a-real-yogi-if-*insert-condition-here* thing.

Ugh. Drives. Me. *Ca-razy.*

Because this thing? It's the opposite of Yoga. Union. This thing creates a divide. And that, in my expert opinion, is BS.

So I had a choice. I could have a pity party for one, wallowing in the Poor Me's, or I could get up and speak my truth.

I got up. Here's how I responded:

"For the first time in my 31 years, I feel comfortable in my own skin. I feel strong, healthy, and okay—full disclosure—there are things I'd like to work on—but overall this is the best I've ever felt and it's taken a long time for me to get to this place of peace. I don't usually comment on negative comments, but hear this. If you have something unkind to say, or have the mindset that only certain body types can practice yoga, then you are a part of the problem and you can leave. We don't need your negativity here. Thick, thin, big, small, whateverthefuckever, yoga is for every single body type. Get on board with that or show yourself out."

Sure, this was me defending myself. And yeah, you could argue that this was me creating a divide between "us" (the true yoga community that is accepting of all body types) and "them" (the people who are not). But this was also me defending any one of my tens of thousands of Instagram followers who might've been questioning their self-worth based on the size of their bodies. This was me standing up for what I consider to be the *true* yoga community, which is inclusive and kind and accepting of all bodies. This was me being authentically myself and saying, "I'm not taking your shit. Bye."

So do that. Lead by confidence, not ego. Take no shit, but do it in a way that serves the greater good.

While the story of my journey and how I've chosen to live my life by these ten Namaslay commandments is woven in throughout this book, my hope is that you see yourself reflected in my experiences. My hope is that you're inspired to dig deep and let your most authentic self shine.

My wish for you is that you live your one precious life with fearless authenticity. That you avoid editing yourself to fit someone else's idea of what you should be. My wish is that you know, from all your days of living in your own body year after year and from all your hard work—all your learning and doing the little things and getting out of your own way—is that you know exactly who you are and honor your greatness.

NOW GO OUT THERE AND SLAY.

Namaslay,
Candace

how to use this book

I wrote this book for two reasons. The first is that people kept asking me the same question over and over again: how do I start practicing yoga?

For some of us who have practiced for years, it seems like such an easy question to answer. You just start practicing. You go to a class, you look up a video online—like Nike says, you just do it.

But I realized that it isn't that easy for most people. Studio classes are expensive, work schedules are demanding, and online videos can be tough to sift through. Sorry, Nike, but it turns out that sometimes we just *can't* do it.

I wanted to help, so I wrote this book for those people—the people who have always wanted to practice but just aren't sure where to begin. And I wrote it for people who have practiced for years, and even for yoga instructors who have a solid foundation but want a modern reference for a deeper understanding of poses and sequencing.

But I wanted to help on a deeper level. Sure, I could explain poses and create sequences to follow, but I wanted to share my story of the darkest time of my life. I wanted to share how sad I was. How scared I was. How much pain I was in. And how I had to dig deep, sift through all the emotions I was dealing with, and decide whether I wanted to dig myself out of the hole I was in or wallow in it.

As you'll read, I decided to dig myself out. But beyond that, I decided that when I got out, I would live my absolute best life. I realized that I'd been ho-humming through life, and I didn't want to do that with my one precious lifetime. I wanted to honor my gifts, do the absolute best that I could, and ultimately help others through the lessons of my struggles.

Use this book not only as a guide to your yoga practice—or, if you're a yoga instructor, as a reference when you're feeling uninspired in your teaching—but also as a guide to living your greatest life. Read it as a testimonial to utilizing the strength that we all have deep within us, and know that the physical, emotional, and spiritual strengths that you have within you are greater and more powerful than any obstacle you'll face during your lifetime. The yoga practice is a way to hone your physical, emotional, and spiritual strengths to help you along your path to living your most authentic life.

The meditation portion of this book demystifies the practice and breaks it down in a way that is easy to implement into everyday life. It goes over useful props for the practice, various ways to sit, and a number of different meditation techniques. You'll learn how to find slow, calm moments in your busy day, confront your demons, and sift through it all, letting go of whatever emotional baggage you're holding onto that you no longer need.

The pranayama practice is about breathing. We breathe twenty-four hours a day without even trying, so you'd think that we wouldn't really need an entire chapter on breathing, but this chapter is about *intentional* breathing. You'll learn different techniques to help you quiet and focus your mind and move through your days with an air of powerful calm.

The physical practice is broken down into three levels in this book: beginner, intermediate, and advanced. But I want to make it very clear that I struggled with this decision because there are some so-called "basic" poses that many "advanced" students can't do. Take, for example, a

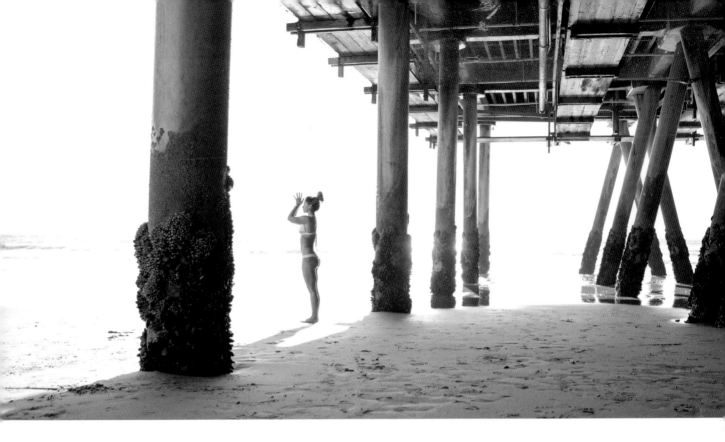

super-strong guy who has never done yoga but has been an athlete all his life. He can likely do a textbook tripod headstand (page 232)—a pose that I consider to be somewhat advanced—but probably can't do a textbook seated forward fold (page 85) due to very tight hamstrings. Does this mean that he is a beginner or an advanced student?

Who cares? Let's set those labels aside and just do what we can with what we have while continuing to work on the areas with which we struggle.

The "levels" in this book are just a way to organize the poses. There are definitely some poses that are best learned in a specific order (like handstand, which came easier to me after I learned crow pose, supported headstand, tripod headstand, and forearm stand, in that order), but try not to get hung up on the idea of becoming advanced or having to be at a certain level. Instead, allow wherever you are in your yoga practice to be just fine with you as you continue to practice.

Years ago, after a very long, hot, sticky day of yoga teacher training in Thailand, I sat in a yoga shala listening to my instructor explain each cue for tree pose. In the thick heat, I drew a stick figure practicing the pose and began drawing arrows all over the page to illustrate the cues. In my exhaustion, I thought, *I wish there was a book that showed each pose with its corresponding alignment cues.* So when I started YogaByCandace, I made sure to bring my vision to life on my blog. I'd have my husband, Greg, take a photo of me in a pose, and then I'd cut myself out of the photo and place it against a white background. Then I'd use Photoshop to draw arrows to point out the various cues that people needed to know. These posts would often go viral on social media, and readers would write in asking if I could put all of the poses together in this way so they could have them for easy reference. Maybe it was my background in education (I have a master's degree in secondary ed), but I understood how useful these images were. As a yoga teacher or an avid yoga practitioner, it is so nice to be able to get the information needed for each pose quickly rather than having to read through pages and pages of description.

I was adamant that the design for *Namaslay* follow the same style that I feature on my blog. I pictured yoga teachers and students alike leafing through the book to find the exact pose they needed and quickly scanning the callouts to find the alignment cue that they weren't totally sure about.

In that sense, this book makes a great reference. However, one thing to keep in mind is that yoga has been around for thousands of years and is constantly evolving. The upside is that there really isn't a wrong way to move on your mat. The downside is that there is so much to the yoga practice that it would be impossible to cover every single pose that exists. So you may notice, for example, that I've included just a couple of variations of a pose that you know has a few others. This is why—there is way too much to fit into one book.

Another thing to keep in mind is that with the practice constantly evolving, it is sometimes difficult to nail down the exact spellings or names of various poses. One school of thought will have a pose spelled one way, and another style of yoga will name it another way. Try not to get hung up on these little discrepancies. Instead, enjoy the journey. What's most important is the alignment, the breath, and how you feel in the pose.

These physical practice chapters break down a number of poses for you so that you can learn the finer points of each pose. Then, at the end of each chapter, there are short sequences that you can follow, with poses pulled from that chapter. Easy peasy. As you become more familiar with the poses, you can start making up your own sequences. Don't overthink it; you literally cannot do this wrong. Allow your body to move and flow, and stay dialed in to how you're feeling.

Following the advanced chapter is a chapter covering restorative yoga poses. People often focus on developing an athletic practice, but it's important to have balance. The restorative practice will calm things down with its intentional sense of ease. Building a strong restorative yoga practice is a wonderful way to increase mobility and decrease tension and stress. This chapter goes over the props that you can use for the restorative practice, but if your budget is tight, just get creative and use what you have at home.

At the end of the book, you'll find a chapter outlining a number of sequences: warm-ups; practices that address different issues, like insomnia; and a few thirty-day programs that you can follow along to. These sequences should help get you on your way to a well-rounded practice. They offer some ideas if you're struggling to make up your own sequences or you just want a no-brainer way to get some good yoga into your life. Feel free to tailor the sequences to work for you. Above all, always work within a pain-free range and honor how you feel.

A WORD ABOUT SANSKRIT

Sanskrit is an ancient language of India and the root of the yogic teachings. Sanskrit words pop up often in the yoga practice because of its Eastern roots, and sometimes students—especially new students—are confused and intimidated by them. I get that. I mean, I sure as hell am not fluent in Sanskrit, and half the time I'm not totally sure I'm pronouncing things right, but at the end of the day, they're just words.

Of course I'd like to learn as much as I can because it's a part of this beautiful practice that I love so much, but I'm not going to be too hard on myself if I mispronounce a word or attend a class and have no clue which posture the teacher is referring to if I haven't learned the Sanskrit word for it, and I urge you to do the same. Let's do ourselves a favor and take the pressure off to be perfect at this. And everything else in life. Life's way too short for that tomfoolery.

In this book, I've included the Sanskrit names for the yoga poses as well as their English names. There are a few poses in this book that don't have a Sanskrit name, and that's because they are newer poses that don't have Sanskrit translations (at least that I could find). As with anything, the yoga practice continues to evolve.

before you begin

So we've covered the principles of Namaslay and how to apply them to life on and off the mat, but if you flip through this book, you'll see that there's a lot more to it than the stories of my struggles. You likely picked up this book because you knew it was about yoga, and yoga is something you're interested in. So what do you need to know before you begin?

where do I start?

People find their way to yoga for a number of reasons. Maybe you're going through something major, like a quarter-life crisis. Maybe your doctor said that you need to de-stress. Perhaps you want to get in shape. Or an annoying friend wouldn't stop talking about how great yoga is and dragged you along to a class. Whatever your reason, you've decided to start practicing, but you may not know where to begin. Even if you do, please humor me and read on anyway.

If you're brand-spankin' new to yoga and you have a little extra money and time, I encourage you to hit up your local yoga studio. A studio should be warm and inviting, with great vibes that make you feel like you've hit the Cool People jackpot. Wear whatever the heck you want (leggings, harem pants, shorts, who cares; just be sure you're comfortable moving in your outfit), avoid eating for two hours prior to class (otherwise it may upset your stomach), and let the teacher know that you're new. Post up wherever you feel the most comfortable (at the back of the room, at the front of the room, by the door; just be sure that you can see the teacher). And do your best. No worries, no expectations. Life is full of stuff to be stressed about—not knowing your yoga basics should not be one of them!

There are a few rules of yoga to keep in mind:

1. **THERE IS NO SUCH THING AS A PERFECT POSE.** The little things, like whether your arm is parallel to the floor or your arm has a beautiful U-shaped arch in dancer's pose (page 179), don't really matter. So don't worry about the little things. Just focus on the important stuff, like proper alignment (such as watching out for your knees and wrists).

2. **IT SHOULD NEVER, EVER HURT.** When it comes to yoga, there is no gain when you're in pain. If you ever feel pain, back off, my friend. But remember that there's a difference between being in pain and being uncomfortable. Discomfort—when you're shaking and sweating and working

hard—is okay. You can do anything for one minute, right? Allow yourself to feel discomfort if it's due to, say, tight muscles, but avoid actual pain at all costs.

3. THE PRACTICE IS FOR YOU, SO DO WHAT YOU NEED TO DO TO FEEL GOOD. Yes, a yoga class is a collective experience, but it's an individual effort. So if you're in the middle of a hot power yoga class and you find yourself feeling tired and mentally worn down, it's your right to take corpse pose (page 136) for the rest of the class. Honoring what you need in every moment is the highest form of yoga. A yoga class is not about the teacher, the studio, or anything else. It's for you, so do what you need to do in order to get what you need out of the class.

Nothing, and I mean nothing, can take the place of a fantastic in-studio yoga class with a real-live teacher who knows his or her stuff and can guide you through a genius sequence that leaves your body feeling like mush in the best possible way. But let's be real: not everyone has a budget or a schedule that can accommodate regular classes at a fancy-schmancy yoga studio. So what else can you do?

You have a couple of options. You can find something (for free!) on YouTube (shameless self-plug: youtube.com/yogabycandace), or you can keep reading. I encourage you to do both.

how often should I practice?

It's important to listen to your body. One of the most incredible lessons I've learned from yoga is that most of the time, I already know what I need. What do I mean by that? Well, one of the most frequent questions that I hear is, "How often should I practice yoga?"

The answer is both simple and complex. In short, you should practice yoga however often you feel you need to.

What's so hard about that? you might be asking yourself. Well, a lot of people struggle with my previous point about feeling like they need to reach a certain level by a certain date. They force themselves to do a strenuous practice when they're overtired or sick. They see yoga as something to cross off their to-do list. Basically, they are getting in their own way with their egos and their hectic lives.

NAMASLAY COMMANDMENT #2:
GET OUT OF
YOUR OWN WAY.

I understand that. Life is tough, and we are busy. I've definitely done it myself. But it's a dangerous thing to do because when you're not listening to your body, you are putting yourself in a position to be injured. So my advice is to really tune in to what you need. If you're tired but have some energy for yoga, do a slow hatha practice (see the next page). If you're overtired and just need some more sleep, roll up your mat and go to bed. Seriously. Listen to your body and honor what it needs, and you cannot go wrong.

what type of yoga is best?

There are so many types of yoga. I recommend incorporating several different styles so that you can build a well-rounded practice. If you have the chance to take a class, the following list should help you narrow down your options:

- YIN YOGA is very, very slow. It incorporates a number of props, and you stay in each pose for three to five minutes (and sometimes longer). It is fantastic for relieving stress and anxiety and developing flexibility because you're meant to sink into each pose, letting your body be effortless. See chapter 6 for more on the yin yoga practice.

- RESTORATIVE YOGA is a very slow yet rejuvenating style. It often uses props, and you hold poses for an extended period, but there is more movement in a restorative class than in a yin class. Restorative yoga is excellent when you're tired, you're feeling under the weather, or you need something uplifting. It is great for developing flexibility as well. See chapter 6 for more on the restorative practice.

- HATHA YOGA is traditionally a slow style of yoga. You pause for a number of breaths in each pose before moving on to the next pose. This style of yoga is ideal for people who are looking for gentle movement and stretching.

- VINYASA YOGA is a much more athletic style. *Vinyasa* is a Sanskrit word that means "flow," so anticipate lots of movement. You can expect to sweat and build endurance with this practice. Don't plan to hold poses for very long, as this class is more about the movement than it is about the stretches. It is effective for developing endurance.

- POWER YOGA is generally a little slower than vinyasa but still involves quite a bit of movement. You can expect to sweat and hold strength-building poses like warrior 2 (page 114) for many breaths. This style of yoga is wonderful for building strength.

Keep in mind that these are just a few of the types of yoga. It would be nearly impossible to name and describe all of them, especially given that many teachers and studios are now branding their own styles.

In this book, I've incorporated poses from all of the above styles, and the sequences at the end of each chapter as well as at the end of the book incorporate both faster, more athletic styles and slower, more restorative styles. *Namaslay,* as the title indicates, gives you the best of both worlds—a yin and a yang so that you feel completely balanced.

what is a vinyasa?

As I mentioned earlier, *vinyasa* means "flow," and if you're taking a vinyasa yoga class, you can expect a moderately paced, constantly moving, flowing style of yoga. This is not the class to take if you're looking for a slow, relaxing, gentle-stretch style of yoga. (If that's you, search for a hatha, yin, or restorative class.)

I have a popular YouTube channel where I release new yoga videos every week. With over one hundred thousand subscribers, I get a lot of comments, and I do my best to respond to them. One of the most common things people write is that my vinyasa classes are "too fast." Here's what I want everyone to know: no, they're not. It's just that if you think they're too fast, vinyasa is likely not the style of yoga you're looking for.

Sometimes in a vinyasa class, the teacher will say, "Go through your vinyasa and we'll all meet in downward dog." If you're like I was as a beginner, you'll look around the room like, "Well, WTF is a vinyasa? Am I supposed to know what that means?" Your heart will race, and you might turn red with embarrassment or panic.

So let me break it down for you: vinyasa is a moderately paced, athletic style of yoga, and it's also a series of yoga poses found in the middle of a sun salutation.

A sun salutation is a series of yoga postures found within a vinyasa class. You start by standing in mountain pose. As you inhale, lift your arms and look up, and as you exhale, hinge at the hips and fold forward into a forward fold. Then, as you inhale, halfway lift and look ahead, and as you exhale, bend your knees, plant your hands into the mat, and step or jump back into chaturanga (or low plank). As you inhale, rise up into cobra pose or upward-facing dog, and as you exhale, roll over your toes and come into downward-facing dog. Breathe here for a few breaths. When you're ready to move on, inhale, rise up onto your toes, and exhale to step or jump to the front of the mat. Inhale to halfway lift and exhale to forward fold. As you inhale, lift your arms and look up, and as you exhale, return to mountain pose.

sun salutation

1. MOUNTAIN POSE

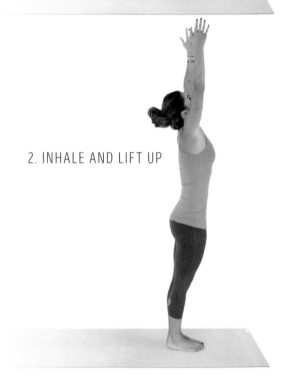

2. INHALE AND LIFT UP

3. FORWARD FOLD

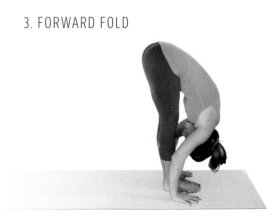

4. HALFWAY LIFT

5. CHATURANGA

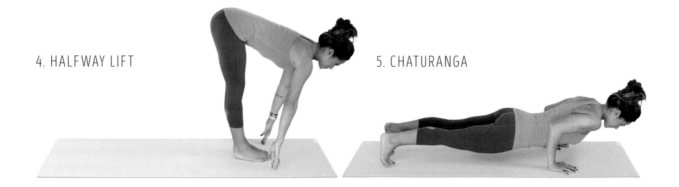

6. UPWARD-FACING DOG

7. DOWNWARD-FACING DOG

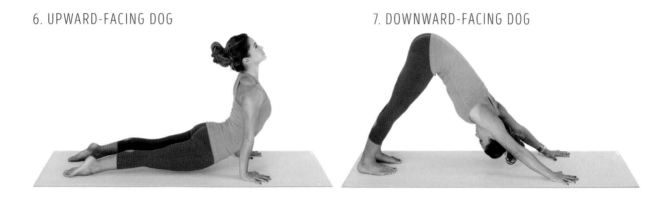

8. RISE UP ONTO YOUR TOES

9. JUMP OR STEP FORWARD

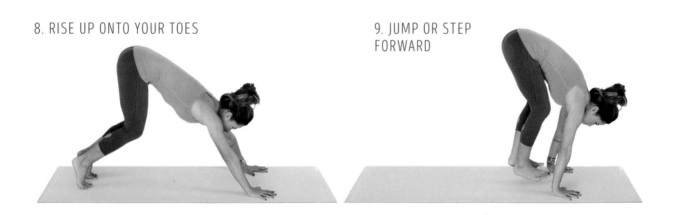

10. HALFWAY LIFT

11. FORWARD FOLD

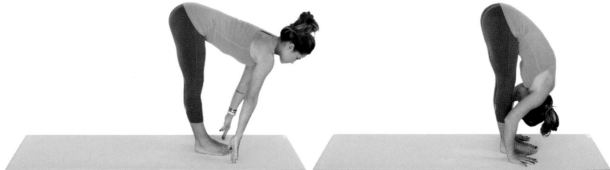

12. INHALE AND LIFT UP

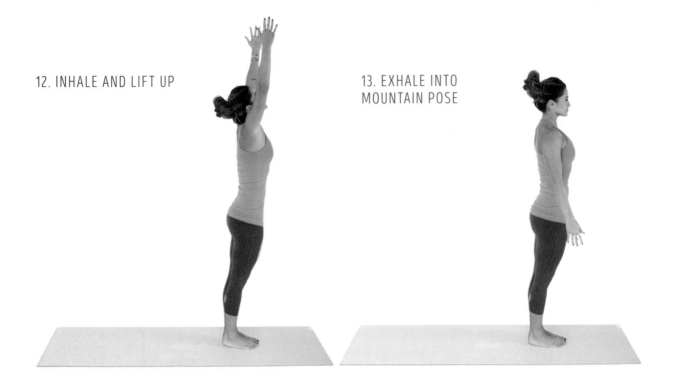

13. EXHALE INTO MOUNTAIN POSE

When you're in a yoga class and your teacher says to "move through a vinyasa," you can do either a half vinyasa or a full vinyasa.

For a half vinyasa, exhale from the pose that you're in and move into chaturanga. As you inhale, come into cobra pose or upward-facing dog. As you exhale, roll over your toes and come into downward-facing dog.

For a full vinyasa, exhale from the pose that you're in and move into chaturanga. Inhale and come into upward-facing dog, then exhale and come into downward-facing dog. As you inhale, rise up onto your toes, and as you exhale, step or jump forward to the front of your mat. As you inhale, halfway lift, and as you exhale, hinge at the hips and come into a forward fold. Then inhale and lift all the way up with your arms overhead, and exhale into mountain pose.

half vinyasa

1. CHATURANGA

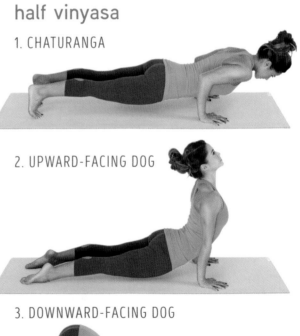

2. UPWARD-FACING DOG

3. DOWNWARD-FACING DOG

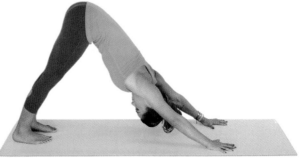

full vinyasa

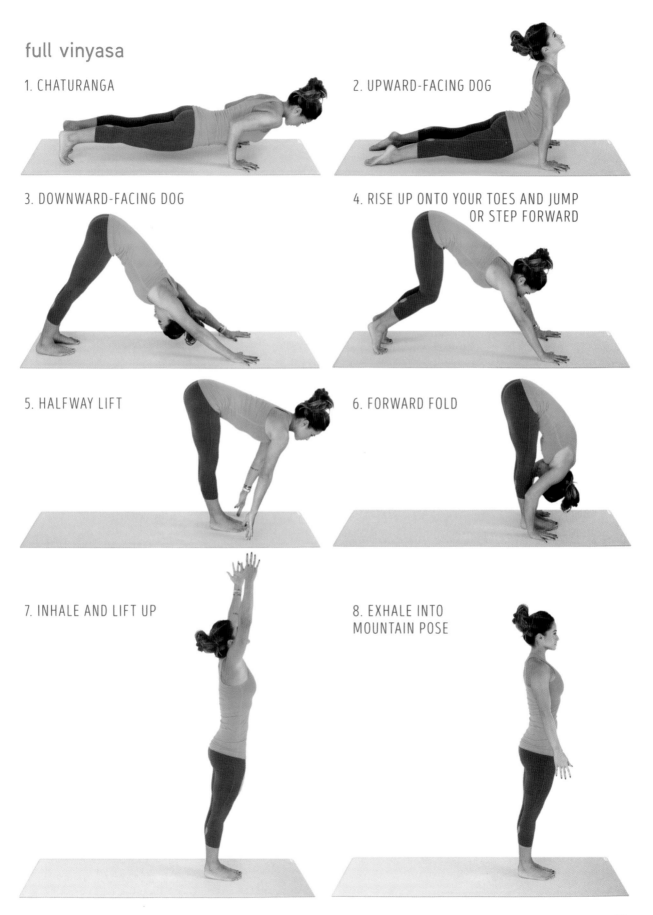

1. CHATURANGA

2. UPWARD-FACING DOG

3. DOWNWARD-FACING DOG

4. RISE UP ONTO YOUR TOES AND JUMP OR STEP FORWARD

5. HALFWAY LIFT

6. FORWARD FOLD

7. INHALE AND LIFT UP

8. EXHALE INTO MOUNTAIN POSE

is this right?

You may see a pose in this book that's done a different way from how your teacher has instructed it, and that's okay. The beauty of yoga is that as long as the alignment is on point, the other things don't really matter so much. For example, some teachers will argue that for triangle pose, you should grab the front big toe. Others will say that the hand should be on the ground in front of the foot. Still others will argue that the hand should be on the ground but *behind* the foot. I say, "Who cares?" As long as your upper body is in line with your lower body and your hamstrings aren't hyperextending, you can put your hand wherever you want. It's your practice, so make it work for you. Don't get too hung up on what's "right," because you're likely to get a different answer from each yoga instructor you ask.

As far as the alignment cues go, I've listed what I believe are the most important ones for each pose. When you're learning each pose, focus on those cues that are listed. The other aspects of the pose will come naturally and will develop as part of your own personal style once you've got the foundation down pat.

foundations of yoga

I consider meditation and pranayama to be the building blocks upon which you can grow a strong personal yoga practice. With meditation and pranayama in place (see chapters 1 and 2, respectively), the intention is there and the mindfulness switch is turned on. Having those blocks in place is hugely important because it cuts down significantly on your chance of injury. With intention and mindfulness as the undercurrents of your practice, you're ready to begin moving.

Whenever you practice yoga, whether you're on your feet or on your hands, it's important to build each pose from the ground up. What I mean by this is that you should check in with whatever part of your body is touching the mat first to set a solid foundation. If you're trying to do a handstand and you're focused on getting your feet up instead of setting up your hands to support you, you're likely to be wobbly, if you're able to get up at all. This can lead to a lot of frustration, so spare yourself and reevaluate.

With the same principle in mind, consider a seated pose like seated forward fold. The inclination is just to fold forward, right?

In each of these examples, tune in to the body part that is touching the mat and start there. For the handstand, you'll want to spread your fingers, grip the mat like a rock climber, and press firmly into the bases of the fingers and fingertips. For the seated forward fold, you'll want to gently pull away the fleshy part underneath each sitting bone. If you build a solid foundation for stability, you're likely to have a much better experience in the pose.

building up from your feet

For upright positions like tree pose (page 105) and mountain pose (page 106), you need to be mindful of your feet:

• Lift, spread, and then place your toes on the floor so that they can gently grip the mat, which helps stabilize the body. Our feet don't get enough attention. We stuff them into socks and shoes for most of the day, so the tiny muscles in the feet are often underdeveloped. At first, you might not be able to spread your toes without bending over and manually pushing them apart with your fingers. Don't worry if this is the case for you. As your feet get stronger, you'll be able to grip the mat with your toes.

• Make sure that your weight is evenly distributed across all four corners of your feet (or foot, if it's a pose that calls for you to balance on one foot). Having equal weight distribution is the key to maintaining balance.

• Feel a sensation of lift in the arch. You're not simply resting your foot on the ground, but intentionally drawing a long line of energy up from the center of your foot. I know this sounds sort of hippie-dippie, but there is meaning behind it, I promise. Imagine that there is a straw going up the center of your leg, much like your shin and femur bones. As you inhale, imagine that through the straw you are able to suck up strength and energy from the earth. What this visualization does is firmly plant your foot into the ground, stabilize your balance, and lift the arch of your foot. It is the difference between being actively engaged and simply resting your weight in the center of your foot.

TIPS FOR A SOLID FOUNDATION IN YOUR YOGA PRACTICE

● SPREAD THE TOES AND FIRMLY PLANT THEM INTO THE MAT

✖ KEEP THIS AREA LIFTED; DO NOT LET IT DROP

★ VISUALIZE A SUCTION HERE THROUGH WHICH YOU LIFT UP

■ REST YOUR WEIGHT EVENLY HERE

building up from your hands

One of the most common complaints I hear in yoga class has to do with painful wrists. And it's understandable; downward-facing dog (page 100) is the pose in which we arguably spend the majority of our class time. If you're doing it improperly, wrist issues are sure to pop up. But with a little attention to proper weight distribution, you can easily avoid wrist pain.

Just as you want to be mindful of your feet and build a standing pose up from there, you want to be mindful of your hands when you place them on the mat.

• Spread your fingers as wide as you can. The wider your fingers, the more stable your foundation. Just like our feet, the little muscles in the hands are often underdeveloped. If they're underdeveloped or tight for you, you may find it difficult to spread your fingers very wide. Just keep working at it every day (I take breaks from working on my computer to give my fingers a little stretch, and I spread them over the keyboard throughout the day), and over time you'll be able to cover more ground.

• Gently grip into the mat like you're a rock climber. This is essential for poses that involve balancing on your hands, because your fingertips will help ensure that you don't tip over.

• Plug the roots of your fingers into the mat. Imagine that your fingers are glued to the mat and commit to not allowing them to lift up. This keeps your weight evenly distributed across your palm.

• Avoid allowing the "arch" of your hand to lift. This ensures that your weight doesn't get dumped into the outside edge of your palm, which can cause serious wrist pain and possibly injury.

AVOIDING WRIST PAIN IN YOGA

IN EVERY YOGA POSE IN WHICH YOU'RE ON YOUR HANDS, FOLLOW THESE GUIDELINES TO AVOID WRIST PAIN:

● FIRMLY PLUG THESE AREAS INTO THE MAT

■ PRESS THESE AREAS INTO THE MAT

▲ NEVER LET THIS PART LIFT UP

✖ AVOID COLLAPSING WEIGHT HERE

★ VISUALIZE THIS AREA AS A SUCTION THROUGH WHICH YOU LIFT UPWARD

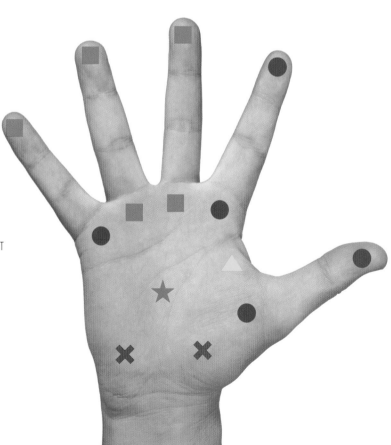

props for yoga

Props are fantastic for meditation, pranayama, and the physical asana practice. They're perfect for beginners, who can use them to access poses that their bodies can't quite handle on their own yet. And more experienced yogis will enjoy the deepening that props provide as they find the fullest expressions of various poses.

yoga mats

I'm going to tell you a secret: I hate using a yoga mat. My personal practice is kind of like a dance, and I don't like being confined to one space. So do you absolutely need a yoga mat in order to practice yoga? No. Does it help? Sure. Mats provide a bit of protection from the hard floor, which can be tough on knee joints, and from a logistical standpoint, they help organize the yoga students in a studio setting.

What kind of mat is best? It depends on what you're looking for and what your budget is. Mats can range in price from $9.99 at a big box store all the way up to $130 at a specialty store.

Here are a few things to take into consideration when choosing a mat:

• **Length:** Are you tall? You may want to look for an extra-long mat that will better suit your needs. There are also extra-wide mats and even giant circular mats if you like to move around a lot during your practice.

• **Traction:** I prefer a mat with open-cell construction, like the Jade Harmony mat. These mats have such excellent traction that no matter how much you sweat, you will not slide. On a mat with closed-cell construction, sweat tends to pool like puddles, and I find myself sliding around a lot more.

• **Thickness:** Do you have creaky knees and wrists? A thicker, firmer mat like the Manduka Black Mat Pro might be something to consider (although it is quite expensive). Be careful not to pick a mat that has too much give, because it can be harder to balance on and tends to irritate the wrists even more. The cushioning makes it difficult to engage the fingertips and take pressure off the outside edges of the palms, which is what you want to do when your wrists are hurting.

• **Weight:** Will you be carrying your mat to and from your car when you visit your local studio or gym? If so, you may want to consider the weight of your mat. Mats can weigh between a pound and a half (those are usually travel mats) and nearly ten pounds (yikes!), so weight is definitely something to keep in mind if you'll be carting your mat around.

yoga blocks

Yoga blocks are useful for everyone, from absolute beginners to the super advanced. They can help a beginner modify a pose or help an advanced practitioner get deeper into a pose. While I wouldn't say that blocks are absolutely essential to the practice, they certainly help, and if it's in your budget, I suggest purchasing two.

types of yoga blocks

Yoga blocks are available in a number of different materials, and to be honest, I don't have a favorite. Asking me to pick a favorite block is like asking me to pick a favorite vacation destination. There are so many great places to go, and they all boast incredible sights, foods, and cultures. When it comes to yoga blocks, they all have awesome attributes, so you just need to decide what you're looking for and go from there.

• **Cork blocks:** Cork is a magical material that somehow manages to be sturdy and hard yet offers a hint of give. For an all-around prop that can be used for anything from an active, strength-building triangle pose (page 185) to a passive, restorative supported bridge pose (page 310), a cork yoga block has my vote.

• **Foam blocks:** I find foam to be quite soft, which works well for seated meditation and restorative yin postures but leaves you wiggling and wobbling when used to give you a boost in a pose like eight-angle (page 226). Foam blocks feel delicious at the end of a practice when you're doing a pose like supported bridge (page 310) or reclined bound angle (page 135).

• **Wooden blocks:** Wooden blocks are quite hard and very sturdy. These types of blocks are excellent for poses like crow (page 222) because they provide an unwavering foundation for your hands, but you'll probably find them too hard for a restorative chest opener like supported reclined bound angle pose (page 321). Wooden blocks also tend to slide a bit on hardwood floors. If you're working on your yoga mat, that shouldn't be an issue, but it's something to keep in mind.

• **Rounded blocks:** I love these ergonomic blocks for any style of yoga, but particularly for restorative practices because they fit flush against the body's curves. They're excellent for poses like pigeon (page 97) and seated forward fold (page 85) because they feel like they become extensions of your body, unlike traditional rectangular blocks. Bhoga makes great ergonomic wooden blocks.

using a yoga block

The trick to using a yoga block correctly isn't so much about the placement of the block, but about what you do once the block is in place. For practices like power or vinyasa yoga, it's important not to rely on the block or rest your weight on it. (The exception is restorative yin poses, where you *should* relax into the blocks.) Instead, draw upon the visualization that I presented earlier about a straw running through the center of your legs (refer to page 25), except this time visualize that straw running through the center of whichever part of your body is touching the block. For example, in triangle pose (page 185), you want to maintain a sense of expansion and length from fingertips to fingertips, so collapsing your weight into the block is not a good idea. Instead, visualize a straw running through the center of your arm, and as you breathe in, imagine that you're sucking up length from the mat to find a long line of energy running through your arm, across your chest, and up the other arm.

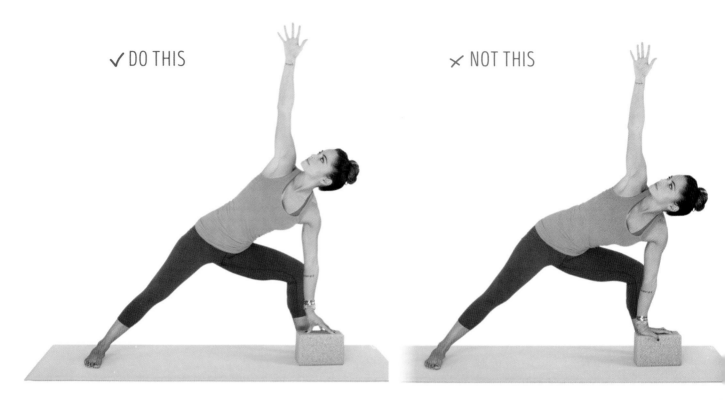

✔ DO THIS   ✗ NOT THIS

There are many ways to use a yoga block, but here are some of my favorites.

SEATED FORWARD FOLD: Sitting on the edge of a block can help people who have tight hips because the height of the block offers extra length in the hamstrings.

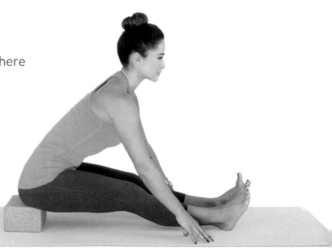

SEATED FORWARD FOLD WITH ROUNDED BLOCK: For more flexible yogis, a block placed against the bottoms of the feet offers a nice place to bring the hands and ensures that the feet stay in good alignment.

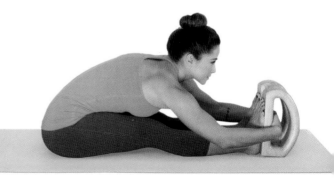

EIGHT-ANGLE POSE: For intermediate yogis working on arm balances, placing a block under each hand gives a bit of extra height, which helps compensate for abs that aren't quite strong enough to lift the body high off the mat.

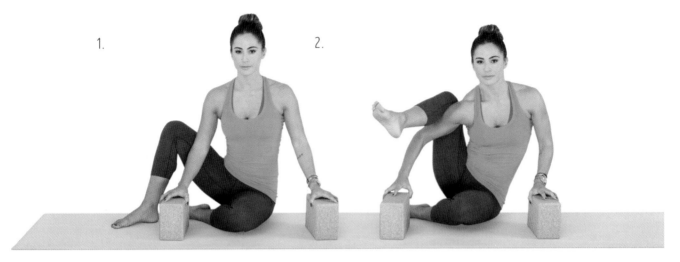

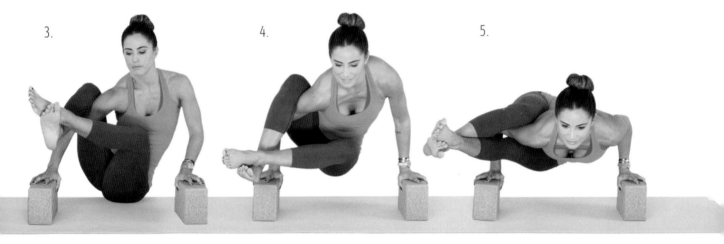

SUPPORTED BRIDGE POSE: Supported bridge is one of my favorite restorative poses because it offers such a nice release for the low back. Place a block under the tops of your hips on the edge that works best for you, depending on your flexibility, and completely relax into the block.

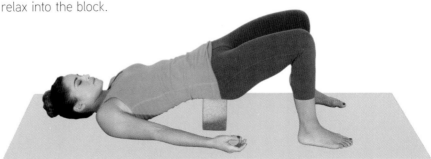

SUPPORTED PIGEON POSE: One of the toughest things about pigeon pose is waiting for those hips to open up. I often see people with hips that aren't facing the front, so sitting on the edge of a yoga block can help position the hips in proper alignment so that they're facing forward.

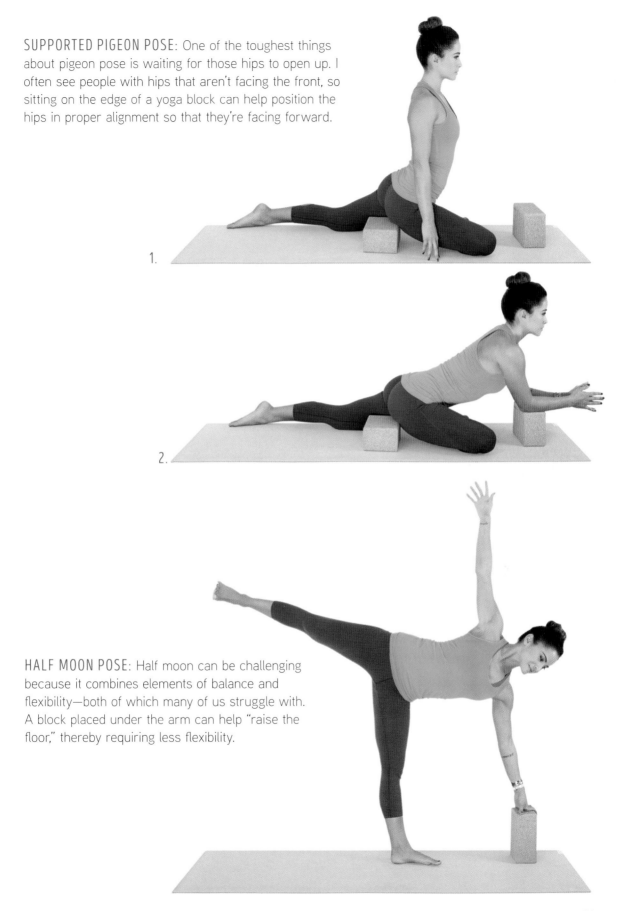

1.

2.

HALF MOON POSE: Half moon can be challenging because it combines elements of balance and flexibility—both of which many of us struggle with. A block placed under the arm can help "raise the floor," thereby requiring less flexibility.

yoga straps

A yoga strap is another excellent tool for yogis of all levels. Just like a yoga block, a strap can offer beginners with limited mobility a way to connect, say, feet to hands in standing forward fold (page 107). On the other end of the spectrum, a strap can help more advanced yogis maintain proper alignment as they work through more advanced poses, like forearm stand (page 273).

types of yoga straps
Yoga straps don't really vary that much. You'll see straps made of hemp or cotton, with the lengths ranging from 6 to 10 feet. The buckle, generally made of either metal or plastic, might be a D-ring, a circle ring, a seatbelt-style buckle, or a tri-bar slide. I prefer a metal D-ring and recommend that you pick a strap length that corresponds to your height. If you're tall, go for a 10-foot strap, and if you're petite, go for a 6-foot strap. If you fall somewhere in the middle, choose the 8-foot length.

using a yoga strap
A yoga strap may seem simple, but here are a few general rules to ensure that you're using it to its fullest potential.

KEEP IT EVEN: First, be sure that the strap is the same length on both sides. When you're in a pose like forward fold, set yourself up for success by putting the center point of the strap around the middle of your feet.

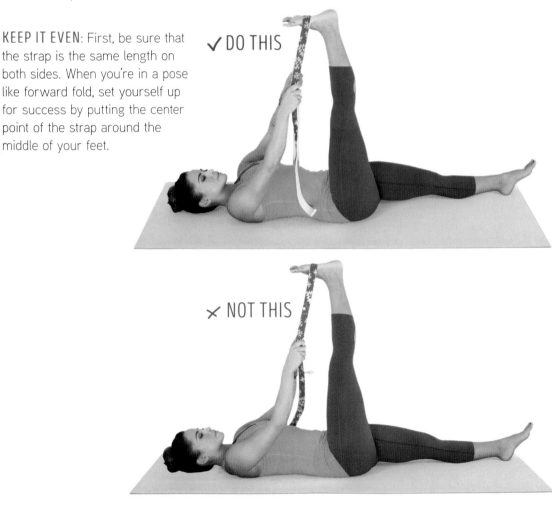

✓ DO THIS

✗ NOT THIS

GRAB AS CLOSE AS YOU CAN: Often, you'll use a yoga strap to help you when you aren't quite as flexible as the full expression of a pose requires. In order to develop flexibility, you need to work at what's called your "edge"—that point between the known ("Oh, I am definitely flexible enough for this") and the unknown ("I'm pretty sure I can't do that"). When you grab as close as you can on the strap, you're working at your edge and developing flexibility.

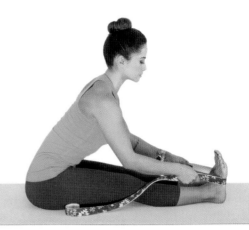

MAKE SURE THAT THE STRAP IS AROUND THE MIDDLE: You want the strap to be wrapped around the middle of the body part in question. For example, in bow pose (page 271), the strap should be against the tops of your feet. If it's too close to your toes, it's liable to slip off, and your chin and upper body could come crashing down to the mat. Placing the strap around the middle of the tops of your feet makes it more likely to stay put and therefore helps prevent injury.

There are many ways to use a yoga strap, but here are some of my favorites.

BABY FLYING PIGEON POSE: This pose is for more advanced yogis who are working on arm balances. One of the common mistakes I see in arm balances is that the elbows tend to veer out away from the body. To prevent wrist injuries, it's important to keep your elbows in line with your wrists. You can do this by using a yoga strap to support your arms. Secure the strap tightly above your elbows, then slowly begin to come into the pose. You'll notice that the tension of the strap prevents your elbows from slipping out to the sides.

POSITION THE STRAP AROUND YOUR UPPER ARMS AND SECURE THE BUCKLE SO IT IS SNUG AND SECURE. THIS WILL HELP YOUR ARMS STAY SHOULDER WIDTH AND HELP PREVENT THE ELBOWS FROM SPLAYING TO THE SIDES, WHICH CAN BE DAMAGING TO YOUR WRISTS.

KING DANCER'S POSE: Talk about a major hip and chest opener! Using a yoga strap makes this gorgeous yet challenging pose more accessible. Place the strap around the center of your foot, grab the strap as close to your foot as you can, and then come into the full expression of the pose.

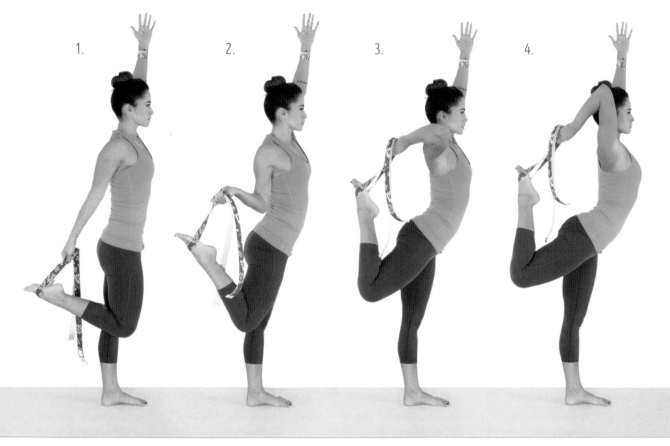

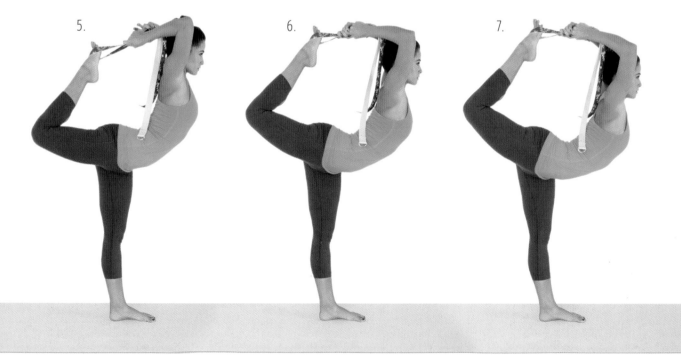

BOW POSE: Another great opener for the hip flexors and chest, bow pose is for beginner yogis who are tight in both areas. Come into the pose by placing the middle of the strap around the centers of your feet, then grab the strap as close to your feet as you can before lifting up into the full expression of the pose.

1.

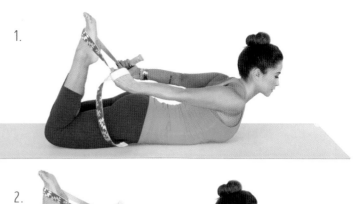

2.

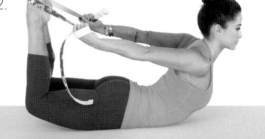

3.

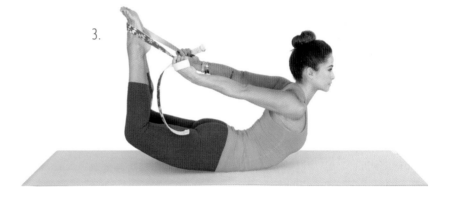

COMPASS/SUNDIAL POSE: This gorgeous pose requires major side-body opening and hip flexibility that isn't usually accessible right off the bat. Begin by putting the middle of the strap around your foot, then grab the strap as close to your foot as you can before lifting your leg and coming into the full expression of the pose

1.   2.   3.   4.

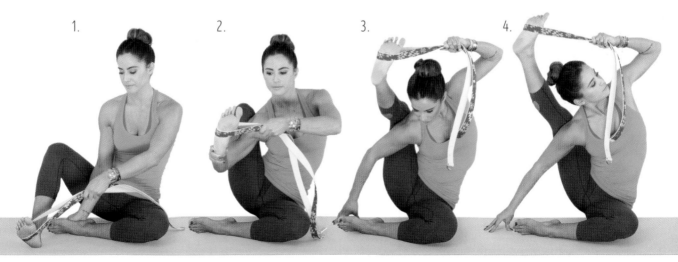

bolsters

A bolster is an excellent prop to have, and I should know because I lived without one for twenty-nine years. When I finally got one, it was life-changing, in the same way that getting your eyebrows threaded for the first time is life-changing. (My threaded ladies know what I'm talkin' about!) The purpose of a bolster is to provide a comfortable place for your body to completely rest. Bolsters are essential for the yin and restorative practices, which are wonderful for developing flexibility and de-stressing. But bolsters are pricey, and I don't understand why. I mean, seriously, they're just like pillows, only firmer and bigger. Anyway, if you can get your hands on a bolster, I definitely encourage you to do so—it is excellent for developing flexibility and will transform your practice. But if a bolster is not in the cards for you, look around the house. Use a couch cushion, a body pillow, or a bunch of pillows wrapped tightly in a thick blanket or towel. Whatever you do, don't let not having the prop keep you from your practice.

blankets

Blankets can aid in savasana (or corpse pose; see page 136) and restorative practices as well as meditation, and they have a few different uses. If you have tight hips, a blanket can provide a firm yet comfortable cushion. Sitting on the edge of a rolled blanket will help tilt your pelvis forward so that you gain a bit more movement in your seated forward fold. You can also place a folded blanket underneath your head for comfort in savasana, or over your body to stay warm during meditation or yin poses. The possibilities are endless.

There's no need to run out and buy one of those fancy-schmancy Mexican blankets that you'll see at yoga studios. Sure, they're beautiful and nice and thick, but really any old blanket that's on the thicker side will do. I recommend a thick cotton or wool blanket, which provides great support and stability. A great substitute is a thick beach towel or two.

GET CREATIVE WITH PROPS

I discovered yoga when I was in high school, but I didn't begin taking it seriously until college. And, as you probably know, when you're in college, you're broke as a joke. And if you've ever been broke as a joke, you know that you'll do anything to save a buck. This is one of the reasons I love college kids and look back on my time as a student with fond memories. I mean, I may or may not have smuggled food out of the dining hall to eat during my study breaks at the library so I wouldn't have to stop by Bookworms, the library's café, and spend a measly $1.50 on a muffin. Hey, $1.50 is $1.50, my friends! I'm not saying that I'd recommend stealing a block from your local yoga studio; I'm just saying that I understand tight budgets. I always tell my students that yoga blocks are so versatile, and if there's room in the budget for only one yoga prop, this is the prop I recommend.

The other thing I love about college kids is that they're so creative. Back in my broke-as-a-joke days, I used to duct-tape two similar-sized books together to create a yoga block. So if a yoga block isn't in your budget, tap into your inner creative self and look around the house for something similar. You're welcome to try my duct-tape-book version if you'd like! I've also used VHS tapes (remember those?) and my brother's Xbox (sorry, Albie!).

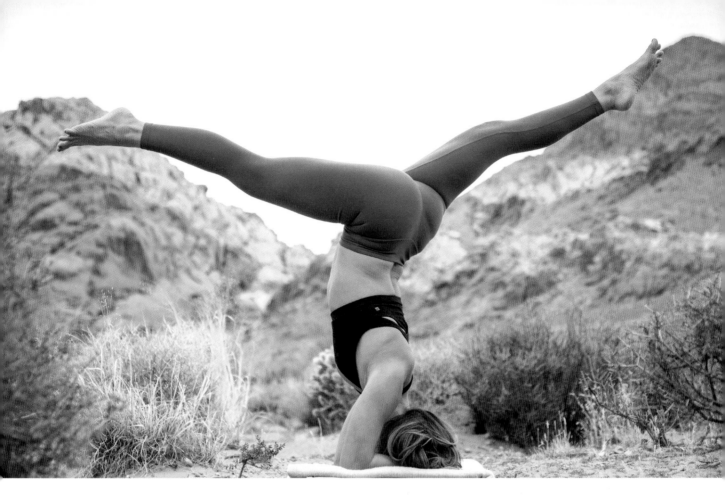

one last tip for your practice: say yes

I've talked about being a Hell Yeah person off the mat, but be sure to be one *on* the mat, too. Sometimes I'll demo a pose that people don't see very often, like baby grasshopper (page 190). It's a pose that looks way more challenging than it is, and more often than not, over half the class will groan and look at each other sideways, and some will even say, "Oh, I can't do that." They say it before even trying! They automatically tell themselves that it can't be done!

I understand it, though, because I used to be just like them. Saying it out loud takes you off the hook. But here's the thing: *there is no hook to be on.* This is yoga. It's not for anyone else but you. So instead of saying no, see what happens when you approach each pose with a "Hell yeah!"—or at least a "well, maybe." Leave yourself open to the idea that anything is possible, and remember that your brain hears everything you say, whether you say it out loud or to yourself. So get out of your own way, say yes, and see what happens. Maybe it won't happen today, but it will happen eventually, if you let it.

the beginning of the end
August 2010

On a heavy August afternoon in 2010, I am making a sandwich. Turkey and cheese, if you really want to know. Yes, I am a meat eater. And a dairy eater. And a bread eater. Don't judge! Remember: Yoga. Union.

Anyway, Greg and I got married a month ago, and I am still riding the post-wedding high. How amazing is it to have everyone you love in one place all at once? My heart is still filled to the brim with the memories of that special day, and my only regret is that it didn't last longer, because I would've loved more time with our guests.

Greg has just left for hockey training camp. He plays professional hockey, and we've been doing this whole hockey song and dance for years. He has a two-way NHL/AHL contract, and he'll go to training camp for a few weeks while I stay back and take care of the dog. Once training camp is over, I'll move to whichever city he's assigned to. Right now I'm staying with my dad in Connecticut. He lives on a beautiful estate that is quintessentially Connecticut—lush, sprawling fields nestled between rolling hills, so far from town that the only sounds we hear during the day are birds and at night, coyotes.

We recently adopted a stray dog, Pasha, and she seems to get along well with my first baby, my Siberian Husky, Buckles. The two dogs complete our little family, since Greg and I are in no rush to have kids. I mean, let's be real, I can barely get *myself* fed and dressed and out the door; I can't imagine having a small human to look after as well.

The dogs scramble at my feet as I cut the sandwich in half and hurry over to the couch. It's 3:59 p.m., and Oprah's about to start. It's her last season, so #priorities, people!

I sit down and so do the dogs, looking up at me with pleading eyes while they not-so-patiently squirm in place. I know I'm supposed to be annoyed with their begging, but they're adorable.

"Oh, come on," I say with a smile, pretending to be irritated but knowing that I would do anything for these pups. I am a certifiably crazy dog lady. I mean, I like my dogs more than I like most humans, and while

I wish I could say I were lying, that in itself would be a lie.

These dogs are my joy. We have conversations. They can't talk back, obviously, but I know what they're thinking. *They* know I know what they're thinking. They know my deepest, darkest secrets and have this innate ability to just *know* how I'm feeling without my having to say a word. How incredible is that? Tell me the name of one human who could do that!

I break off two small pieces of crust and feed one to Pasha, who gobbles it up like she's never had food in her life. Then I hold out the other piece to Buckles, who has waited patiently but who, I can tell, can barely contain his excitement. I hold out my hand and he gingerly takes the crust in his mouth, but before I can blink, Pasha attacks him. With blood-curdling growls and a rage I've only seen depicted in dogfights in the movies, she goes for his neck, and I instantly drop my plate to break them up. Buckles starts defending himself, and I try to grab the scruffs of their necks, but it's useless—they are going to the death. I yell and scream and try to grab them again, but they are like wild animals.

It's weird the things that pop into your head in the middle of a crisis.

Years ago, we used to take Buckles to a dog park, and once a fight broke out between two other dogs. One of the owners had an iced coffee, and she poured it on them, which stunned them just long enough that the two owners could pull the dogs apart.

This is what I'm thinking about as I see these two dogs go at it.

I run to the kitchen and fill a huge glass with water. My heart is racing as I yell at the dogs to stop and will the water to come out of the tap faster. When the glass is about three-fourths of the way full, I quickly shuffle back to the living room, careful not to let any water splash out. When I get to them, I tip the glass over. It has no effect. I am humiliated that I've wasted time filling a glass of water for nothing, and I feel hot tears sting my eyes.

"Stop it!!!!" I scream at the top of my lungs, as if that's going to do anything.

My heart races as I get as close to the dogs as I can and reach out, but they're moving in circles as they jab at each other with their mouths, like fighters in a ring going in for the knockout punch. Pasha, who is all white and likely part Akita, shows no signs of blood on her fur, but Buckles has blood coming from his head and two front paws, and they are still viciously going at one another. I am crying hard now and yelling for my dad, who is outside mowing and surely cannot hear me.

Again I grab the scruffs of their necks and manage to pull them apart. I hold them away from each other, my arms burning, and Buckles seems to settle. But Pasha, her lips curled, snarls and lunges at him one more time. I shift Buckles away from her, and Pasha's teeth sink into my right forearm like a knife through butter.

I howl in pain and let both of them go as I grab my arm. The bite sends Buckles into a frenzy, and the two resume their fighting. The room starts to spin, and I feel hot as a wave of adrenaline washes over me. My breathing is too quick, and I'm starting to feel dizzy. I press my left hand harder into the bite and try to assess the situation. It feels like everything is moving in slow motion.

Think, goddammit! I tell myself.

I do a quick mental assessment. *How much blood have I lost? Enough to pass out? Can I get up and get these dogs away from each other again?*

I yell for my dad as if my life depends on it.

Your life does depend on it, you idiot!

Through sobs of pain, I peek at the wound. A large strip of flesh flaps opens to reveal a deep bite. I can see the fatty layer of tissue that protects the tendons. It looks like salmon roe. I immediately cover it with my left hand and make my way to the stairwell next to the entryway, where I collapse on the bottom step, my breathing labored. I can barely see through my tears, but I notice that the dogs have stopped fighting and are just staring at me from the other room with big, blinking eyes.

I throw my head back and scream bloody murder for my dad. As if by some force of God, he bursts through the door, and I start to feel like I'm having an out-of-body experience.

Do you ever have moments when you're going through something terrible but simultaneously feel like you're not really in the moment? As if you're operating your body with some remote control while sitting across the room? There I was, lying on the stairs sobbing, feeling faint, like I was losing a lot of blood, and at the same time I was engaging in all sorts of crazy self-talk.

Oh, please, you're not dying, Candace. Pull it together, a little voice inside snickers.

Another voice chimes in: *Well, you might be. Stranger things have happened.*

"I thought I heard you," my dad says softly as he kneels down next to me.

My dad is the kind of person you want to have around when something goes wrong. He has an uncanny ability to remain calm. Actually, it's almost maddening how perpetually calm he is. He is the opposite of an alarmist, and even that is an understatement. I can count on one hand the number of times I've seen him angry or even overly excited about something.

Okay, so Dad's not worried. You're probably overreacting, I think. A part of me starts to believe that maybe I've screamed for nothing and that none of this is a big deal. I have a tendency to be, shall we say, a bit dramatic.

"I think we'd better get you to the ER," he says evenly, soothingly. "You're going to need stitches."

So Dad's worried. You're not overreacting.

I cry harder. I have never needed stitches before, and the thought of someone sewing my skin together scares the hell out of me.

He helps me stand, walks me to his car, and drives me (faster than his normal 30mph) to a nearby walk-in clinic.

This was the beginning of the end for me.

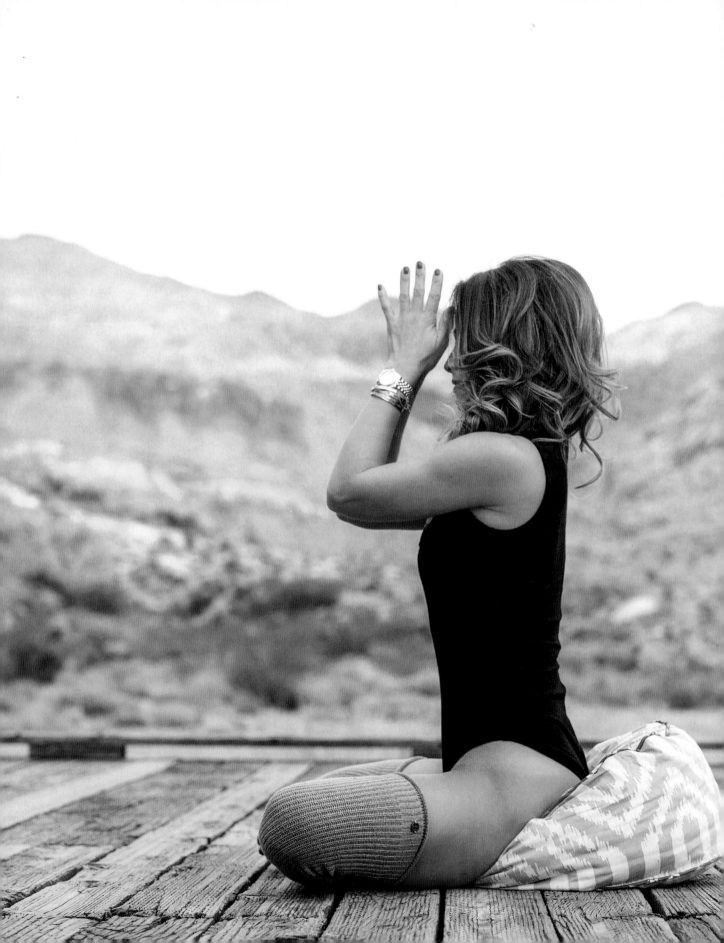

CHAPTER 1:

everything you need to know about meditation

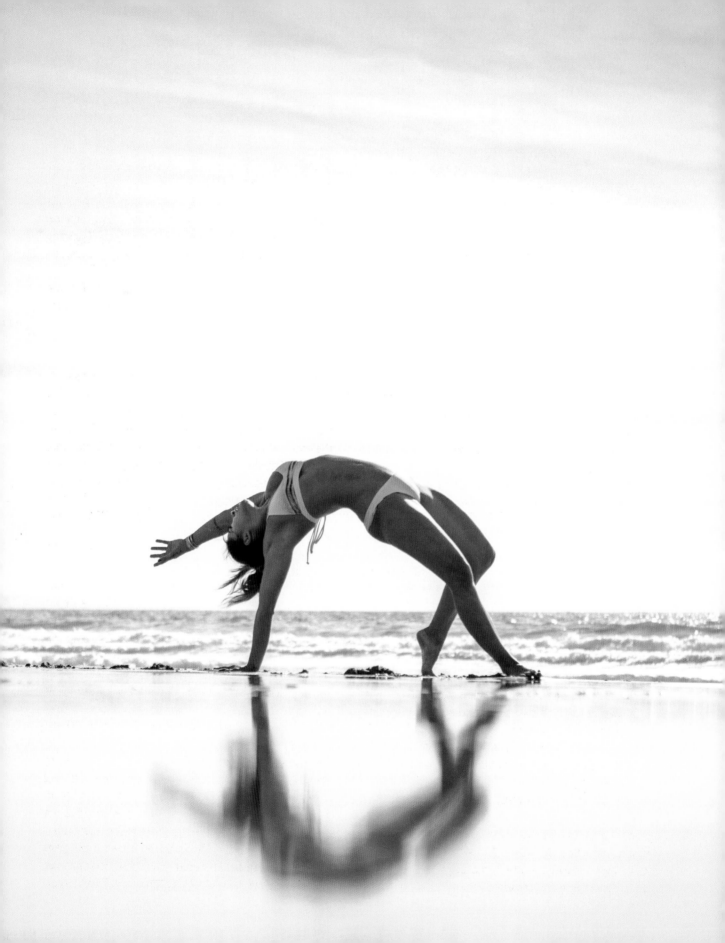

first meditation
September 1999

My mother has always marched to the beat of her own drum. If you have a parent like that, I can guarantee that it has simultaneously embarrassed you (have fun explaining to your fellow fifth graders that your mom's homemade "chocolate chip" cookies—which look like shapeless little turds—are actually made with carob chips) and made your heart burst with pride, like the time a total Cool Girl came up to us at TJ Maxx.

You know the Cool Girl when you see her—she is effortlessly beautiful in that "what-do-you-mean-I-woke-up-like-this" kind of way, with tousled hair that smells like the tropics and perfectly worn-in jeans that hang just right. She knows a little bit about everything and isn't afraid to start a conversation about things that matter. She laughs without holding back and is kind and thoughtful and totally at ease in her own skin. Pretty much everything I was not at age fifteen.

"Excuse me," she breathes as she runs up to my mom. "I saw you get out of the car earlier," she laughs, "and I had to follow you in here to ask about your sweater. It's incredible! Where did you get it?"

I look from her to my mom skeptically, because there is no way on God's green earth that my crunchy granola mom is wearing anything even halfway cool, and I'm certain the Cool Girl must've followed the wrong woman.

My mom's sweater is something she's had forever and wears on repeat every fall and winter. For the first time, I cock my head to the side and really *look* at it. It's a chunky handmade Fair Isle sweater, ivory with a brown design. It's oversized and sort of shapeless, and my mom wears it with a turtleneck underneath.

"Oh, this?" my mom says, looking down, equally surprised. "I got this at a consignment shop in the seventies."

The girl lets out a wistful chuckle. "Of course you did."

She sighs as she reaches out to lightly run her finger over the shoulder. "All the best stuff comes from consignment shops," she says, looking each of us in the eye and giving us the kind of smile that warms your soul before she turns and walks away.

My mom looks at me pointedly and makes an "I told you so" face with a smile she can't conceal, because she owns a consignment shop—something I'd always been moderately embarrassed by, because as a high schooler, having a mom who sells other people's clothes for a living feels so awkward. But at that moment, my heart swells with pride.

Yeah, Cool Girl, I think. *That's my mom! Wearing the sweater you love and will not be able to borrow. Because she's* my *mom. Boo-yah.*

****

The first time my mom drags me to Kripalu, a converted monastery nestled in the Berkshire hills of Massachusetts, it's a crisp, sunny Sunday in September. These days, Kripalu, in case you're not in the know, is a world-renowned yoga center. Back then, though, Kripalu was just a big old gorgeous building for patchouli-smelling new-school hippies who did a weird thing called yoga. There were no New Yorkers to be found—just a bunch of patchouli-smelling new-school hippies.

See, my mom discovered Kripalu before doing yoga was cool (which, now, is one of those things that ranks right up there with the Cool Girl sweater day). Back then, you could spend the day at Kripalu for $25 per person. (For the record, I just called, and now it costs $120 for the day.) You'd get access to the whirlpool and sauna area and the meditation room, a delicious meal, and a yoga class, and you'd pretty much just hang out there, soaking up all the good vibes.

So why did my mom have to *drag* me there? Let's get back to the story.

As a sophomore in high school, I wear a veil of teenage angst. I date a boy who drives a motorcycle, and my mom can't stand it. She and I are at odds all the time because she's so strict and so worried about me. And like the naive, self-centered teen that I am, I don't realize that she's doing the best she knows how, and instead I'm convinced that she's out to make my life a living hell, so really? The last thing I want to do

43

on the weekend is be with her at some hippie-dippie commune.

"Just go and check the place out," she says as she curls up in one of the wooden rocking chairs lined up in front of the bay windows that overlook the rolling Berkshires.

I scowl and turn on my heel. *The sooner I pretend to explore the place,* I think, *the sooner we can leave.*

The hallways of Kripalu are long, and thanks to the oversized windows and skylights, the entire place is flooded with natural light. It's so beautiful that it's hard to be angry here, I notice with annoyance. I pace down the carpeted corridors and pass by the gift shop. It's situated next to a set of five wide steps that lead to a huge empty room.

Noting the sign, I take off my shoes and walk in. It's the largest room I've ever been in, and it feels infinitely bigger because it is completely empty. The ballroom-sized space has wall-to-wall plush carpeting—the kind that you sink into with each step—and I feel miniature as I look up at the sky-high ceilings. The tall, wide windows that frame the room make it seem like the walls are made of glass, and a soft yet vibrant light drenches the space in a golden glow. Candles are lit and the lights are dimmed, giving the room a warmth I've never felt before. I take a cushion from the back of the room, set it in a corner, and have a seat. The clock strikes 4:59pm, and suddenly people begin pouring in. It's the strangest thing—despite the mass of people, the space is silent. I almost wonder if I've gone deaf because I hear nothing. With quiet yet determined faces, each of them silently takes a cushion and places it on the ground with intention.

What is happening? What are they going to do? I wonder.

Then a small man in nondescript baggy pants and a thin white T-shirt heads to the front of the room. He picks up a huge mallet, stands next to a gong that's larger than he is, and strikes it.

Ah, I think, looking around and noticing that people have adopted the traditional meditation setup. *It's a meditation session.*

Meditation is weird to me. *Like, what am I supposed to do?* I wonder. I sit there, glancing around the room for clues. *Is this like praying? Am I supposed to bow my head? Should my eyes be closed? Am I supposed to do something with my hands?*

My heart starts to beat a bit faster because I feel like I shouldn't be here. Like I'm intruding. And, if I'm being honest, I would rather not be here. If I had a choice, I'd be at home, listening to Nirvana, talking on the phone with my friends. But here I am.

I assess the situation. *Can I leave?* I wonder. *No,* I realize. I'm not about to walk out, because what if the gong man calls out and tries to stop me and then there I am, being called out for skipping out on meditation in front of, like, three hundred people?

So I stay and try to blend in. To act like the Cool Girl, who always knows what to do in this sort of situation.

I notice that everyone is sitting in different ways and doing something different with their hands, so I feel like I can do what comes naturally and not risk having the gong man yell at me. I sit tall on my cushion, cross my legs like a kindergartner, and fold my hands in my lap.

Now what?

I sit there. The gong guy bangs the gong, which echoes throughout the room so powerfully that it feels like the sound is reverberating inside me.

For a few minutes, there's nothing. Nothing at all. I feel my lungs inflate as I inhale. I think nothing. My brain's switch has turned off. I breathe. In. Out. In. Out.

Then, out of nowhere, my thoughts start up. *I wonder what homework I have due for tomorrow. I wish I knew when picture day was; I need something to wear.*

The gong sounds again and brings me back to the present moment. I peek around and then close my eyes and breathe, feeling that gong sound echo inside me, and there's nothing but breath for a few moments.

Silence.

And breath.

I hope Mom is going to make cookies tonight. Do I have a field hockey game this week? Did our uniforms come in yet?

The gong sounds again, nipping my thoughts in the bud, and I'm brought back to the massive room and the immense resounding tone of the gong. I get lost in that powerful yet comforting sound. I dive in, imagining that I'm swimming in its warmth.

The next time the gong sounds, I notice with delight that I've managed not to have one distracting thought since the last gong.

This time, though, I sense movement, and I open my eyes, finding that people are beginning to get up and return their cushions to the back of the room. Feeling a twinge of disappointment that the class is over, I reluctantly get up.

I make my way back down the corridors, going slower this time. I notice everything on the walk back—the smell of lavender in the air, the way the hallway carpet gives just slightly less than the carpeting in the meditation room. I glance outside, realizing that I can't find a word to describe the beautiful cool gray color outside as dusk arrives.

When I find my mom, I can feel my face harden a bit as I put on a mask of indifference. While I liked how I felt and actually enjoyed the meditation class, I'm not about to give her the satisfaction of knowing it.

"You did the meditation?" she asks as she closes the journal she's been writing in. "How'd it go?"

"Meh, it was whatever," I mumble and look away. I hate myself for being so mean to her. It physically hurts my heart when I'm so cruel. *Why am I so awful to her?* I wonder. I can't answer the question and struggle to push the guilt aside.

On our way out to the car, we notice a sign advertising a tag sale in one of the guest rooms. Back then, people stayed at Kripalu for extended periods practicing Seva, which means "selfless service" but is basically Sanskrit for "you work for us for free and we'll give you a place to stay and throw some kale and beans your way." My mom, Cool Girl–approved consignment shop owner that she is, is always on the hunt for unique things to sell at her store and suggests that we check it out before we leave.

"Okay," I try to say pleasantly, because I still feel bad for being so rude.

No one is at the tag sale when we arrive—not even the owner of all the stuff—so I feel like we are snooping around someone's private things. And then I notice a sign that says "Honor System" with a little cash box below it.

I pick up a cassette tape (remember those?!) and read its handwritten label, "Angry Music."

"We should get this," I say to my mom with a grin. I'm on a mission to prove to her that these hippie-dippie happy-go-lucky people aren't all rainbows and kombucha all the time, and I can't wait to hear what's on this angry mixtape. Pleased that I'm not being a little brat for, like, once in my life, she tucks a dollar into the cash box and we leave.

Back then, I'd never have admitted it to my mom (#teenagerproblems), but I loved it at Kripalu. Yes, it was sort of out there and attracted all sorts of wild and free types, but I felt safe and accepted there.

In the car, I pop in the cassette. Rage Against the Machine, a rap-metal band popular in the 1990s and early 2000s, comes on. The song is "Killing in the Name," an expletive-driven manifesto that was released six months after the 1992 Los Angeles Riots, which were triggered by the acquittal of four white police officers in the brutal beating of Rodney King, a black taxi driver.

I turn it up and grin. "Well, Mom," I say with a smirk, "let's see what your weirdo Kripalu people are listening to these days," and I turn up the volume just loud enough to irritate her. (She's the type who needs to lower the volume to see where she's going , and ironically, these days so am I.) The song repeats "Fuck you, I won't do what you tell me"—a lyric directed at corrupt government officials— sixteen times before finishing with a hate-filled "motherfucker!!!" that seems to go on for six syllables.

"Well," my mom says with a laugh, "This certainly is 'angry music'!" She turns up the volume just a bit higher, flicks the high beams on, and relaxes into her seat as we drive down the dark, twisting Berkshire roads with the rap-metal blaring.

I look at her incredulously, and for the first time in my life I realize that two seemingly opposite things can exist: a gentle, quiet, peaceful sense of self, like the one I experienced at Kripalu in my first-ever meditation class, and a driven, powerful sense of self that questions our experiences and strives to create something better, like the Rage Against the Machine song describes.

That drive home was the beginning of the formation of Namaslay: the idea that we can move through life being kind, warm, and loving on the surface but also be fueled by an undeterred drive to tap into our fullest potential and live our greatest life.

Okay, listen. I'm going to just come out and say what no one else will: meditation is freaking weird.

Like, you just sit there.

That's it!

How weird is that?! To just sit there. In silence. Doing nothing.

In a world of Instagram and hashtags and trending topics, where information is constantly blasted out like T-shirts shot into the crowds at basketball games, it's pretty bizarre.

When I first started practicing yoga, in high school, these were the things I was interested in:

- clothes (new ones, not consignment ones)

- friends (the more the merrier)

- boys (bad boys, to be exact)

- singing (I was in this kickass a cappella group called The Sweethearts—don't you dare laugh)

- working out (my first "real" job, if you don't count babysitting, was at a gym)

- English, woodworking, and music classes (my favorites, in no particular order)

- instant messaging (real embarrassment lies within your first IM name, am I right or am I right?)

Meditation, as you can see, did not make it onto the list of things that I cared about.

Yoga, as in the poses and the one-handed handstand on your fingertips (not yoga as in union), fell under my "working out" category, and that was about all I had to say about it at the time. I did power yoga because the movements reminded me of my days of doing gymnastics as a kid. I really liked the class. Plus, the teacher was a total Cool Girl from The City (New York, which is really the only city that matters when you're from Connecticut). She was tall and had this choppy, piecey short haircut that she pulled off because she rocked it with confidence. She wore funky clothes and layers of incredible jewelry that I never had a prayer of finding around my small rural town, and she was warm and kind without being all chakras-and-crystals about it. She was just a nice Cool Girl who happened to come up from the city to teach yoga on the weekends. I was always sad that I wasn't old enough to go out with the class afterward to drink wine and eat cheese at the local bar, which was their Sunday night ritual.

She didn't incorporate a lot of meditation—just some corpse pose nonsense at the end of the class, which, if I'm being honest and you promise not to tell anyone, was slowly becoming one of my favorite parts of the class.

It was weird to just lie there for no apparent reason. On the one hand, I thought, we're done, right? Can't we just go home? But on the other hand, at the end of a tiring, sweaty class, lying there pretending to be dead was the most welcome, albeit strange, thing. Plus, the Cool Girl would come around with these lavender eye pillows and place one over my eyes and then press down on my shoulders, and it just felt nice, so I ignored my teenage instinct to scoff and rolled with it instead.

NAMASLAY COMMANDMENT #3:
CONTINUE TO LEARN.

WTF is meditation?

When I considered the idea of traditional meditation, I pictured some old man wrapped in robes levitating with his hands in prayer position.

Not only could I not do that, I didn't *want* to do that. Hello, this is crazy person with swirly eyes type stuff! Meditation seemed like a joke, and so far from my reality as a stressed-out, insecure high school kid just trying to make it through the day without having a mental breakdown. Taking time to "sit in stillness" felt so foreign that it seemed completely unattainable and, if I'm being honest, it seemed like a waste of my precious time.

So if you're on the fence about meditation, or even if you're vehemently against it, I 100 percent get you, and not just from my own personal experience as a student. In my years of teaching yoga, I've encountered so many people who immediately dismiss meditation. It's like they're intimidated by it because the idea of doing nothing is so unbelievably foreign. But their intimidation is often masked by annoyance.

"What exactly am I supposed to do?" they ask with an exasperated sigh. "Like, just sit there?"

As it turns out, yes. Meditation is choosing to be fully present in your body and sitting with whatever it is you're going through. It sounds so vague, so crunchy granola that sometimes I want to barf when I hear myself explain it, but I promise I am not getting all hoo-hoo weird on you. That's truly all it is—simply being present in the moment.

I know what you're thinking. Being present in the moment? What does that really *mean*?!

It's like this. Have you ever gotten into your car after a long day at work and driven home and then realized that you have no idea how you actually got home? You weren't paying attention to the route you took. You have no idea how many stoplights there were. You didn't notice the old lady who sits on her porch day after day, or the fact that you pass the same group of kids walking home from school, hunched over from the weight of their oversized backpacks. You were just going through the motions and not paying much attention.

And there's nothing wrong with that, really. But things could be better. You could be psyched about your drive home from work! You could sing in your car and smile and wave at the old lady on the porch (which would totally make her day, by the way). You could smile as you reminisce about your days as a middle schooler (but I don't recommend stopping to chat with them because strangers pulling over to talk with kids is generally frowned upon). But, in all seriousness, that drive home could be the best part of your day!

With meditation, it's about waking the eff up and paying attention, not so much to the world around you but to what's happening *within* you. I know this sounds like mumbo jumbo, but I promise it's not.

Meditation is about taking a second to do a sort of internal body scan. It's looking at yourself and saying, "Self? How *you* doin'?" It's running through the checklist of what you're dealing with and how you're feeling, acknowledging that, and then seeing if you can flick off the thought switch, set the to-do list aside for five minutes, and just breathe.

Meditation is about being fully aware in the moment. When we are fully aware, we are more in tune with ourselves, and we are able to reach deep and tap into that innate sense of calm that we're born with.

TAP INTO YOUR GREATNESS.

Okay, now that we're clear on the fact that meditation is just sitting there and breathing (#weird), what does it mean in terms of the yoga practice?

Well, the kind of meditation that shows up in the yoga practice is often a seated meditation, but there are many different types. You could do a walking meditation, a music meditation, a silent meditation...the list goes on. But really, it doesn't matter what you're doing—you could be playing golf or walking a tightrope between two skyscrapers. What's important is your breath and your focus. The goal with meditation is to unplug the tube in your mind that enables thoughts to stream through and see if you can think nothing and just breathe.

This is where things get really hard, because we're pretty much thinking stuff from the second we wake up until the second we fall asleep. And if we're not thinking stuff, stuff is thrown at us in the form of social media timelines and those scrolling newsfeed thingies along the bottom of the television screen. Actually, when you stop and think about it, going through your day is pretty much just figuring out how to duck and miss all the *stuff* that's thrown at you. Oof. With all the stimuli, it's *tough* to think nothing. But I urge you to try.

Think nothing, and instead be an observer. Imagine that you're outside your body and you're quietly looking at this person before you, seated and breathing. It's a little strange, yeah. But I'll tell you a secret: all the best things are. Like avocados and the fact that they seriously go with everything. (I'm not kidding. Try avocado mixed with a teaspoon of maple syrup and a teaspoon of cacao powder. Don't say I never gave you nothin'!)

So yeah, meditation is *hard*. And in theory, it shouldn't be. Because you just sit there and breathe. I can't think of anything simpler. So why is it such a struggle for so many people?

This is where I wish I could drop some mind-blowing wisdom to magically enlighten you, but the truth is, I haven't got a clue. Sorry about that.

But I can help you if you're finding meditation to be a huge pain.

If you're frustrated because your brain is having diarrhea of the thoughts and there's no such thing as Imodium for your brain (except for maybe Xanax, which I don't recommend taking on a whim), here's what to do:

First, don't get frustrated. So your brain won't STFU. Who cares? There's no one to impress right now. There's no test after your meditation session. Stop beating yourself up.

Second, take a deep breath. Let go of expectations. Get out of your own way. Forget the idea of needing to be able to do everything (or at least this meditation) perfectly. Let. It. Go. If you're a visual person like me, you can do what I do: visualize your thoughts as fluffy white clouds against a bright blue sky. When you look up at the clouds in real life, they don't piss you off. They're just clouds. And you watch them go by and then get on with your day. Do the same here. Watch your thought-clouds go by without giving them any energy, and then get back to focusing on your breathing. Pretty soon, the thoughts will slow down and come less frequently. Before you know it, your sky will be bright blue, and if a cloud happens to roll through, you'll just watch it go by without being disturbed.

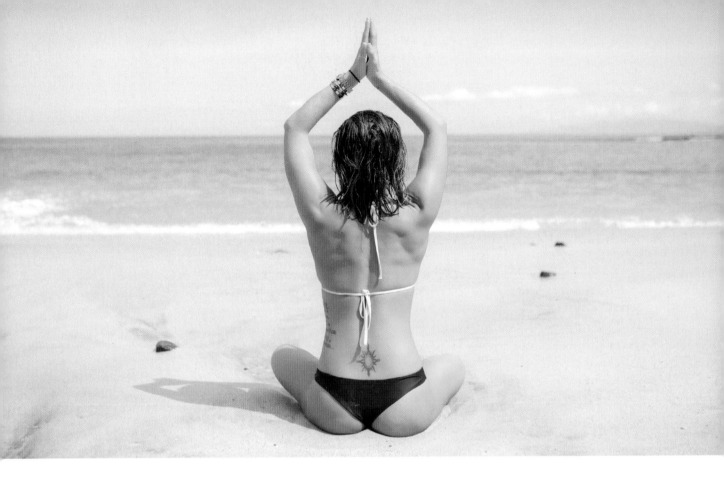

what is meditation good for?

When I was in college, I lost three family members right in a row, unexpectedly: to suicide, old age, and a motorcycle accident. The second I found out about the first death, the suicide, I was in Costa Rica for spring break, and it felt like my whole world came crashing down around me. Then sweet Sittee, my grandmother, died. And then a motorcycle accident claimed the life of an uncle. I was shaken to the core. It felt like the universe had taken my world, shoved it into a blender with some broken glass, blended it on high, and force-fed it to me. I was a walking lunatic.

The deaths in my family triggered anxiety and depression within me that were so profound, I felt paralyzed. It started with anxiety, which would swoop down out of nowhere like an eagle catching its prey. My body would sweat uncontrollably, a pit would form in my stomach, and waves of adrenaline would wash over me again and again, making me feel like I was drowning. My throat would begin to tighten, and no matter how hard I tried, I couldn't breathe normally. I was always gasping for air, struggling to stay afloat. I felt like nothing was within my control.

Back on campus, I felt like I was going crazy. Loud noises and bright lights frightened me, and I had to stop eating at the larger dining halls. I felt debilitating anxiety from the moment I woke up until the moment I went to sleep. I lost a worrisome amount of weight and suffered from multiple panic attacks on a daily basis.

I stopped hanging out with nearly all of my friends. I skipped classes. I felt like I was suffocating all the time. All. The fucking. Time.

Depression followed on the coattails of the anxiety. It pulled me down into a deep, dark, cavelike place—echoing, scary, dangerous, and cold. I felt alone and lost and afraid.

I was transferred from a triple to a single dorm room, and I lay in bed all day, every day, staring at the ceiling, unblinking, with tears dripping from eyes that felt like a faucet with a perpetual leak. I felt empty, without words to express the hollowness that gnawed at me. My thoughts seemed slow, cloudy, and muddled, and I felt like I was going crazy. I never opened the windows because the outside noises—the laughter and chatter of the people whose lives were going on—made my heart race. I started eating in my room because being around other people made my throat tighten up. My room was dank and stale-smelling, reeking of old soy milk and body odor, and I didn't care. When you're that low, nothing really matters to you.

With the help of a shrink, I got my hands on some trazodone, an antidepressant and sedative that numbed me and slowed my speech and reaction time. I felt like my life was in slow motion. One day, when I couldn't take the smell of my room or myself anymore, I summoned enough energy to walk halfway down the dorm hall to the showers. I put my forearm against the gritty, dirty taupe tiles, rested my head against my arm, and stood under the scalding water, wishing it were hotter so it could burn away the pain. I imagined the lava-hot water melting my skin, muscles, and bones away to nothing. Fat tears rolled down my face. I felt half immobilized by immense sadness and half immobilized by the trazodone, and I prayed to just disappear.

It felt like five minutes, but I cried in the shower for over an hour that day, feeling like these deaths were insurmountable. They made me realize that everyone I loved in my life was going to die at some point. And I felt terrified that I would be left here on earth to grieve them, feeling small, frightened, and alone.

I enlisted the help of a psychologist, who diagnosed me with PTSD. In addition to twice-daily talk therapy sessions, some Prozac and Klonopin, and a cutback on the trazodone, he recommended meditation.

"You're going to think I'm crazy," he warned me, "but I want you to just sit there and breathe. Don't let any of the thoughts that have overtaken your life creep in. If they do, just let them go as easily as they came without worrying about the fact that they came at all."

I rolled my eyes and sort of scoffed at the fact that he thought that "a few deep breaths" were going to save me from the crippling panic attacks I'd been experiencing, but we'd been working together for over a month, and he was the first shrink I'd seen (and believe me, I've seen far more than my fair share) who wasn't all "and-how-did-that-make-you-feel" phony. He wasn't the type who looked at his watch while I was talking. He didn't take notes with a raised eyebrow when I told him my crazy thoughts. He didn't laugh or tell me that I should go to church or suggest that I was making my problems up (all three of which actually happened at one point). He just listened and talked with me. He treated me like I was a normal person going through some really hard shit. And I will forever be grateful for that.

Anyway, if I hadn't had so much respect for him at that point, I would've abandoned the therapy, because meditation? It seemed like a joke solution for some very serious problems. Under other circumstances, I would've walked out of the room.

But I stayed.

"Okay, let's practice it together," he suggested from his chair across the room. "Close your eyes, sit tall, and we'll breathe for just one minute." Sensing my irritation, he said gently, "You can do anything for a minute."

I considered this. *I can do anything for one minute,* I affirmed. It became a mantra that I would use repeatedly throughout my life, and I always think of my shrink fondly when I use it.

"Okay," I said meekly. And we began. With the first breath, I felt my throat start to constrict, as if I were about to have yet another panic attack. The bright, airy room started to feel like it was suffocating me, and I inhaled sharply, feeling my heart begin to race.

"Um," I interrupted, alarmed. "My heart is racing." Tears lined my eyes, and my hands began to shake. I was frustrated and angry that I *couldn't even do one minute.*

"That's because this is something new," he said gently. "If you want, try keeping your eyes open—a soft gaze—and see if you can breathe through the newness."

NAMASLAY COMMANDMENT #4:
GET COMFORTABLE
BEING UNCOMFORTABLE.

So I did.

And I didn't feel an immediate shift. But I did feel marginally better after one minute. The completion of one full minute and the fact that I felt just the slightest bit better illuminated a ray of hope. Maybe I *did* have the power to help myself.

A few days later, my mom sent me a CD (remember CDs?) of guided meditations that she had picked up at Kripalu. The dynamic of our relationship had evolved, as it does when you start to let go of being a little high school know-it-all, and I had been open with her about my struggles. Because depression runs deep in our family, I think she was more worried than she let on. She made me promise to call her whenever I needed to, no matter the hour. I think she could hear in my voice that I was scared of my thoughts. I wasn't about to admit it to her (listen, I said the dynamic had changed; I didn't say that I'd turned into a model daughter), but I was grateful for her support, and I put the CD on immediately after I opened up the package.

There were a number of guided meditations, and as a total beginner—and someone in the middle of a quarter-life crisis—it was exactly what I needed. A guided meditation was far easier for me than meditating on my own. I found that listening to someone talk me through the meditation offered a distraction from the crazy thoughts that would pop up when I tried to do it on my own.

Over the next few weeks, I scrambled to play that CD whenever I felt a panic attack coming on, and for those few minutes during and a few minutes after the meditations, I'd feel something that resembled normalcy. My heart rate would slow to a more regular rate, my hands wouldn't shake, and that pit in my stomach would melt away. I wish I could say that meditation completely healed me from the anxiety, depression, and panic attacks, but I'd be lying. I had a strong support system and a couple of prescriptions (hey, just speaking the truth here), but meditation was a key component of my healing, and it remained the one thing that I kept returning to over the years whenever my life would get too chaotic. The support systems wavered, the prescriptions ran out, but meditation was always there.

These days, completely off all medication and no longer (that much of) a walking disaster, I incorporate morning and evening meditation every single day because I find that it starts my days off on the right foot and ends them just as beautifully.

Should I meditate more often? Yeah, probably. But I do what I can. And do you know what that is? Ten breaths in the morning and ten breaths at night.

Right now, that's all I can manage, and I've gotten sick of judging myself for not doing more. What I'm doing is my best, and I've made a commitment to let that be enough. And that feels so, so good.

So ten breaths, morning and night. And let me tell you, ten breaths is enough.

Sure, I'd probably feel a difference if I took a hundred breaths, but ten really does a good job. Ten sets the foundation for a beautiful day. Ten helps me unwind before bed. Ten offers clarity and calm and a sense of gratitude, all of which drive my day. So yeah, I love ten. And I think if you gave it a shot, you would, too.

There are so many benefits to meditation. When we slow down our thought process (or manage to turn it off completely), we become calmer and more self-aware. But scientifically, what's happening inside is pretty fascinating.

So what does this mean for you? It means that if you're struggling with major anxiety and depression, there is hope. Along with professional help, meditation offers a tremendously effective healing component to whatever it is you're dealing with.

And even if you're not going through a serious life crisis, but are just generally ho-humming through life with a moderate level of stress, anxiety, and heaviness, I still recommend meditation. Think of it like a daily multivitamin that can support and enhance the quality of your life.

A consistent meditation practice can help balance stress levels. When we lower our stress levels, we're able to lower our cortisol levels. Cortisol is responsible for a number of issues that we may experience, including inflammation, stress, and exhaustion. High stress levels may also contribute to digestive issues, impact metabolism, and increase anxiety and depression, so when we lower those stress levels, other health issues we're dealing with may begin to diminish. A meditation practice may also help boost immunity, improve focus, and increase productivity. So basically, start meditating and boom! You've just served yourself a piping-hot cup of health. Drink up.

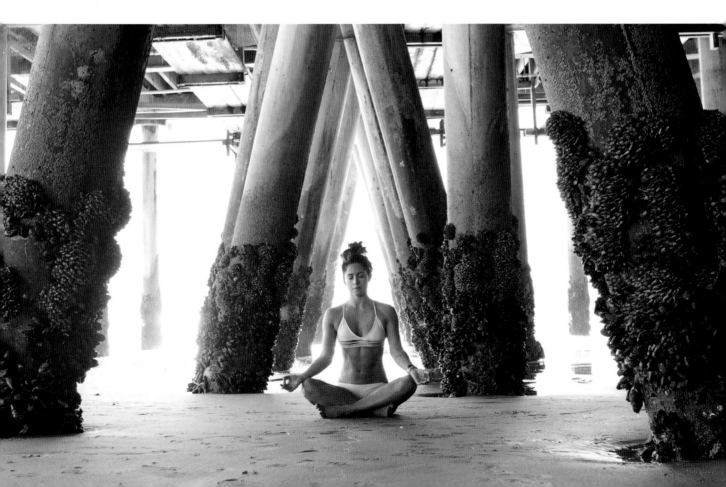

meditation 101

In yoga, the type of meditation you generally hear about is seated meditation, but really, there are a number of different types (see "types of meditation" a little later in this chapter), and no matter what anyone might tell you, no one type is better than the others. You may find that you are more successful with meditation when you're taking a walk in the woods than when seated at home in a quiet room. Whatever floats your boat, my friend.

But for the purposes of this book, I want to shine the spotlight on seated meditation. It's pretty basic and we're talkin' basics, so here goes.

choosing props for meditation

For a seated meditation (and pretty much anything else in life), all you truly need is yourself. That being said, having a few props makes it much more comfortable.

meditation cushion

A meditation cushion is like morning coffee. You won't die without it (okay, some people might argue with me on that one), but it certainly helps a sista out. I recommend getting one if it's in the budget and you have limited mobility and/or plan to practice meditation for long periods at a time.

Meditation cushions vary in material, shape, and size. For people who have tight hips, I like a cushion that mimics the shape that the legs make when seated in meditation because its outer points offer a bit more support for the legs and knees than its round counterparts do. For people who are more open in the hips, I recommend a simple round cushion. Whatever the shape, I suggest getting something that has a medium firmness to it. A cushion that is too soft won't offer a solid foundation of support when used for an extended period, and a cushion that is too firm will simply be uncomfortable.

bolster

Bolsters can be used in a number of different ways for meditation. Like yoga blocks (see below), they offer good support for people with limited hip mobility. I like a bolster when seated in hero pose because it sits pretty high and offers a significant amount of support, which is excellent for people who have touchy knee joints. You also have the option to sit on the edge of a bolster in lieu of a meditation cushion. This option is best reserved for those with slightly more open hips and healthy knees. And if you happen to have three bolsters at your disposal, then holy smokes, you've really hit the yoga prop jackpot, and you can put them to good use by placing one under each knee for support and sitting on the edge of the third one.

yoga blocks

Foam blocks are a good alternative to meditation cushions and bolsters because they offer the slightest bit of give, which I find to be the perfect amount of firmness. For seated meditation, a block provides good support for people with limited hip mobility.

You can sit however you'd like while you meditate (hero pose is great, or you can sit cross-legged), but if you use a block to make it more comfortable, the key is to sit on the very edge of the block so that your pelvis is tilted slightly forward. This will help you maintain a long spine and support good posture.

meditation bench

A bench made specifically for meditation is another option. Meditation benches are designed with comfort in mind, so they usually are just high enough that your shins can comfortably come down underneath and rest on the ground while you sit on the bench cushion. They are often pretty pricey and range anywhere from $25 to $300.

blankets

There are a number of ways to use blankets for meditation. You can wrap one around yourself while seated, you can roll one up tightly and sit on the edge of it as you would a yoga block, or you can fold two and place one underneath each knee for support when you're seated cross-legged on a block.

preparing your meditation space

For nine years, my husband's job as a hockey player had us moving twice or sometimes, when he was traded, three times per year. Let me just put my Captain Obvious hat on for a second and state for the record for anyone who may not know: moving sucks. No matter how often you do it, it doesn't get easier.

Moving is stressful and labor-intensive in a way that makes you feel like you're running a marathon alone and barefoot—so basically you've accomplished nothing that counts, and all you have to show for it are some blisters, a sweaty T-shirt, and a serious case of hanger: the unfortunate state of being so hungry that you're liable to cut someone if you don't get food in you *now*.

Now imagine doing that two or three times a year. Good times!

With the constant moves, I wanted to maintain some sense of normalcy and keep up my personal yoga practice, but I felt like I never had the time. I mean, really, who has the time to drop everything and Om out?

The truth is, we all have the time, but I was just too lazy to clear a little space on the floor and set up the mat and cushion for meditation. After one particularly good practice around year five of our moves, I found a solution. Because I was absolutely famished—I mean, approaching hanger status—I decided to make a quick snack before picking up my yoga practice area.

Like I said, I was kind of lazy, and I didn't get around to cleaning up the area. The next morning, during breakfast, I thought to myself, *I think I'll just leave it there. I'm more apt to practice when things are all set up.* And I did. My practice went from once every other week to a few times a week. Why didn't I think of that before? See? Sometimes being lazy pays off.

Do you need a dedicated meditation room in order to have an effective meditation session? No. But if you can spare a corner of a room, it's nice to have. Not only does it make meditation one step easier (if your stuff is already set up, all you have to do is take a seat—doesn't get easier than that!), but it also creates a great ambiance for a successful meditation. Here's how I like to design my meditation area:

• **A place to sit:** I put down a cushion or bolster as a place to sit for my meditation. You could also use a rolled-up thick towel or blanket.

• **Ambiance:** To create a calming atmosphere, I decorate the space with beeswax candles (they also purify the air!), live plants (they, too, purify the air), incense, and inspiring little trinkets that I've collected on my travels, like an elephant statue I bought in India and a rhinoceros statue I got in Morocco.

• **Music:** Music and sound meditations can be really calming, so I outfit my meditation area with portable speakers and a Tibetan singing bowl. See "types of meditation" a little later in this chapter for more on music meditations.

• **Aromatherapy:** Essential oils can be a beautiful complement to meditation. Some of my favorites are lavender to de-stress, peppermint to wake up, and lemon to uplift.

positioning your body for meditation

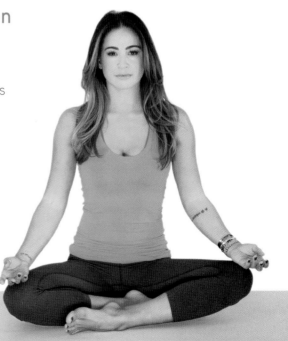

There is no "correct" way to position your body for meditation. I suggest that you try out the following poses a few times and see what feels best for your body.

EASY POSE
Easy pose is what my friend Jenna, a kindergarten teacher, calls "crisscross applesauce." Basically, it's how we sit on the floor as kids. But as adults, we have more flesh than we did back in kindergarten, so it's important to set up correctly. To do this, gently pull the fleshy part of your bum away from the sitting bones so that when you sit down completely, your sitting bones are firmly rooted into the ground. Then, as you breathe in, lengthen from the base of your spine up through the crown of your head. Your hands can rest in your lap.

HERO POSE

To be honest, I've always thought that this pose must be named hero pose because if you can get into it without ruining your knees, you deserve a gold star for being the hero that you are. I have great knees, but this pose is not my fave, and that's an understatement. Hero pose is not recommended for people with knee issues. If your knees are good, though, feel free to give it a try.

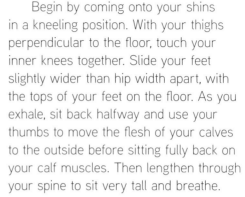

Begin by coming onto your shins in a kneeling position. With your thighs perpendicular to the floor, touch your inner knees together. Slide your feet slightly wider than hip width apart, with the tops of your feet on the floor. As you exhale, sit back halfway and use your thumbs to move the flesh of your calves to the outside before sitting fully back on your calf muscles. Then lengthen through your spine to sit very tall and breathe.

If regular hero pose places a little too much pressure on your knees, you can use a yoga block to help you. Just set the block down and sit on the very edge of it.

LOTUS POSE

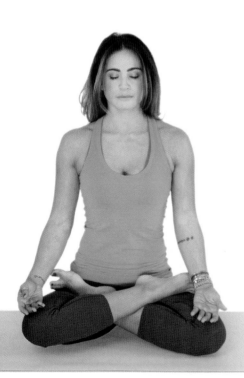

Lotus is the pose that I envisioned I had to get myself into before levitation when I first learned about meditation, so it always brings a smile to my face. This is another pose that's not recommended for people with finicky knees. If you're in the clear, though, you can give it a try.

Begin by sitting on the floor with your legs out in front of you. Bend your left leg and send your left foot to the right, across your torso. Take your left foot in your right hand and hold your left knee with your left hand. With the left ankle and knee joints even, slowly flex your left foot and spread the toes. This helps prevent ankle sickling (the hyperextension of the lateral ankle ligaments, or the outside edge of the ankle). Then slowly guide your left foot into your right hip crease (where your leg attaches to your torso). Keep your left foot flexed as you bend your right foot out to the left. Lift your right foot with your left hand and hold your right knee with your right hand. Then slowly flex your right foot, spread the toes, and guide your right foot into the left hip crease, with your right ankle and knee joints even. Sit very tall and breathe.

If the full expression isn't quite accessible to you yet, you can do half lotus. Begin by sitting on the floor with your legs out in front of you. Bend your left leg and send your left foot to the right, across your torso. Take your left foot in your right hand and hold your left knee with your left hand. With the left ankle and knee joints even, slowly flex your left foot and spread the toes. This helps prevent ankle sickling. Then slowly bring your left foot into your right hip crease (where your leg attaches to your torso). Bend your right leg with your right foot out to the left, but keep the leg on the ground instead of pulling it up and putting your right foot into your left hip crease. Sit tall and breathe.

CORPSE POSE

Corpse pose (page 136) is usually the very last pose in a yoga class. It's a great way to give your body time to absorb all the movements you just did and totally relax. Begin by lying on your back on your mat with your feet about mat width apart. Bring your arms to your sides, with your palms facing up. Close your eyes and let your eyes sink into the sockets. Close your mouth, but part your teeth as you relax your jaw. Breathe in and out through your nose and relax completely.

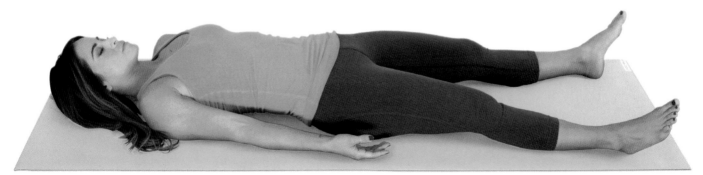

mudras for meditation

With that out of the way, let's talk mudras (pronounced "moo-dras"). *Mudra* is a Sanskrit word meaning "closure" or "seal," and it refers to the numerous hand gestures used during meditation and yoga practice. Each of the mudras has a different purpose or focus. Many people believe that incorporating mudras into the meditation or yoga practice helps complete the energy circuit inside us rather than letting it "escape" through the tips of the fingers. I know that sounds a little nutzo, but just roll with it. Here are a few mudras I love that you can use in meditation:

• ANJALI MUDRA: This is one of the most common mudras you'll see in yoga class. Simply bring your hands together in prayer position at the heart center. This mudra can be used for grounding and centering in every aspect of the practice—meditation, pranayama (breathing exercises—see chapter 2), or yoga poses [think high lunge (page 112) or warrior 1 (page 113)]. It's a good alternative to arms overhead, which can be tough for newbies in a flow setting.

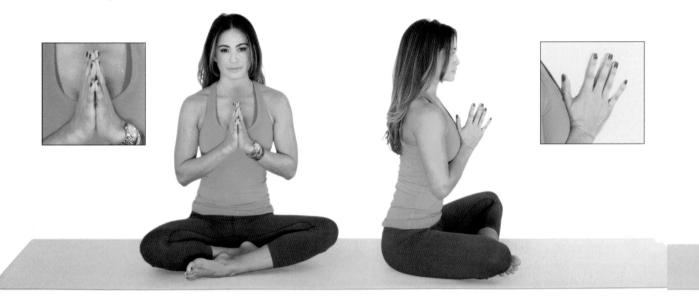

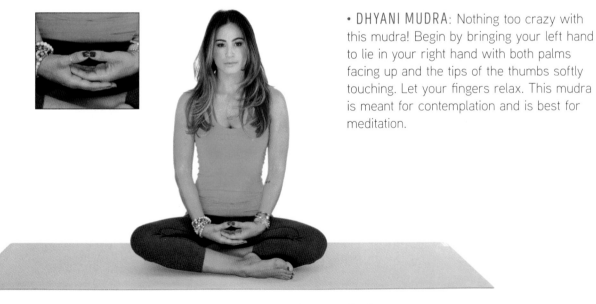

• DHYANI MUDRA: Nothing too crazy with this mudra! Begin by bringing your left hand to lie in your right hand with both palms facing up and the tips of the thumbs softly touching. Let your fingers relax. This mudra is meant for contemplation and is best for meditation.

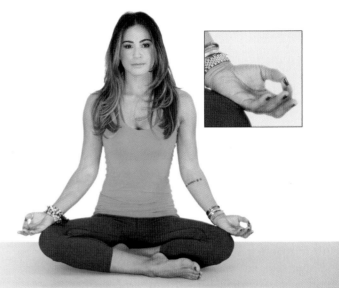

• CHIN MUDRA: I laughed at chin mudra when I learned it in teacher training because I try to remember things using various word associations, but this one has nothing to do with the chin (and that's probably why I remembered it so clearly). To perform chin mudra, touch your thumbs to your index fingers lightly. The thumbs are said to represent the supreme soul and the index fingers the individual soul, so the intention of joining the two is to connect those energies. The other fingers can stay relaxed or outstretched. This mudra can be performed during meditation or pranayama or in asana [think reverse warrior with one arm extended (page 116)].

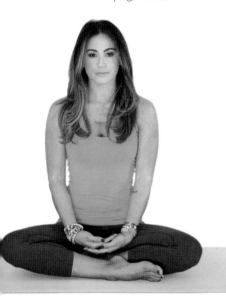

• BHAIRIVA AND BHAIRAVI MUDRAS: These two mudras are pretty much the same; the name changes depending on which hand is on top. For Bhairiva mudra, begin by placing your right hand on top of your left with both palms facing up. For Bhairavi mudra, place your left hand on top of your right with both palms facing up. Both mudras symbolize the innate union of the individual and supreme consciousness.

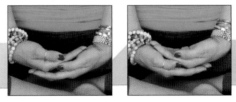

• ADHI MUDRA: Adhi mudra is another one that makes me laugh because the shape is a fist you'd make if you were going to punch someone (see how Zen I am?), and "ahhhh!" (the first syllable) is the sound I think I would make if someone were to punch me! Don't judge, friends; that's how I remembered this one. Except I later learned that if you were really going to punch someone, you wouldn't want to tuck your thumb in like this because you would risk breaking your thumb. See? You learn something new every day. Anyway, begin by tucking your thumbs into your palms with the tips of your thumbs touching the base of your pinkies, and then fold your four fingers over the top. Many people use Adhi mudra during pranayama, with the hands pressed into the body just below the ribs to aid in complete exhalations.

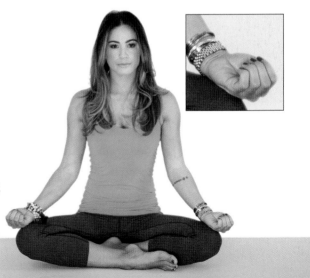

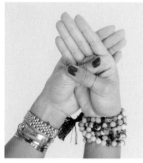

• NAGA MUDRA: Naga mudra is called the mudra of deeper insight, as the hand positioning is meant for clarity and wisdom in dealing with everyday problems or larger issues. Cup your right hand in your left and position your thumbs over one another so they form an X, with your right thumb on top. Keep your fingers together.

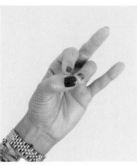

• RUDRA MUDRA: This is easily my favorite mudra, admittedly because the rhyming name is fun to say. I never claimed to be mature! Rudra mudra is said to activate the solar plexus and is good for relieving stress, fatigue, and exhaustion. Place the tips of your index and ring fingers on the tip of your thumb. Keep your middle and pinky fingers extended and breathe.

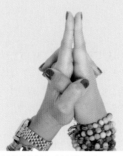

• KSPANA MUDRA: This mudra is said to alleviate negativity, and since I think we can agree that we could all use a little clearing of negative energy, I'm a big fan of incorporating this mudra into the meditation practice. Put your hands together and interlace your fingers. Extend your index fingers and cross your thumbs over one another in the shape of an X, with your left thumb on top.

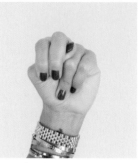

• KASHYAPA MUDRA: The kashyapa mudra is said to bring about balance and protect against negative energy. Place your thumb underneath your index and middle fingers, letting the tip of your thumb poke out as you make a fist. Breathe fully and deeply as you rest your hands on your thighs.

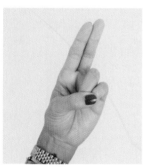

• PRANA MUDRA: Prana means "breath," so the prana mudra is said to awaken dormant energy and help you feel revitalized and energized. To do it, place the tips of your ring and pinky fingers against the tip of your thumb and extend your index and middle fingers.

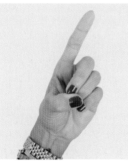

• VAJRA MUDRA: Vajra mudra is said to improve blood circulation, so it's ideal to try when you're feeling chilly or dealing with low energy. Place the tips of your middle, ring, and pinky fingers against your thumb and extend your index finger.

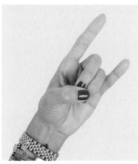

• APANA MUDRA: Apana mudra is meant to create inner balance and cultivate patience, confidence, and a sense of grounding. To do it, place the tips of your middle and ring fingers against the tip of your thumb and extend your index and pinky fingers.

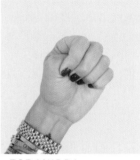

• TSE MUDRA: Tse mudra is said to help alleviate mild depression. To give it a try, place your thumb against your palm and cover it with your fingers.

types of meditation

One of the most confusing things for beginners is the big question of what exactly we do during meditation. As someone who is constantly on the go, wanting little more than to end the day with my to-do list completed, I get it. We're so used to being productive that the idea of sitting and literally doing nothing but breathe confuses us. It's so simple, but we're perplexed. It's kind of funny if you think about it.

So, if you find yourself in this position, don't worry. It's normal. But meditation is so transformative and beneficial. I mean, you know that already. We read studies about its impact on athletes and CEOs. We know it's important, right? So set aside the confusion, give it a try, and you may find yourself one of the many benefiting.

One of the key aspects of yoga is self-study, and meditation is an excellent vehicle for cruising down this path. There are a number of different types of meditation that you can do to ease into an effortless meditative practice, each with its own focus.

breath awareness meditation

With a breath awareness meditation, you basically just want to observe the flow of your breath. Close your eyes and begin to tune in to how you breathe naturally. Go through a mental checklist:

• **Pace of the breath:** are you breathing fast or slowly?

• **Quality of the breath:** is it shallow or deep?

• **Temperature of the breath:** do you notice a difference between the inhale and the exhale?

After you go through this checklist, try to slow down your breathing and make your inhales and exhales of equal length. Begin with one minute. You can do anything for one minute, right? Then work your way up to two minutes and see if you can eventually expand to a twenty-minute practice. Or an hour, if you really want to go for it.

body scan meditation

The body scan meditation is one of my favorites because it forces you to take time to pay attention to yourself and take inventory of what's going on inside, which is something I often forget to do. It's excellent for stress and pain management.

Begin by sitting tall and closing your eyes. Take a few deep, clearing breaths. Then begin scanning your body, starting at the top of your head, moving slowly down to your neck, to your shoulders and chest, to your belly and back, through your hips, and so on. Take a mental inventory of where you're feeling tension, stress, and tightness and where you're feeling openness, movement, and relaxation. As your breathing slows down and becomes more controlled, you may notice a shift in your overall stress or pain levels.

music meditation

A music meditation is another way to switch up the meditation practice. Choose calming music without lyrics. Begin by taking a clearing breath, then breathe fully in and out through your nose. Empty out your lungs completely with each exhale and fill them up fully as you inhale. Let the music carry you throughout the meditation, and when thoughts come, just let them go without giving them any energy.

Music meditation is great for anyone, but I particularly like it for beginners or those who find themselves easily distracted. You can create a playlist based on how much time you have for meditation, and you know that at the end of the playlist the music will stop and you'll be finished. Knowing this means that you won't get distracted by wondering how much time is left, which allows you to be more fully present.

mantra meditation

Mantras are just inspiring words or phrases. Mantra meditations are excellent when you're dealing with something out of the ordinary in your life. For example, if I'm feeling particularly distracted, I'll do a mantra meditation for focus. If I'm feeling rage (hey, I'm only human!), I'll do an Om Shanti mantra, where I will think "om" on the inhale and "shanti" (which means "peace") on the exhale. I recommend mantra meditation for beginners, because having the distraction of repeating the same thing over and over means that there isn't room for any other thoughts, making it effective and easy to practice.

Begin by sitting tall and take a clearing breath in and out. Then close your eyes and breathe in and out through your nose, making sure that your lungs completely fill up on the inhale and completely empty on the exhale. Then repeat the first part of your mantra on the inhale and the second part of your mantra on the exhale. So if your mantra is "calm, focused," you would say "calm" to yourself as you inhale and say "focused" to yourself as you exhale. I generally use two words or a phrase and break up the phrase for the inhales and exhales.

Suggested mantras for various purposes

- I am energized, I am focused. I use this mantra when I hit an afternoon slump and am feeling sluggish and distracted by every little thing. I take five minutes—sometimes less—and breathe in as I say to myself, "I am energized," and exhale as I say to myself, "I am focused."

- Be here now. I once heard someone say that if we're anxious, we're living in the future, worried about things that haven't happened yet. Whenever I feel like this, I like to remind myself of whatever it is I'm doing at the moment. I know this sounds crazy, but bear with me. If I'm anxious as I'm driving to a meeting, I'll literally say to myself, "Relax, all you're doing right now is driving." As I pull into the parking lot, I'll say to myself, "There's no need to be anxious. All you're doing is parking the car. All you're doing is getting out of the car. All you're doing is walking into the meeting. All you're doing is shaking someone's hand." It's a good tactic to distract yourself from the what-ifs when taking five minutes to meditate isn't feasible because you're driving or otherwise occupied. When you *do* have five minutes, however, this small but mighty "be here now" mantra is especially effective when you are experiencing anxiety and stress. Repeat "be here" on the inhale and "now" on the exhale.

- Inhale the good, exhale the bad. This mantra is perfect for inviting the good into your life and letting go of the bad. As you inhale, say to yourself, "Inhale the good," as you visualize good energy entering your life. As you exhale, say to yourself, "Exhale the bad," as you visualize all negative things you're holding onto leave your body and your life.

- Inhale and lengthen, exhale and release. This is an effective mantra for people who are feeling tense, stressed, or in pain. Pay particular attention to the lengths of your inhales and exhales and try to go as slowly as you can, making sure that the inhales and exhales are the same length. With the inhale, try to lengthen anywhere you are feeling stress, and with each exhale intend to release that tension and stress.

- Thank you. I love this mantra for manifesting a sense of gratitude. As you inhale, think the word *thank*. As you exhale, think the word *you*. Breathe fully and deeply, keeping your face calm and your shoulders away from your ears, and let go of any thoughts aside from "thank you."

symptoms

There is something very, very wrong with me. Eight months after the dog bite, I am in so much pain that I can't think straight. My whole body aches deep to the bone, like I have the worst flu of my life. I have shooting pains in my chest and down my legs, complemented by pins and needles so severe that I don't feel like I can support myself if I stand up too quickly. My toes, ankles, knees, hips, wrists, and fingers are inflamed, and I can barely walk. I have a persistent, painful rash along my jaw. My heart races, and the rhythm seems unpredictable. The sun hurts my eyes, and even the slightest subtle background noise hurts my ears. I have debilitating insomnia, and when I *am* able to fall asleep, I have intense, vivid, violent nightmares and bolt awake in the middle of the night, out of breath, terrified, and soaked in sweat.

But I don't look sick. I look like my normal self—my brown eyes are almond shaped from my Ecuadorian heritage, and my skin has a warm olive glow from my Lebanese background. I look vibrant and healthy, but I feel like I'm trapped inside a body that is betraying me.

I have been to eight doctors in the last eight months, and nobody can figure out what is wrong with me. My rapid decline terrifies me.

It's a quiet April evening and I am in the bath, crying. I think to myself, *How is it that not one single doctor of the eight (eight!) that I've seen knows what is wrong with me? What if I never get to the bottom of this? What if the trend continues and I become increasingly worse?*

Depression runs deep in my family, and I have felt the pull of that anchor many times throughout my life. I've worked with a number of therapists and have taken my fair share of antidepressants. But this bleakness, this hopelessness, this black hole that I am staring into is something new.

I submerge my head under the hot water. The uncontrollable tears disappear into the bathwater, and I hold my breath, wondering if I can hold it just long enough to stop breathing and escape this pain. *Is it possible to drown yourself?* I wonder. Then I think of the hairdryer in the cabinet. For a flash of a second I allow myself to consider whether I could plug it in. Turn it on. Put it in the water. I want to run away from these thoughts, but I am simultaneously ashamed and curious and desperate.

Greg knocks on the bathroom door and opens it. I bring my head to the surface, feeling humiliated by my thoughts and worried that he can see what I'm thinking. Hot tears continue to roll down my cheeks.

"I heard you crying," he says softly, clinging to the door, unsure of what to do, whether to enter or leave me alone. We are newlyweds but haven't been able to enjoy the typical newlywed stage. You know, the blindly happy phase. The phase where you've got the too-big grin plastered on your face and your heart skips a beat when you get to introduce him as your husband. We haven't gotten the newlywed stage because I've pretty much ruined it by getting sick.

Greg hasn't once complained, but I know it's been hard for him. My mystery disease has stumped doctor after doctor, and I can sense that he is just as scared as I am.

I sit up and pull my legs into my chest. The pain in my aching knee joints rips through my body like an electric current. I sob uncontrollably like a three-year-old having a tantrum, letting it all out. I am scream-crying in agony because I just don't know anything. I don't know what the *fuck* is wrong with me. I have gone to every doctor I can think of and *they* don't know what the fuck is wrong with me. I am getting worse each day, and I can feel my brain starting to become affected. I don't even know how to explain this brain part, but I've started, um, *seeing* things. Really strange things. Like aliens and zombies—things that look human but *aren't*, and I know what you're thinking because I am thinking the same thing—*that's* crazy talk. Rein it in, Candace. Get it together, girl.

But I can't. My heart races and I rub my eyes and I'm scared to even breathe, because the visions of zombies and alien creatures are still there, pretty much anytime I am in a room alone, staring at me with warped, raw, bleeding skin and eyes that are too big for their heads. I am terrified all. Of. The time.

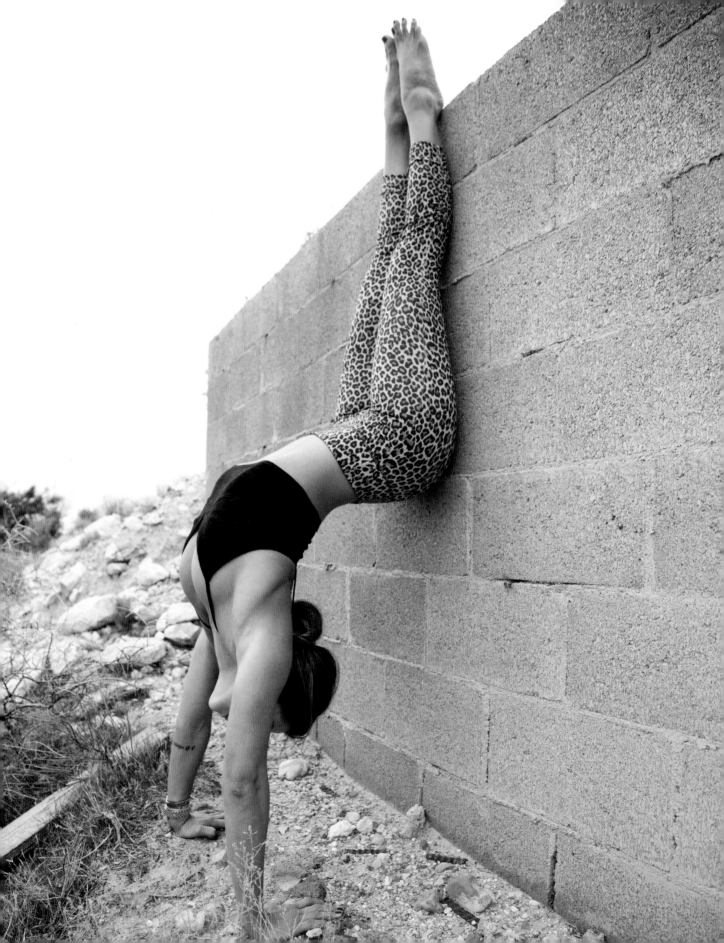

I haven't told anyone about this, for obvious reasons. I mean, would you?

"Candace," Greg says gently as he sits on the side of the tub and puts his hand on my wet back. He doesn't know what to say, and I don't blame him, and through his gentle touch I can feel his heart breaking for me.

"I don't want to die," I whisper once I've caught my breath. "But I can't live like this. I don't want to live like this." I breathe in sharply, startled by my own truth, and feel a new wave of hot tears come to the brim of my eyes. "I would rather not live than feel this pain."

"Please don't say that," he breathes. I consider telling him about the hairdryer, but I don't want to worry him any more than he already is.

A week later, my mother-in-law arrives to take me to my ninth consult, with a Lyme Literate Physician (LLMD)* in upstate New York, on a hunch that I might have Lyme disease. My mother-in-law's demeanor has always been ruled by a steady, quiet calm. If she is worried, I can't tell. She makes small talk as we zip down the twisting New England roads, and I close my eyes and try not to cry. Another brain thing is happening. Not the alien thing, but something else. This is also new, and it is equally terrifying. I can't focus on a *word* she is saying. Not one word. I know she is speaking in a normal, even tone of voice, but it sounds like the volume is turned way, way up and the speaker is broken, distorting the sound of her voice. I can hear what she's saying, but it is deafeningly loud, and I can't compute the meaning. My ears feel like they might bleed, my heart is racing uncontrollably, and my breath quickens. Yes, I can hear what she is saying, but it's like my brain is having trouble processing it. I can't find the words to explain this to her, so I offer mm-hmms and yeahs where it seems like they might fit. Spring has sprung, and the shadows falling across the road let us know that the buds on the not-so-bare trees are about to bloom. I want to crawl into a hole, cover myself with cool, heavy soil, and disappear. Decompose. Rot.

*A Lyme Literate Physician is a doctor who closely studies Lyme disease and treats Lyme patients. Lyme is a relatively new disease, first appearing in the 1970s, and appropriate treatment is hotly debated and very controversial. If you'd like to learn more, there is an interesting documentary called Under Our Skin that talks more about the issues.

After we park, I shuffle into the building. Having lost weight, I am swimming in my sweatpants. On a normal day, I would feel naked without my makeup. I love makeup. In that sense, I am a girl's girl. But I don't have the energy for anything, not even a five-minute makeup routine. Just the shuffle in makes me feel weak. I want to ask for a wheelchair, but I feel ashamed.

I do my best to fill out the forms, but the words are blurred and I can't focus. We are ushered into a quiet office, where my intake is recorded for scientific purposes because Lyme, having been discovered in the early 1970s, is a relatively new disease. From what they can tell, it varies widely on an individual basis. So much is still unknown, so these Lyme Literate doctors record everything, collecting data, trying to make sense of it all. It's like a mystery straight out of the movies, and in New England, everyone knows someone who has Lyme disease.

The intake process lasts more than three hours, and by the end I am once again in tears. The doctor speaks to me, but I can't figure out what she is saying. I stare at her, seeing and hearing words come out of her mouth, but it's like she's speaking in a dialect that I can't understand. I feel like I'm having an out-of-body experience. I see myself sitting in the chair, squinting at the doctor's mouth and trying to decipher her words. The doctor is kind in a no-nonsense sort of way that they must teach in med school, and I observe her mouth moving. I try to associate the shape of her mouth with words I know. The sounds of her words enter my ears, but I am behind on processing them, almost like a movie with audio that's off by a few seconds. It is terrifying because I cannot explain this. I can't put the words together in my own head well enough to speak them. I can't make sense of what's going on, and I literally cannot tell anyone. I feel trapped in my own body.

My mother-in-law and I are escorted to an exam room, where a nurse draws seventeen vials of blood. I am poked and prodded. I am told that I'll need to see my OB/GYN to rule out all STDs, including gonorrhea and HIV. I am given antibiotics and told that "it can't hurt to take them" until we get the test results back.

I leave feeling exhausted.

I go to my OB/GYN. They draw twelve more vials of blood, tell me I don't look sick, and suggest that I go to church. If I had been able to lift my arm, I might've raised it to lash out. But I am too weak for that, so I laugh halfheartedly through my tears and hobble out the door.

A week later, they call to say that I am clear of all STDs and there is nothing wrong with me that they can tell.

About six weeks after that, I get another phone call. It is the Lyme doctor. I have tested positive for Lyme disease.

I am overjoyed to finally have a diagnosis and get on a solid treatment plan so that I can get back to my old self.

"It's a long road ahead," the doctor says with a clipped warning tone. "You'll likely experience a Herxheimer Reaction from the medication. This means you'll get worse before you get better. It's just how things work," she says matter-of-factly.

The warning goes in one ear and out the other because I'm just happy to have a plan.

I buy a small notebook. I take my medication religiously, at the same exact time every day, and record it all in my notebook. I'm taking over ten pills a day, so it's important to keep track.

NAMASLAY COMMANDMENT #5:
DO THE LITTLE THINGS.

I am doing everything right. I've stopped eating gluten and sugar, and although I haven't had a drink in months (I just don't like how drinking makes me feel), I won't be drinking any alcohol anymore either—all doctors' suggestions while I'm on these heavy-duty antibiotics.

For the first few weeks, it's all good. But I'm supposed to continue to work my way up on the dose because we are trying to "be aggressive" with the treatment. Although the doctor has warned me about the possibility of the Herxheimer Reaction— where you feel way worse before you feel better—I up the dose and don't care. I am ready to weather any storm if it means that I can be well again.

But one month in, all twenty-two of my symptoms worsen. They become angry and volatile. I am seeing even more gory visions—aliens and zombies that look so real and so hideous that I am terrified to be away from Greg for even a second. He can't even be in a different room. I'm like a toddler clinging to her father's leg as he cooks dinner. The anxiety is at an all-time high. I know it sounds absurd, but I am petrified to try to sleep. The nightmares are so violent that I try to stay awake at night so that I can sleep during the safety of the warm morning light, when it seems less likely that something bad will happen.

My inflamed joints worsen. For a period of time I cannot leave my bed. My joints hurt so badly that I cannot dress myself, cook for myself, or fold the laundry. I can't walk. Greg carries me to and from the bed. I feel like a small child as he dresses me. I am so out of it, I feel drugged, and I cannot carry on a coherent conversation for longer than a few minutes. I haven't left our small apartment in weeks. I fall into a deep, dark, lonely depression.

It's summertime, and Facebook shows me that my friends are out there enjoying life. They are living it up, kayaking and traveling and spending the day at the beach, and while I know that all social media timelines are really just highlight reels, scrolling through them makes me feel sorry for myself. Looking at the posts both exhausts me and gives me the worst case of FOMO (fear of missing out) of my life. I feel excluded and inadequate because I can't be a part of their good time. Worse, I'm worried that my health will continue to decline. The what-ifs scare me. What if I never get better? What if I lose the ability to walk for good? Lose my eyesight? Continue to have these weird fucking visions?

I call the doctor, who suggests that we back off the antibiotics and up the dose again after a few weeks. Because she is the expert, I trust her.

Lying in bed one day, after watching three full-length documentaries (my current time-killing vice), I stare at the ceiling. Buckles is asleep at my feet. Like most dogs whose humans are sick, he just seems to know. Pasha is long gone. The day after the dogfight, we took her back to the woman who rescued her. I still feel guilty about that, although the woman ended up adopting her and giving her a good life.

In the months since I began taking the antibiotics, I have gotten progressively worse, and I have every reason to believe that I won't get better. I have watched a number of documentaries about the seriousness of this disease. I am haunted by the image of one woman with chronic Lyme whose tongue has recoiled into the back of her mouth. She can no longer speak. She can barely move. She is wheelchair bound. Having suffered from Lyme for years, she is the living dead.

I have read many articles that describe the controversy surrounding this disease. Doctors have been stripped of their licenses to practice because of how long they're prescribing antibiotics, but there is apparently no other way to treat Lyme disease. Insurance companies won't cover the cost of the treatment, and I have racked up tens of thousands of dollars' worth of medical bills. I feel hopeless and helpless and like a burden to everyone I know.

I am sweaty in my bed, having lain here for two weeks straight, unable to get up. I feel dirty and tired and weighed down by sadness and guilt. A big part of me wishes that, poof, I could evaporate into thin air, because what kind of a life is this? I'm so sick of being sick. I just can't do it anymore.

My eyes sting as tears well up. I want to give up.

But then I hear a small voice deep within me. It is so small that I can barely hear it, but it's begging not to be ignored. I listen closely.

You can do this, it says. *Yes, you can.*

My eyes soften. The welling tears go away like a wave that never got to break. That little voice is like a ray of soft light. It brightens my bleak outlook just the slightest bit, and as I breathe in, I close my eyes and will myself to feel that light grow. The warmth that spreads within me feels like a blanket of calm.

What if I can do this? I think. *What would I do if I made it through this?*

I allow myself to start daydreaming, escaping my current situation. I dream up all the things I will do if I get better. No, scratch that. Not *if* I get better. *When.*

BELIEVE IN YOURSELF.

I get out my journal and write.

Take yoga teacher training, I scrawl. I envision the people I would meet. The things I would learn. The environment—somewhere warm. No, somewhere hot. Where the sun always shines. A place where the people are kind.

Travel more, I write. I envision my plane ride, my first solo flight in ages. The goal would be not just to travel, but to travel alone. To prove that I can be the girl I was at sixteen, fearlessly heading off to Costa Rica with an open heart and a willingness to welcome whatever the universe offered.

I smile, remembering that girl. *You're still that girl,* I tell myself.

After writing just those two things, I'm tired and my eyes hurt, so I set the journal aside and close my eyes, picturing myself strong, healthy, independent, and thriving in the most magical, tropical place.

This is where you can go, the voice inside me says. I hear the sounds of the jungle; I feel the warmth of the sticky, humid air; and if I listen closely, I can hear the roar of the ocean in the distance as I drift off to sleep.

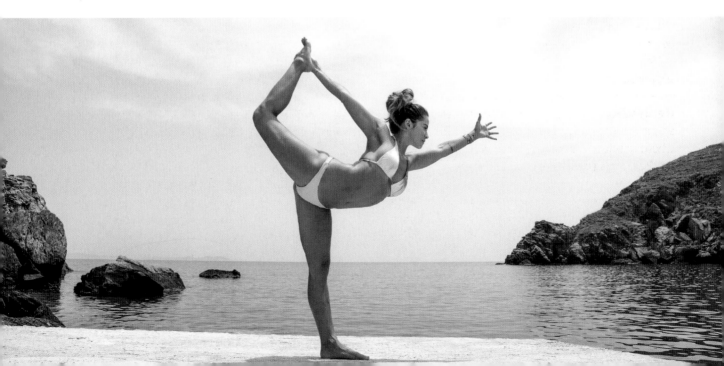

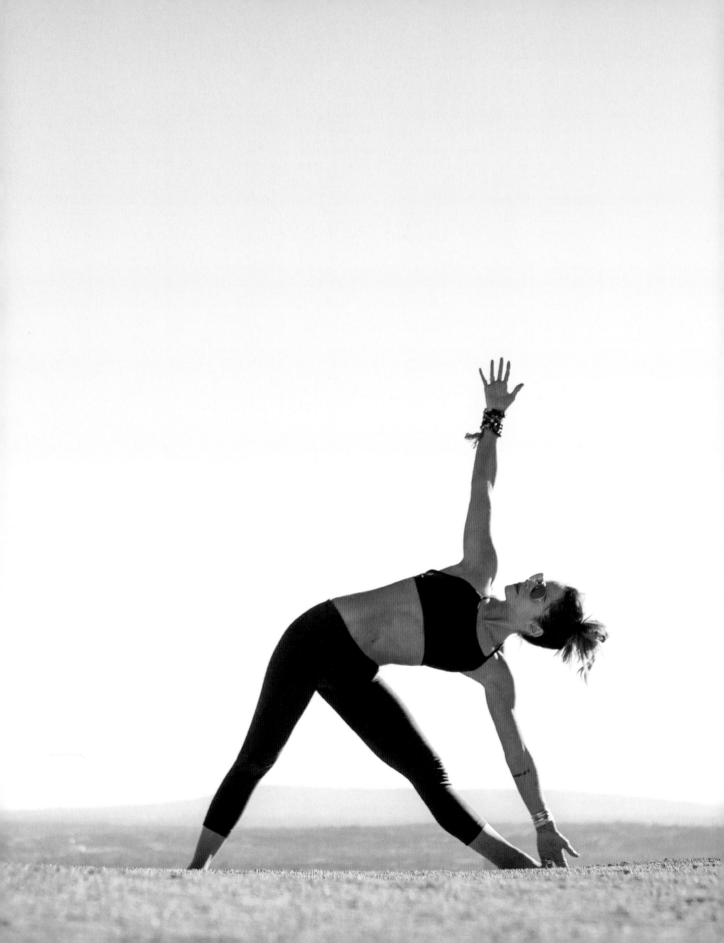

CHAPTER 2:

everything you need to know about pranayama

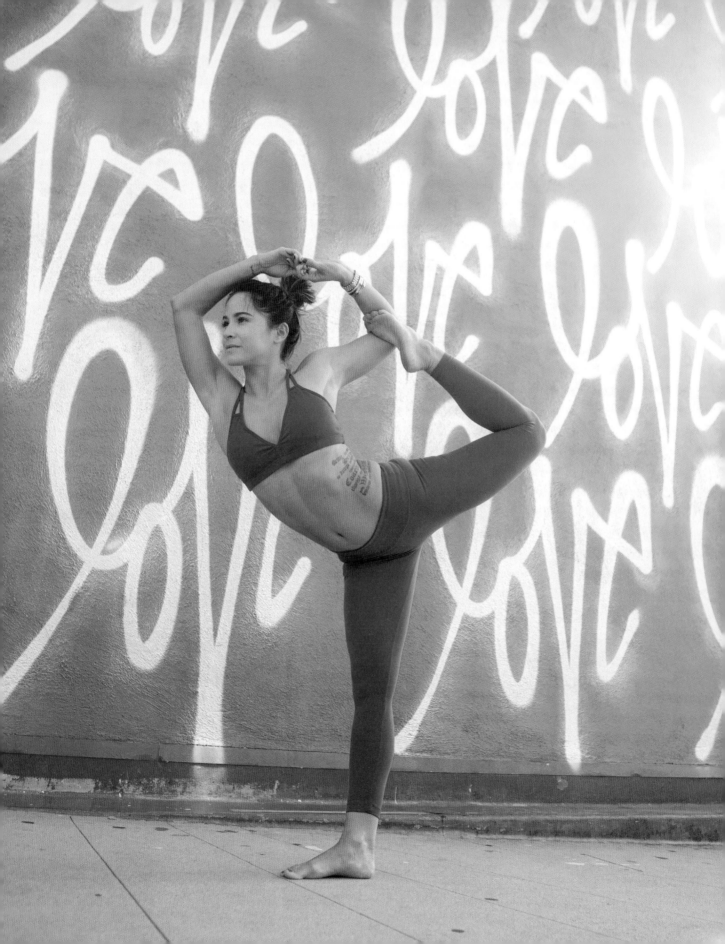

"What the hell," I hiss under my breath as the light turns red. It's 4:58 p.m. and I'm racing from my job as a teacher in an inner-city school to the neighboring town, trying to make it to yoga class on time.

I'm clenching my jaw as I tap the steering wheel impatiently, waiting for the light to change. Finally it flashes green, and the car in front of me, maddeningly, infuriatingly, just sits there. Like, to test me.

"Go!" I snap as I lay on the horn. The driver flips me off, and I am right on his tail as we both turn left. I pass him at the first chance I get and glance his way as he flips me off again.

At last I reach the yoga studio, five minutes after class is supposed to have started. I park and race up the stairs like a bat outta hell, nearly tripping over myself to get to the front desk.

"Hi," I say, juggling my bag and mat while slipping my shoes off with my feet and digging around for my wallet.

"I know I'm late," I exclaim, "but I'll sneak in quietly, I promise!" I look up, flashing my most charming smile, and dive back into my bag in search of my elusive wallet. The woman behind the counter looks at me calmly and asks for my name.

"Take a deep breath," she says softly as she looks up my account. "You're here now."

I stop and look at her, furrowing my brow and narrowing my eyes, half irritated and half realizing that she is right. I've been going through life on fast-forward. It's the whole reason I come to yoga class: to slow the heck down. My student loans bills are arriving in the mail. My car is a rust bucket and needs to be repaired. My students come from tough backgrounds, and my days are long and exhausting and stressful. It's my first year teaching at this school, and I often feel like I'm running around like a chicken with its head cut off.

I take a deep breath, stop searching for my wallet, and bring my entire body to stillness. As I exhale, the wallet topples into my hand. I smile and hand my credit card to the receptionist.

"You're in luck, anyway," she smiles as she hands my credit card back. "The teacher arrived a bit late, so I don't think they've even started."

I walk across the hall, put my stuff in an empty cubby, open the door, and settle in on my mat.

"We'll start with a breathing exercise," the teacher says. "Relax your hands in your lap and sit tall."

My mind is still swimming with thoughts from the day. There was a drive-by shooting that afternoon, and the bullets ricocheted off the windowpanes of my classroom. Heartbreakingly, all the students immediately sank down under their desks, like they expected it. Like it was no big deal. A student threw a chair at me. The stupid guy at the light flipped me off as I drove here. I'm so *tired* and my mind is racing, but I try to do what she says.

"Now we'll breathe the three-part breath. This means we'll start from the base of the diaphragm, and as your inhale builds, you'll breathe into the lungs to the point where you can almost feel your ribcage widen, and then at the top of the breath, almost when you feel like you can't breathe in any more air, take one final sip into the chest."

The entire room inhales in sync.

"As you exhale," she says gently, "see if you can let go of any of the baggage you've toted in with you."

I exhale, noticing that gravity is gently pulling my shoulders away from my ears, and as the day's stressors fade away, tears of gratitude brim my eyes.

We breathe in again, simultaneously, and I am moved by the collective effort of the people around me. We exhale in sync, and the tears silently roll down my cheeks. I am so, so stressed out. I feel broken and exhausted and like I'm barely keeping my shit together 98 percent of the time, but right now I am so grateful to have this second to just *breathe*.

NAMASLAY COMMANDMENT #6:
MANIFEST GRATITUDE.

Let's talk pranayama. Many beginners get nervous when it is brought up because it's a big ol' Sanskrit word that leaves people scratching their heads, like, "Pranawhaaaaaaaat?!"

If this is you, fear not. I'll break it down for you. Pranayama is just about breathing. The word itself is made up of two words: *prana,* which refers to the breath and means "life force," and *yama,* which means "control." The combination of the two words just means "breathing exercises." I know that the idea of breathing exercises sounds intimidating, but there's good news. Since we literally breathe 24/7, none of us are beginners. In fact, since we've been breathing our whole freaking lives, we should be champions at it. Pranayama, therefore, shouldn't be too hard for us, right?

Well, technically, yes. But the difference between breathing how we naturally breathe and practicing pranayama is that how we naturally breathe usually reflects how we're feeling in the moment.

Think about it: When you're angry, your heart starts to race and your breath can be shallow and rapid. When you're nervous or scared, your breath can be sharp and uneven. When you're stressed out, you may hold your breath or breathe unevenly without realizing it. When you're profoundly sad to the point that you're crying, your breathing can be erratic and interrupted.

Pranayama practices offer a number of different ways to breathe. You can think of it as a way to train your lungs to breathe to their fullest capacity so that it'll become second nature in your life off the mat. During pranayama practice, you breathe with intention and reap the benefits, which include increased lung capacity, increased blood flow, better circulation, and decreased stress, anxiety, and tension. And this can impact so many different aspects of life. If you're an athlete, pranayama practice may help make you a more efficient runner, weightlifter, and more. It's also likely that much of the sport you practice is mental. Pranayama can help "get your head in the game," if you will. If you have a high-stress job or home life, a solid pranayama practice may help you control your stress levels. If you're prone to anxiety attacks, a consistent pranayama practice may help you keep them at bay. And if none of those apply to you but you know that your life would benefit from an element of calm, developing a pranayama practice is the way to go.

Pranayama is a separate practice from meditation and asana, but it's also a complementary part of the meditation and asana practice. That is, you'll have a practice that focuses on breathing (pranayama) and a practice for meditation and movement, but you'll obviously need to breathe through each. The idea is to train your lungs to implement the lessons learned from pranayama into your meditation and asana practices.

In the yoga practice, pranayama traditionally comes before and/or after the asana to warm up or cool down the lungs. Just like with meditation, you'll want to sit tall so that your lungs aren't compressed or otherwise hindered by your posture. If you're just starting a pranayama practice, set a small, attainable goal, like one to five minutes for each session, and slowly work your way up. Remember, there's no required amount of time—do what feels right for you and works with your schedule. Some people practice pranayama daily for five minutes, twenty minutes, or an hour. Whatever works best for you is the right amount.

types of pranayama

There are a number of different types of pranayama. These four will get you started on the right foot.

UJJAYI BREATHING   ocean breath

Ujjayi breathing is both a type of pranayama that can be practiced on its own and the style of breathing that should be used when practicing yoga asana. Known as the "conqueror breath," it helps keep the mind calm and focused and helps diminish anxiety, stress, and tension. It is an excellent exercise for the lungs, as each breath brings the lungs to their fullest capacity. The sound you make when practicing ujjayi breath is like the sound of a seashell put to your ear, which is made by constricting your throat.

Begin by inhaling and exhaling normally, then slowly begin to breathe deeper, trying to match the length of each inhale to the length of each exhale. Bring your awareness to your throat and constrict the throat to create that ocean-in-a-seashell sound.

TIP:
If you're having trouble developing that sound, hold your hand in front of your mouth and imagine that it's a mirror. Then open your mouth and fog up the mirror as you make the sound "ha." Then inhale, maintaining that sound and fogging sensation. From there, close your mouth and continue to breathe the same way you were breathing to create the "ha" sound, and you should hear the seashell noise.

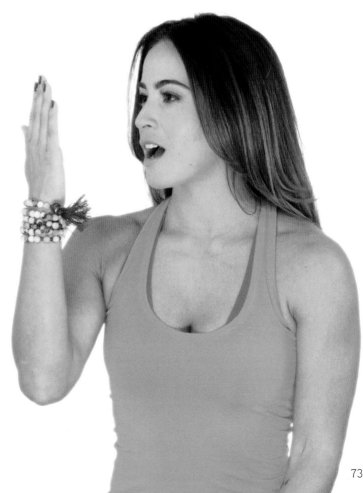

NADI SHODHANA alternate nostril breathing

Begin by resting your left hand in your lap. Then take your right hand and bring your peace fingers down to your palm so that just your thumb, ring finger, and pinky are extended.

From here, place your thumb gently under your right nostril so that it is plugged. Breathe in through your left nostril.

At the top of the inhale, gently place your ring finger under your left nostril, unplug your right nostril, and begin to exhale.

When the exhale is complete, breathe in through your right nostril. At the top of the inhale, plug your right nostril with your thumb and exhale through your left nostril. At the end of the exhale, breathe in through the left, then plug the left, unplug the right, and breathe out through the right. Continue in this fashion for five to ten minutes.

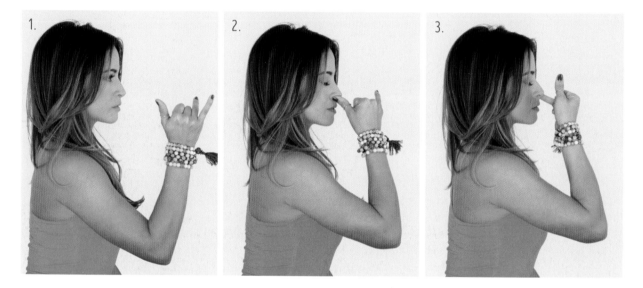

ALTERNATE VIEW

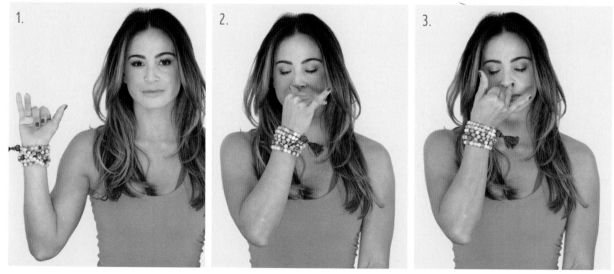

DEERGHA SWASAM three-part breath

This exercise is an excellent way to develop full lung capacity. Begin by taking a clearing breath in and out through your nose. Then imagine that each inhale and exhale you're about to take is split up into three parts. For the first third of the inhale, visualize the air filling up your belly. Then, for the second third, visualize the air filling up the sides of your torso as your ribs expand wide, and finally, visualize the air filling up your chest. At the top of the inhale, you should feel like you aren't able to take in even one more sip of air. As you exhale, do the same thing but in reverse: at the top of the exhale, visualize the air exiting your chest area, then your rib area, and finally your belly. At the end of the exhale, you should feel like it isn't possible to empty out any more air from your lungs. You can continue like this for anywhere from three to 300 (or more!) breaths.

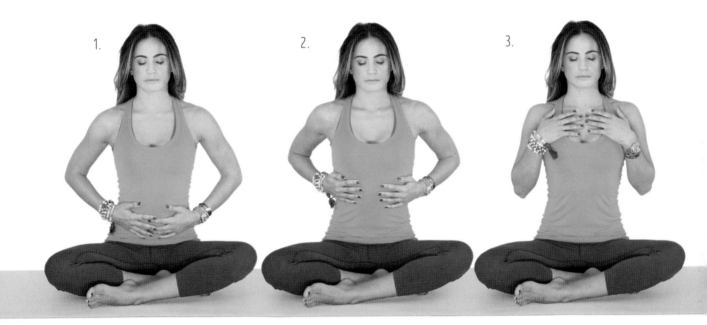

KUMBHAKA PRANAYAMA breath retention

This exercise takes the three-part breath a step further. Perform the three-part breath and explore breath retention: at the top of the inhale, hold your breath inhale for a count of three, five, or ten, then exhale slowly. Repeat this process a few times, then explore holding your breath at the bottom of the exhale for a count of three, five, or ten before inhaling slowly. Practice often; it's great exercise for the lungs.

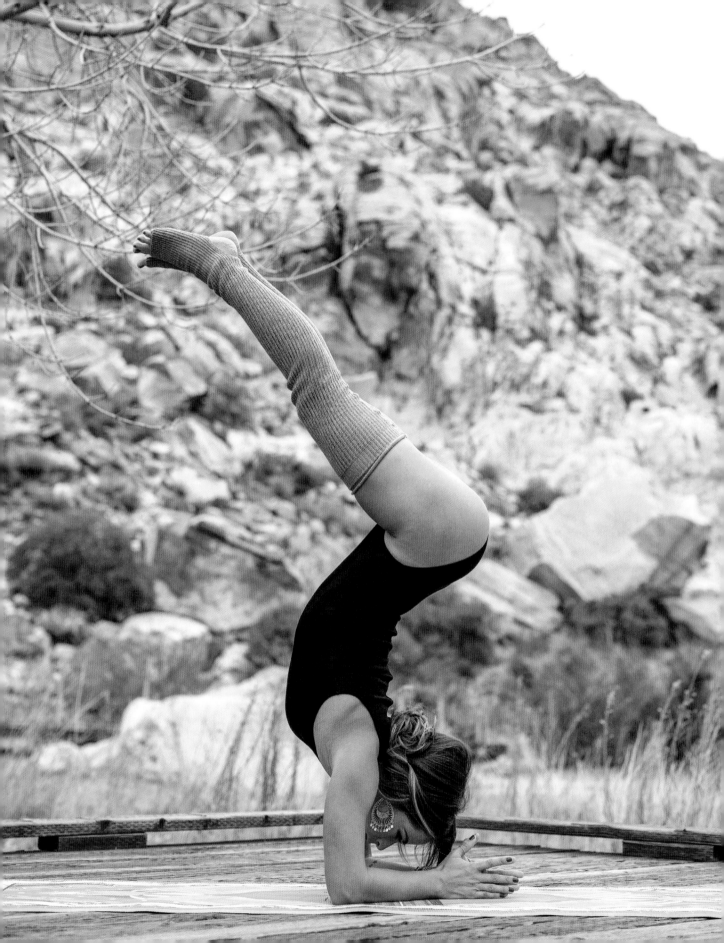

NAMASLAY COMMANDMENT #9:
DEFY YOUR LIMITS.

For some reason, it seems like everything in Paris is a little bit special. Like everything has a certain *je ne sais quoi* that its American or even fellow European equivalent just doesn't have. Even the fresh orange juice served at the restaurant next to our hotel, which surely can't be much different from the fresh-squeezed juice we would find in the U.S., tastes like a little bit of magic.

Greg and I have been here for three days, and it is the first time in fifteen months that I've felt great.

"Oh. My. God. You need to try this," I say, holding out the other half of my salted caramel macaron.

He agrees it's the best macaron we've tried so far. It's also the first bit of sugar I've had in over a year, but I don't care. This trip is a cause for celebration. It's the first trip we've taken that hasn't been ruled by the state of my health. Instead, we've been frolicking around the city like the newlyweds we never got the chance to be, and I'm the happiest I've been in months.

"Come on," he says, lifting his bike upright. "Let's keep going. I think the main road is up this way." He catches my eye and hides a smile.

"Oh, really?" I ask, raising my eyebrows and playing along. "What's the name of that main road again?"

It's our inside joke that he butchers the French language like no other.

"Champs something, whatever," he laughs as he gets on the bike.

"Champs-Élysées. It's pronounced 'shomsee-lee-zay.' How many times do I have to tell you?!" I fake-scold and hop on my bike.

"Yeah, yeah," he says, jokingly rolling his eyes, and he starts pedaling.

The sun is shining, and as we ride along, I'm overcome by a sense of gratitude so huge that I feel like my heart could burst. It's a simple thing, really, to ride a bike down a street, but this is a ride I will never forget. Just one year before I literally needed someone else to dress me because I couldn't lift my hands over my head due to excruciating pain, and now here I am riding a bike. A bike! Down the Champs-Élysées, of all places.

I vow never to take my health for granted.

"Hurry up," Greg says over his shoulder as we approach an intersection. "Let's try to make this green light."

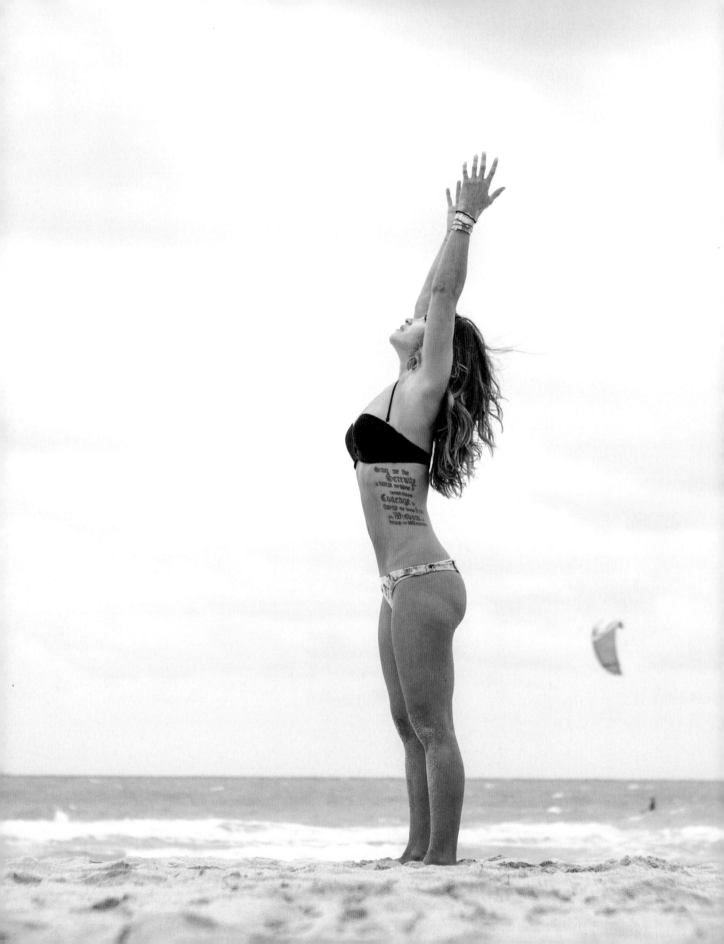

CHAPTER 3:

yoga for beginners

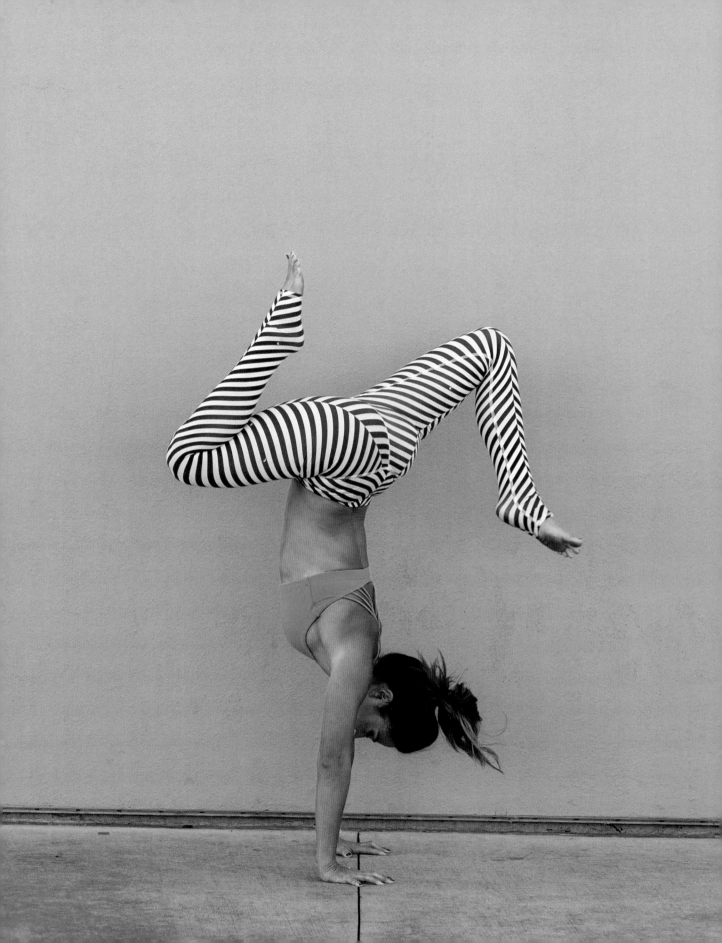

It's a frigid February evening and I can hear the wind howling outside, but I'm so hot in this yoga studio that I feel like I could scream. My body is shaking, and we've been in downward-facing dog for what feels like ten minutes.

The teacher is assisting one of the students with her alignment, and I am indescribably angry about her blatant disregard for the rest of the class. *We. Are. Suffering!* I silently scream, trying to telepathically deliver the message that all is not Zen in this sweltering studio. *Did you forget about us?!*

I am angry at the whole world because this teacher has left us in downward dog for far too long and my arms are shaking and I can feel the sweat pouring out of orifices from which sweat should not pour. I glance at the person next to me, hoping to catch her eye so I know I'm not alone in my irritation, but her eyes are closed as if she's actually enjoying this particular form of torture.

"Okay, class, as we take a big Buddha belly breath in, we'll slowly lift our right legs up for three-legged dog," the teacher says, her smile actually audible in her words.

My arms are on fire and I want to murder someone. What is it about being in physical distress that makes me rage?

"And from here, we'll step the foot to the top of the mat and gently perch the left leg on the left arm in preparation for crow pose."

Ughhh, I mentally grumble. Arm balances are, uh, "not in my practice," which is yoga-talk for "I can't do them." I collapse to the ground and sit there, not sure where to look because I don't want to be called out for not trying a pose I *know* I can't do.

For the most part, I love power yoga because I work up a good sweat, and at this point in my life the practice is mostly physical to me. It kills two birds with one stone: it's a challenging workout, and it does something for me mentally as well. But I don't want to waste my time with poses I can't do, so I'm irritated.

I make a mental note to avoid this teacher in the future.

"Now, remember," the teacher says with her annoying little smile, "attitude is everything. If you approach it with an open mind, you might be surprised at what you can do. I'll break it down for those of you who may be new to the pose," she says pointedly as she walks by me, the only person not doing crow pose.

Ugh, she is the worst.

She breaks down the pose. To humor her, I follow suit. I bend my arms and lean forward like she says. I put one knee on my arm and start to put the other knee on my other arm before I realize, *OMG, I'm actually in it! I'm in crow pose!!! No way!!!!!!*

I verbally pat myself on the back. *Candace, you're a freaking genius,* I tell myself. *You're a golden goddess sent from the heavens to do glorious and complicated pretzel poses! You can literally do anything you put your–*

And splat! I've fallen, but I'm laughing.

It happened! I *can* do this!

NAMASLAY COMMANDMENT #7:
BE A HELL YEAH PERSON.

I realize that when I stop approaching challenges with the idea that I can't, I'm a lot stronger than I think I am. We all are.

Now that we've gone over meditation and pranayama, we're ready to dive into the meat of the yoga practice: the asana. Don't let it scare you; *asana* is just a fancy Sanskrit word for "posture." When we discuss asana, we're talking about the glittery physical poses that we see sprinkled throughout social media, photographed in mystical lands against gorgeous backdrops. Now, I'm not going to lie; I think those pictures are pretty to look at. But I know, and now you do, too, that yoga is so much more than the postures. That being said, there's no denying that yoga is quite physical.

As explained on page 19, the physical practice has a number of different styles to choose from. For example, you can practice a slow, gentle style like yin, which is excellent for restoring the body and building flexibility. Or you can practice a more athletic style like Bikram, which helps build strength and endurance. Or you can practice a flow style that marries the two to develop both flexibility and endurance. Whatever style you choose to practice, it's important to start at the very beginning: with a solid foundation.

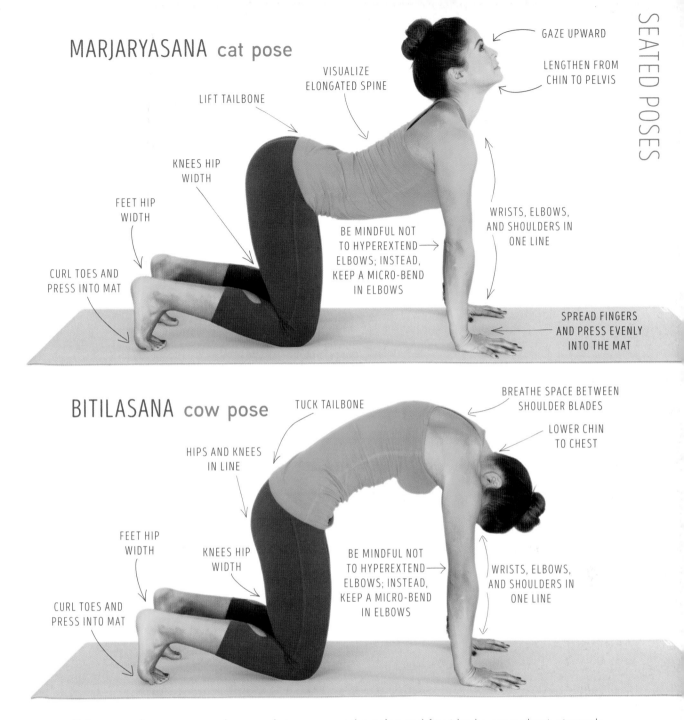

MARJARYASANA cat pose

GAZE UPWARD

LENGTHEN FROM CHIN TO PELVIS

VISUALIZE ELONGATED SPINE

LIFT TAILBONE

KNEES HIP WIDTH

FEET HIP WIDTH

CURL TOES AND PRESS INTO MAT

WRISTS, ELBOWS, AND SHOULDERS IN ONE LINE

BE MINDFUL NOT TO HYPEREXTEND ELBOWS; INSTEAD, KEEP A MICRO-BEND IN ELBOWS

SPREAD FINGERS AND PRESS EVENLY INTO THE MAT

BITILASANA cow pose

TUCK TAILBONE

BREATHE SPACE BETWEEN SHOULDER BLADES

LOWER CHIN TO CHEST

HIPS AND KNEES IN LINE

FEET HIP WIDTH

KNEES HIP WIDTH

CURL TOES AND PRESS INTO MAT

BE MINDFUL NOT TO HYPEREXTEND ELBOWS; INSTEAD, KEEP A MICRO-BEND IN ELBOWS

WRISTS, ELBOWS, AND SHOULDERS IN ONE LINE

Cat pose and cow pose work as a pair to warm up the spine and front body—your chest, stomach, hip flexors, and all the muscles and parts that run along the, well, front of your body. These are perfect poses to incorporate at the beginning of the day or after you've been sitting for a long time.

Begin by coming up onto all fours, with your wrists, elbows, and shoulders in one line and your knees underneath your hips. Curl your toes. As you inhale, lift your head and your tailbone and breathe into your entire front body. This is cow pose. As you exhale, press into the mat, round your back, tuck your chin, and breathe into the space between your shoulder blades. This is cat pose. Inhale and come into cow pose, then exhale and come into cat pose, moving as slowly or as quickly as feels good for you. You can do this for a few breaths or a few minutes—whatever feels right.

PARIGHASANA gate pose

Gate pose opens up the side body, which runs from the top of the hip bone, up the sides of the ribs, and in through the underarm area.

    Start by sitting on your shins with your thighs perpendicular to the floor. Stretch your left leg out to the left. Rest your left hand on your left leg and lift your right arm up and over your head until you feel a stretch in your side body. As you breathe for three to five breaths, visualize your inhales creating space in the intercostal muscles (the muscles between your ribs). It feels delicious. Then switch sides.

    This pose can aggravate touchy knees. If it doesn't feel so hot for you, fold your mat a few times to create a little extra padding, or place a folded blanket underneath your knee.

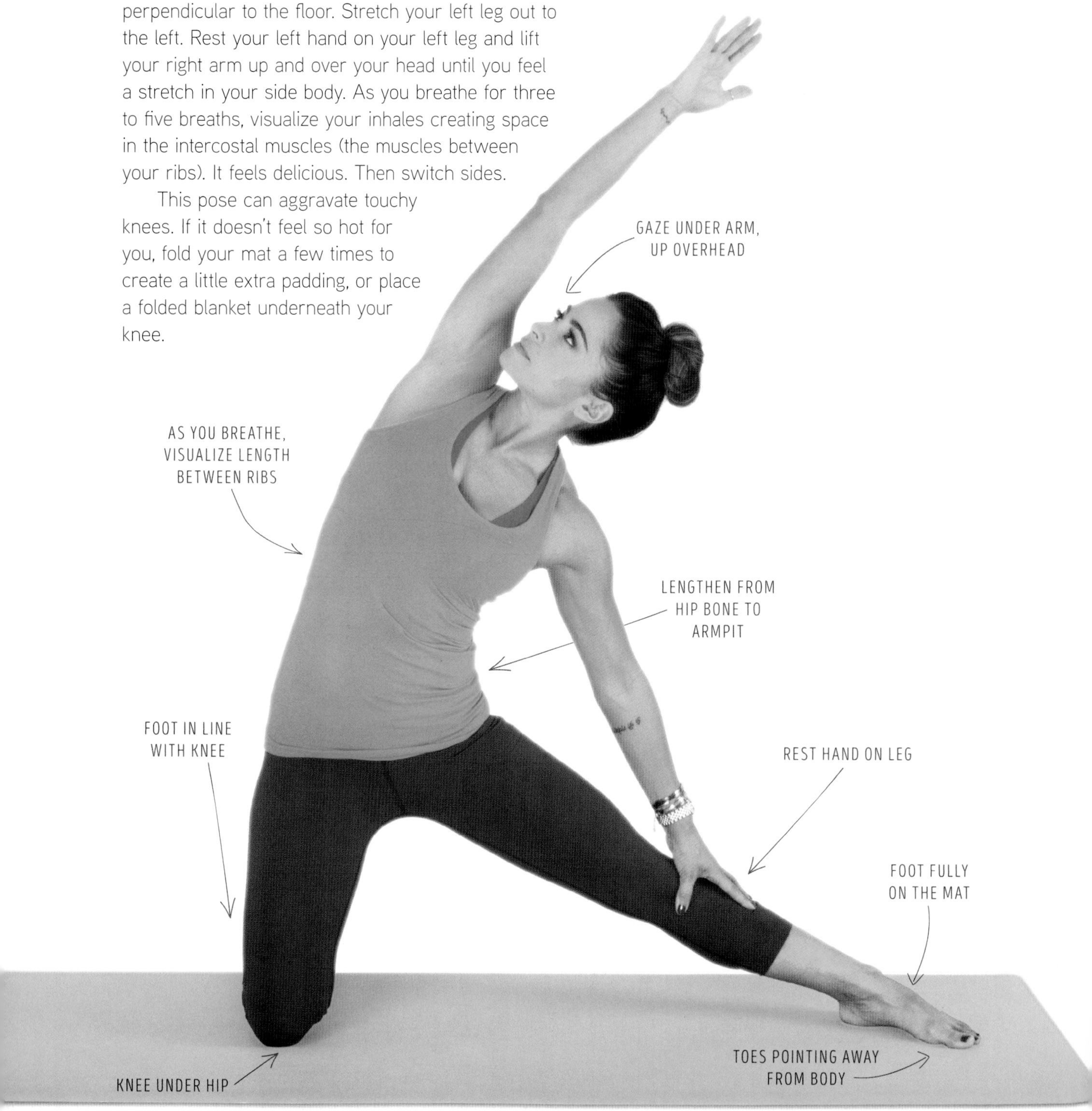

GAZE UNDER ARM, UP OVERHEAD

AS YOU BREATHE, VISUALIZE LENGTH BETWEEN RIBS

LENGTHEN FROM HIP BONE TO ARMPIT

FOOT IN LINE WITH KNEE

REST HAND ON LEG

FOOT FULLY ON THE MAT

KNEE UNDER HIP

TOES POINTING AWAY FROM BODY

PASCHIMOTTANASANA seated forward fold

This pose is good for opening up the hamstrings.

Start by sitting with your legs straight out in front of you. Gently pull the flesh from underneath your sitting bones so that your sitting bones are firmly rooted into the mat. Then gently flex your feet and spread the toes. This engages your leg muscles, which helps prevent hypermobility (extreme flexibility in the joints) and protects your hamstrings.

As you inhale, follow your breath from the base of your spine to the crown of your head. Maintain that length in your spine as you exhale and slowly come forward. A lot of people just want to get their head to their knees. Despite popular belief, this is not the point of this pose; it actually stretches the back rather than the hamstrings, which is not what you want. Instead, aim to have your thighs and stomach meet as you keep your low back long (not rounded). You have a couple of options for your hands, which will depend on your flexibility. While maintaining the connection between your thighs and stomach, you can either grab hold of your shins, wrap your peace fingers around your big toes, or interlace your fingers around the bottoms of your feet. With each exhale, aim for a little more movement and breathe through any tension you feel in the backs of your legs. Breathe for three to five breaths or more, and gently release the same way you went in.

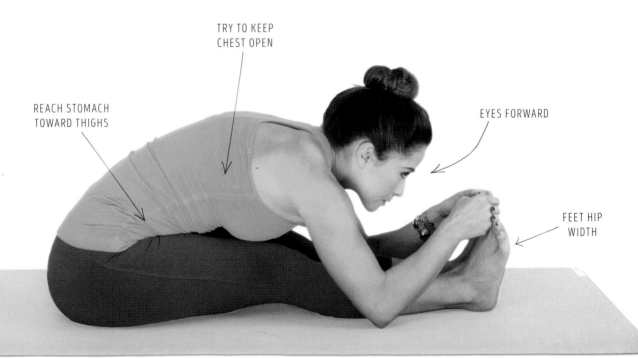

TRY TO KEEP
CHEST OPEN

REACH STOMACH
TOWARD THIGHS

EYES FORWARD

FEET HIP
WIDTH

MODIFIED VERSION

If your hamstrings are tight, you may not be able to reach your toes. If you need to, use a yoga strap to help you, grabbing hold of the strap as close to your feet as you can.

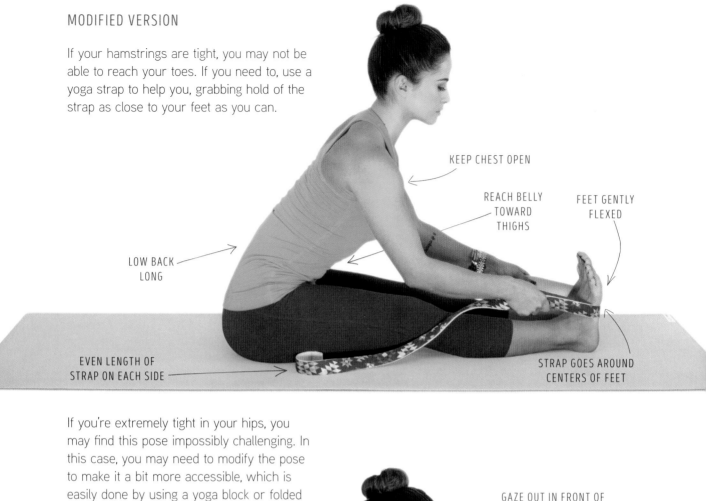

KEEP CHEST OPEN

REACH BELLY TOWARD THIGHS

FEET GENTLY FLEXED

LOW BACK LONG

EVEN LENGTH OF STRAP ON EACH SIDE

STRAP GOES AROUND CENTERS OF FEET

If you're extremely tight in your hips, you may find this pose impossibly challenging. In this case, you may need to modify the pose to make it a bit more accessible, which is easily done by using a yoga block or folded blanket. Slide the prop underneath you and sit on the edge of it so that your pelvis tips slightly forward. Remember to keep your toes spread and your feet and leg muscles engaged to protect your hamstrings, then follow the steps above to come forward.

GAZE OUT IN FRONT OF YOU ON THE GROUND

KEEP CHEST OPEN

LOW BACK LONG

REACH BELLY TOWARD THIGHS

FEET HIP WIDTH

SITTING BONES ON EDGE OF BLOCK

BREATHE LENGTH THROUGH HAMSTRINGS

AGNISTAMBHASANA fire log pose

Fire log is one of the best poses you can do to open up your hips. It's excellent for people whose jobs require them to sit for the majority of the day, and it's vital for athletes—especially runners, skaters, and Olympic weightlifters.

To begin, sit on your mat and bend your left leg. Place your left shin on the ground so that it is parallel to the edge of the mat. You're going to make an upside-down triangle, and your shin will be the top of that triangle. Your pelvis will be the apex, so you may need to shift to put your pelvis in the right spot. From here, lift your right leg and stack the right shin on top of the left so that your right ankle is on top of your left knee and your right knee is on top of your left ankle. Read that sentence again if you need to; I know it sounds like a confusing game of Twister!

If your hips are extremely tight, you might find that your right knee doesn't seem to want to touch your left ankle. In fact, your right knee might be so high that it's nowhere near your left ankle. If this is the case, it's no big deal. It just means that you're tight, and you can fix that with patience and consistency. Do not—I repeat, *do not*—attempt to press or shove that knee anywhere but where it wants to go. With time and lots of practice, your hips will open up and that knee will come down onto the ankle. Until then, roll with it, take a few deep breaths, and then switch to the other side.

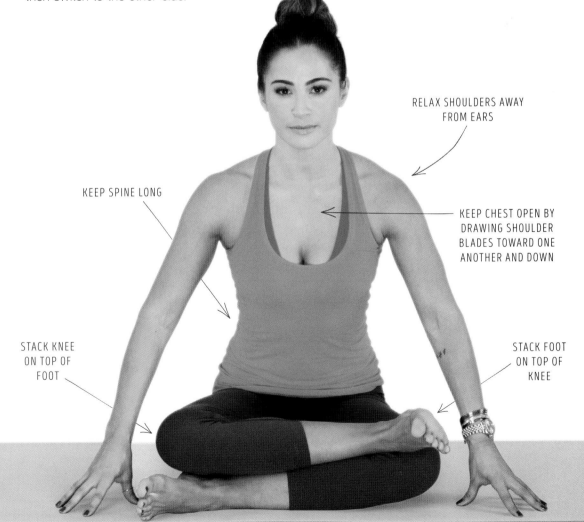

RELAX SHOULDERS AWAY FROM EARS

KEEP SPINE LONG

KEEP CHEST OPEN BY DRAWING SHOULDER BLADES TOWARD ONE ANOTHER AND DOWN

STACK KNEE ON TOP OF FOOT

STACK FOOT ON TOP OF KNEE

BADDHA KONASANA cobbler's pose / bound angle pose

If tight hips are a pain in the butt for you (see what I did there?), you're gonna want to get down with cobbler's pose. It's a must-have for kicking tight hips to the curb.

Begin by sitting on your mat with your knees bent and your feet together, as close to your pelvis as you can get them. Open up your knees so that the bottoms of your feet touch. Then wrap your hands around your feet so that the thumbs lie across the arches and peel your feet open like a book. As you do this, keep your shoulder blades drawn back so that your chest stays open. Then exhale and bring your chest forward.

If you're very tight through the hips, then your knees might be very high. In this case, just press your elbows into your inner thighs to help open them up. If you're more flexible through your hips and groin, your knees won't sit up as high; they may even go right to the ground. What's important is that no matter how flexible you are through your hips, you keep your back long and your chest broad. With each exhale, come forward as far as you comfortably can while maintaining the integrity of the pose through your alignment.

Please don't think I'm nuts, but I love this visualization: imagine that your knees have sprouted fingers (I know, I know) and you're trying to reach through your knees to grab something just out of reach. This visualization will help keep the stretch in your inner thighs and remind you to keep opening up, working to loosen up those tight hips.

BEGINNER VARIATION

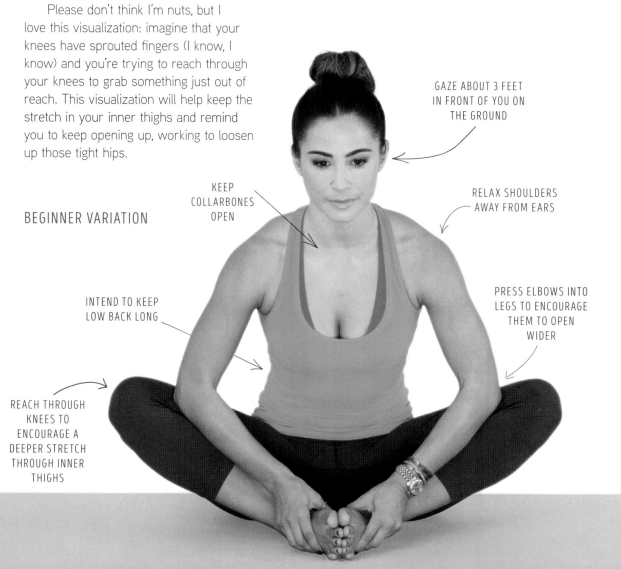

GAZE ABOUT 3 FEET IN FRONT OF YOU ON THE GROUND

RELAX SHOULDERS AWAY FROM EARS

KEEP COLLARBONES OPEN

PRESS ELBOWS INTO LEGS TO ENCOURAGE THEM TO OPEN WIDER

INTEND TO KEEP LOW BACK LONG

REACH THROUGH KNEES TO ENCOURAGE A DEEPER STRETCH THROUGH INNER THIGHS

FULL EXPRESSION

KEEP ENTIRE BACK LONG, PAYING PARTICULAR ATTENTION TO LOW BACK

KEEP HIPS ROOTED INTO THE MAT

GAZE ON THE GROUND OUT IN FRONT OF YOU

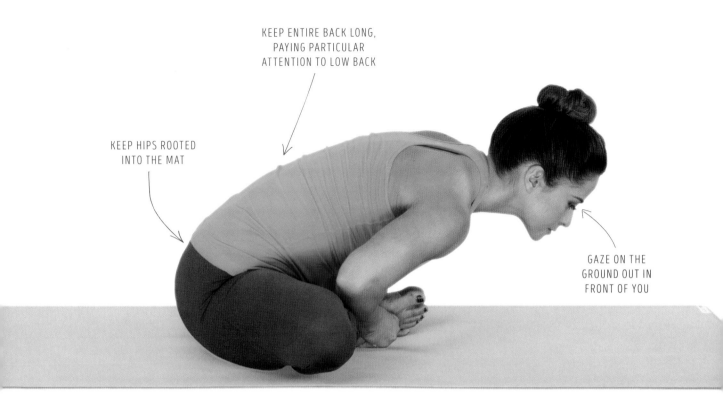

KEEP SHOULDERS RELAXED AWAY FROM EARS

DRAW SHOULDER BLADES TOWARD ONE ANOTHER FOR AN OPEN CHEST

REACH THROUGH KNEES FOR A DEEP THIGH STRETCH

PRESS ELBOWS INTO KNEES TO ENCOURAGE A DEEPER INNER-THIGH STRETCH

WRAP FINGERS AROUND TOPS OF FEET

USE THUMBS IN ARCHES OF FEET TO OPEN FEET LIKE A BOOK

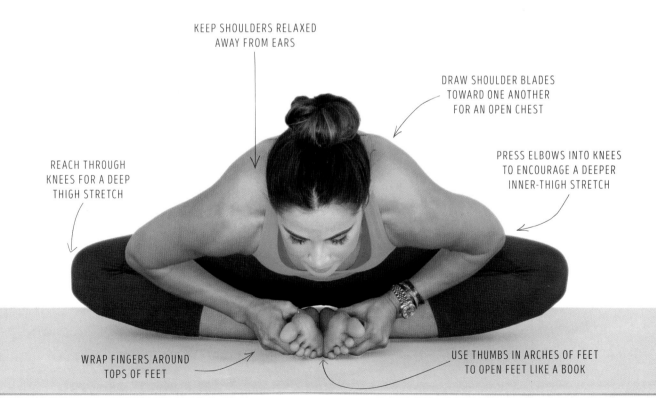

SUKHASANA easy pose

This is called easy pose because it's easy peasy. It's my go-to pose for seated meditation, and I like to do it at the beginning of my yoga practice because it's nice and gentle.

To begin, sit on your mat with your knees bent and out to the sides. Bring your left foot in toward your pelvis and take your right foot slightly in front of your left foot so that they're not touching. As you inhale, lengthen through your spine. If you find it difficult to sit tall here without your lower back wanting to round, sit on the edge of a folded blanket or yoga block.

You can rest your hands on your legs or bring them to prayer position—there's really no right or wrong way to position your arms. Breathe fully and deeply for as long as you like.

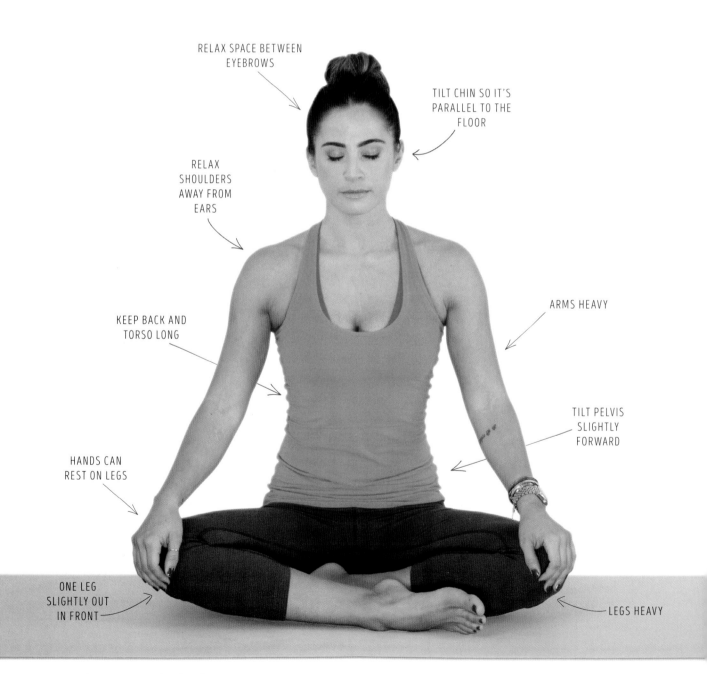

RELAX SPACE BETWEEN EYEBROWS

TILT CHIN SO IT'S PARALLEL TO THE FLOOR

RELAX SHOULDERS AWAY FROM EARS

ARMS HEAVY

KEEP BACK AND TORSO LONG

TILT PELVIS SLIGHTLY FORWARD

HANDS CAN REST ON LEGS

ONE LEG SLIGHTLY OUT IN FRONT

LEGS HEAVY

SUKHASANA variation
seated side-body stretch

This pose is so delish, like drinking hot chocolate on the coldest day of the year after an afternoon of sledding. It's the simple things, am I right? With a nod to the simple things, we've got this easy-breezy side-body stretch that feels wonderful any time of the day or night.

Begin by sitting in easy pose (page 90). Reach your right fingers to the right, placing them on the ground about 18 inches away from you. Then inhale and lift your left arm up over your head as you lean to the right. Keep your left palm facing down and see if you can bring the arm in line with your ear as you look out from underneath your left arm. As you inhale, visualize the spaces between your ribs widening ever so slightly. Use your breath to cultivate this sense of openness. Breathe for five to seven breaths (or more if you like) before switching sides.

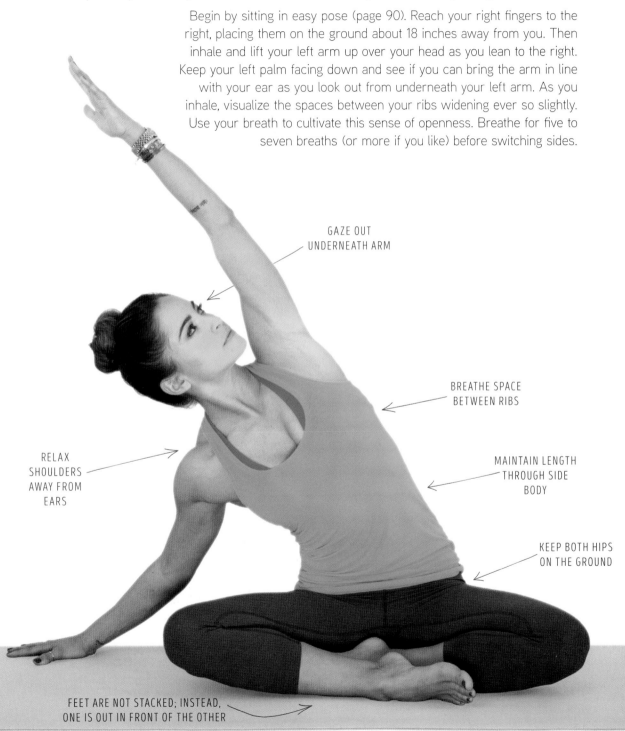

GAZE OUT UNDERNEATH ARM

BREATHE SPACE BETWEEN RIBS

RELAX SHOULDERS AWAY FROM EARS

MAINTAIN LENGTH THROUGH SIDE BODY

KEEP BOTH HIPS ON THE GROUND

FEET ARE NOT STACKED; INSTEAD, ONE IS OUT IN FRONT OF THE OTHER

PARIVRTTA SUKHASANA revolved easy pose

This is a great little twist that I think is perfect first thing in the morning because it's gentle enough to get the blood flowing but impactful enough to wake the body up.

Begin by sitting tall on your mat with your legs bent, your right foot in toward your pelvis, and your left foot slightly in front of the right. As you inhale, lengthen through your spine. As you exhale, gently initiate a twist to the right from your belly button, taking your gaze over your right shoulder with your left eye. Bring your left hand to your right knee and, if you feel you need to go deeper, use the knee as leverage to deepen your twist. Keep your chest broad by drawing your shoulder blades gently toward one another. Take three to seven breaths here before switching sides.

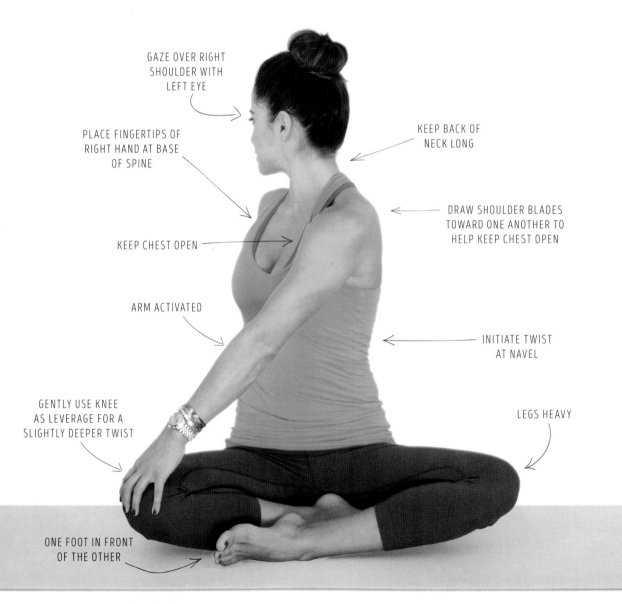

GAZE OVER RIGHT SHOULDER WITH LEFT EYE

KEEP BACK OF NECK LONG

PLACE FINGERTIPS OF RIGHT HAND AT BASE OF SPINE

DRAW SHOULDER BLADES TOWARD ONE ANOTHER TO HELP KEEP CHEST OPEN

KEEP CHEST OPEN

ARM ACTIVATED

INITIATE TWIST AT NAVEL

GENTLY USE KNEE AS LEVERAGE FOR A SLIGHTLY DEEPER TWIST

LEGS HEAVY

ONE FOOT IN FRONT OF THE OTHER

BALASANA child's pose

Child's pose feels great if you've got open hips. It's touted as a resting pose, and it's the one you're advised to go into if you need a break in yoga class. You start on all fours and then shift back so that your arms are outstretched in front of you, your head is on the ground, and your hips are resting on your Achilles.

The problem is that if your hips are tight, child's pose feels like the opposite of a resting pose. In fact, it can be such a (literal) pain-in-the-ass pose for tight-hipped people that I wouldn't put it past them to curse its existence and demand their yoga class money back. If you're nodding along in agreement based on past experience, fear not. I have a solution for you, my friend: a blanket.

See, the problem is generally that the hips don't reach the Achilles tendons due to tightness. To connect the two, just roll up a thick blanket and place it between your calves and hamstrings. Boom, done.

Once you're in child's pose, you can stay there for three breaths or three minutes (or longer!)—it's totally up to you.

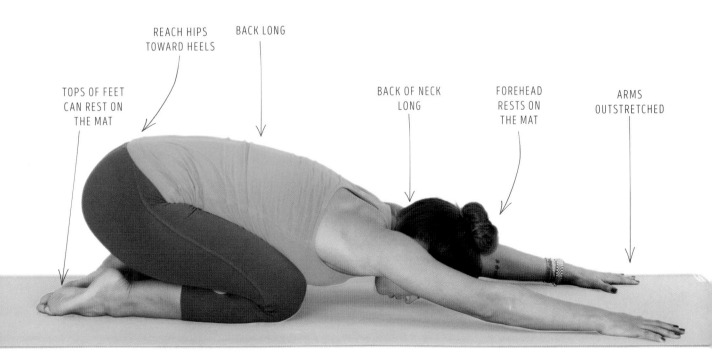

TOPS OF FEET CAN REST ON THE MAT

REACH HIPS TOWARD HEELS

BACK LONG

BACK OF NECK LONG

FOREHEAD RESTS ON THE MAT

ARMS OUTSTRETCHED

VIRASANA hero pose

I covered hero pose in the meditation section (see page 56), so you already know that this pose is tough for people with creaky knees. If that's you, avoid it at all costs. If your knees are healthy, you can go ahead and give it a shot.

Begin by coming onto your shins in a kneeling position. With your thighs perpendicular to the floor, touch your inner knees together. Slide your feet slightly wider than hip width, with the tops of the feet on the floor. As you exhale, sit halfway back and use your thumbs to pull the flesh of your calves to the outside before sitting fully back on the calf muscles. You can stay here for five breaths or five minutes (or longer!)—it's totally up to you.

If sitting back on your calves places a little too much pressure on your knees, you can use a yoga block to help you. Just set the block down between your calves and sit on the very edge of it.

MODIFIED VERSION

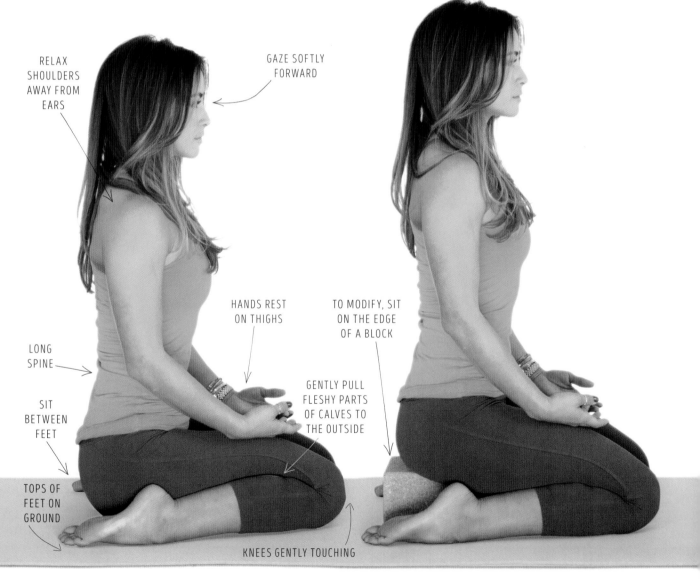

RELAX SHOULDERS AWAY FROM EARS

GAZE SOFTLY FORWARD

HANDS REST ON THIGHS

TO MODIFY, SIT ON THE EDGE OF A BLOCK

LONG SPINE

SIT BETWEEN FEET

GENTLY PULL FLESHY PARTS OF CALVES TO THE OUTSIDE

TOPS OF FEET ON GROUND

KNEES GENTLY TOUCHING

BHARADVAJASANA half-bound lotus twist

This isn't a pose that I often see integrated into classes, but it's a lovely little hip opener that also incorporates a gentle stretch through the chest. The twist is also detoxifying, making it an appropriate pose to combat midday weariness.

Begin by sitting on the floor with your legs straight out in front of you. Shift to the right, bend your knees, and swing your legs to the left, letting your left foot lie next to your left hip. Bring your right foot into the left hip crease. On the next inhale, place your left hand underneath your right knee, with the fingers pointed in toward your body. Then, as you exhale, reach your right hand behind you to take hold of your right foot. Look over your right shoulder with your left eye as you intend to breathe length through your torso. Take three to five breaths before switching sides.

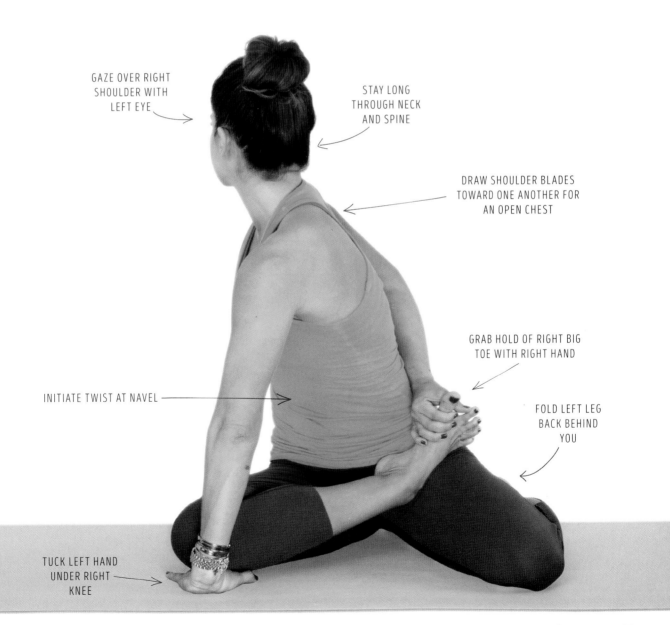

GAZE OVER RIGHT SHOULDER WITH LEFT EYE

STAY LONG THROUGH NECK AND SPINE

DRAW SHOULDER BLADES TOWARD ONE ANOTHER FOR AN OPEN CHEST

GRAB HOLD OF RIGHT BIG TOE WITH RIGHT HAND

INITIATE TWIST AT NAVEL

FOLD LEFT LEG BACK BEHIND YOU

TUCK LEFT HAND UNDER RIGHT KNEE

ARDHA KAPOTASANA half pigeon pose

I love this pose, but I know many people who want to pull their hair out when they're in it. It's a deep hip opener, and I recommend it to everyone, but especially those who sit for the majority of the day, as it offers a fantastic stretch for the piriformis and hip flexors.

Begin in downward-facing dog (page 100) and step your left leg forward to the front of your mat, bending your knee and placing the outside of your left calf muscle on the ground. A lot of people ask me if the front leg needs to be bent 90 degrees. The answer will vary based on who you ask, but my answer is no. Yes, this pose is traditionally done with a 90-degree bend in the front knee, but knees can be finicky, and in my opinion it simply isn't worth forcing the knee into a 90-degree bend and then placing pressure on it with hips that aren't "perfectly" open. I suggest that you forget about the angle of your knee and focus on the angle of your hips. You want your hips to be facing the short edge of your mat.

Your left leg should reach the floor. If it doesn't, place a yoga block or folded blanket underneath your left sitting bone. This will also help your hips face forward if they aren't facing forward already.

Extend your right leg behind you, then turn around and look at your right foot. It often tends to splay out to the side, so bring it in line with your leg if it's not in line already. Then face forward and breathe in. As you inhale, lengthen through your spine and puff out your chest. It's called pigeon pose, so puff it out like a pigeon—you want to create a little backbend, but focus on length through your bend so you don't compress your spine. Roll your shoulders back, allowing the shoulder blades to melt down the sides of your back. Bring your fingertips on the ground in line with your shoulders.

TO MODIFY, SIT ON THE EDGE OF A BLOCK TO GUIDE HIPS TO FACE FORWARD

Imagine that your knees are like magnets. You should feel them gently pulling toward one another, which helps lift the pelvic floor. Breathe fully and deeply for three to seven breaths before moving into pigeon pose (opposite).

GAZE FORWARD

PUFF CHEST OUT; VISUALIZE LENGTH FROM CHIN TO BACK TOES

BREATHE INTO HIP FLEXORS

BEFORE YOU LOOK FORWARD, GLANCE BACK AND ENSURE THAT YOUR FOOT IS STRAIGHT BACK. THE TENDENCY IS FOR IT TO SPLAY TO THE SIDE, WHICH CAN COMPROMISE THE ANKLE.

HIPS FACING FORWARD

BEND LEG OUT IN FRONT (IT DOES NOT NEED TO BE AT A 90-DEGREE ANGLE)

USING A DRISHTI

We're visual people and we get distracted easily. If you're in a yoga studio, maybe you can't help but notice the cute top the student next to you is sporting. If you're at home, maybe you're distracted by the paint that's chipping in the corner of your ceiling. A drishti is a focal point, and it's meant to limit our distractions while we're practicing. It's the place where you'll softly gaze and focus your energy. By maintaining a soft fixed gaze, you'll be able to tune out the periphery and go inward.

If you were to put two people next to one another during a yoga practice—one who had a drishti and one who did not—it would be very obvious to you which person was which. The person without one would be easily distracted, agitated, unstable in balancing postures, and easily frustrated and would tire quickly. The person with a drishti would be moving effortlessly and powerfully, with a calm, quiet expression. Of course, there are other factors to consider: a drishti isn't this magical thing you do to have perfect focus and clarity while practicing, but it is the one thing you can do to make the most out of what you're working with.

The beautiful thing about a drishti is that you can apply it to your life off the mat as well. Next time you're in the gym or in the office, look around at who is using a drishti and who isn't. The people who are, are generally calm and focused. The people who aren't are struggling. Interesting, right?

KAPOTASANA pigeon pose

This pose targets the back of the hip and is ideal for people with very tight hips like runners and desk dwellers. Remember that you can always use a block if you're extremely tight. Simply place it under your hip and sit on the edge as you move into the pose.

Begin in half pigeon pose (opposite). Take a deep breath and lengthen through your spine. As you exhale, come forward, walking your forearms out in front of you. If you feel incredibly tense as you start to come forward, you can place a yoga block under each forearm and stay there. If you're very open, you can continue to walk your arms all the way out. Try to keep your hips even. Breathe fully and deeply into the back of the hip of your forward leg. Take three to seven deep breaths before gently coming up.

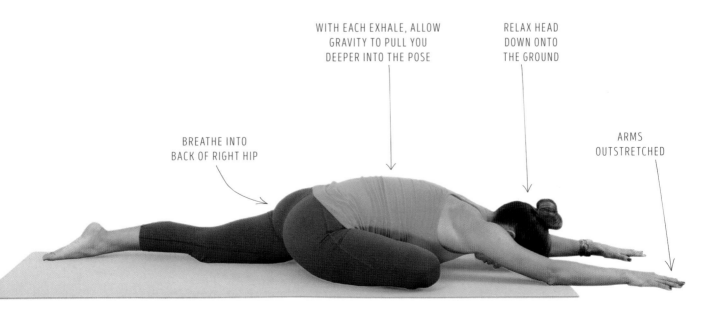

WITH EACH EXHALE, ALLOW GRAVITY TO PULL YOU DEEPER INTO THE POSE

RELAX HEAD DOWN ONTO THE GROUND

BREATHE INTO BACK OF RIGHT HIP

ARMS OUTSTRETCHED

DANDASANA staff pose

Story time! When I first learned this pose in teacher training, it was the hardest thing for me. I was baffled by it because it doesn't look like much, but keeping yourself upright like this for more than a few breaths is no joke for the core and chest muscles. If you're struggling with staff pose, you can modify it as discussed below. If you're not struggling, then I salute you, my friend.

Begin seated on your mat with your legs straight out in front of you and your feet hip width apart. Gently flex your feet and spread the toes. Engage your quads by lifting your kneecaps. Draw your navel in and up to activate your core, and roll your shoulders back as you plug your hands into the mat (if they reach!). If you're struggling to remain seated in this 90-degree angle due to tight hips, place a folded blanket underneath you and sit on the edge. This will help tilt your pelvis slightly forward, making the pose a bit more accessible. Gaze out in front of you on the mat and breathe fully and deeply in this position for three to seven breaths before releasing.

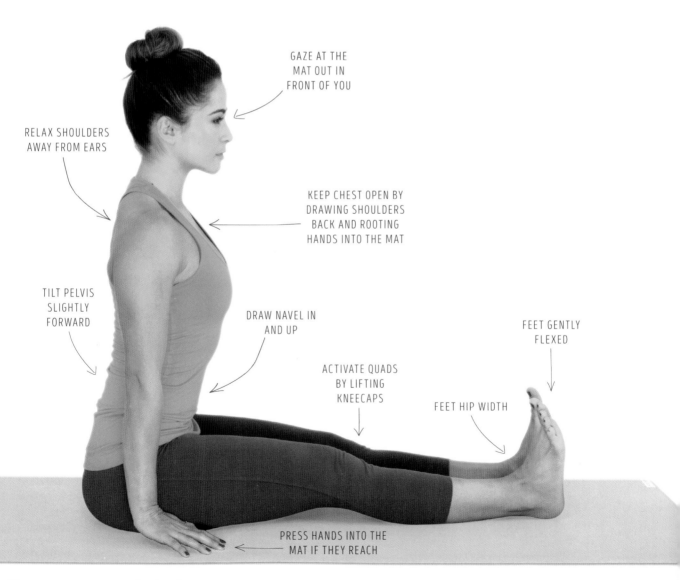

GAZE AT THE MAT OUT IN FRONT OF YOU

RELAX SHOULDERS AWAY FROM EARS

KEEP CHEST OPEN BY DRAWING SHOULDERS BACK AND ROOTING HANDS INTO THE MAT

TILT PELVIS SLIGHTLY FORWARD

DRAW NAVEL IN AND UP

FEET GENTLY FLEXED

ACTIVATE QUADS BY LIFTING KNEECAPS

FEET HIP WIDTH

PRESS HANDS INTO THE MAT IF THEY REACH

UTTANA SHISHOSANA extended puppy dog pose

This pose is fantastic for opening up tight chest muscles, armpits, and shoulders. It is particularly beneficial for people who sit for long periods and for athletes like Olympic lifters, golfers, baseball players, hockey players, and skiers.

Begin on all fours, with your knees directly underneath your hips. On your next inhale, walk your arms out in front of you, keeping your legs in the same position. If you need to modify, place blocks underneath your forearms. Once you're in your expression of the pose, gently press into your forearms and breathe into your armpit and shoulder area to loosen any tightness you feel. Stay in this position for three to seven breaths before moving on.

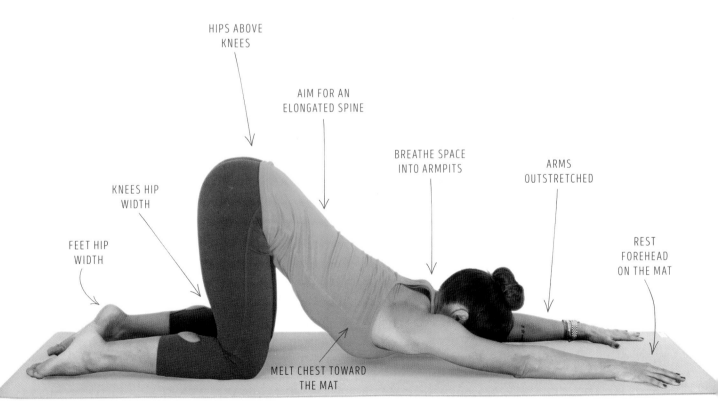

HIPS ABOVE
KNEES

AIM FOR AN
ELONGATED SPINE

BREATHE SPACE
INTO ARMPITS

ARMS
OUTSTRETCHED

KNEES HIP
WIDTH

REST
FOREHEAD
ON THE MAT

FEET HIP
WIDTH

MELT CHEST TOWARD
THE MAT

ADHO MUKHA SVANASANA downward-facing dog

Confession: Downward dog used to make me very, very angry. When I'd be in class and the teacher would leave us in the pose for too long, my body would shake and I'd start to rage inside. The good news is that I hear this same complaint from a lot of newbies, so I guess that means we're normal. The bad news is that the rage doesn't usually go away until we build up enough strength to hold the position comfortably for a number of breaths. The *great* news, however, is that with practice you'll get stronger, and any less-than-stellar feelings you have about downward dog will go away eventually. This is true for any pose, by the way. Just stick with it!

Begin on all fours with your wrists, elbows, and shoulders in one line, your knees directly underneath your hips, and your feet in line with your knees. Look down at your hands and spread the fingers as wide as you can. Then actively do what I refer to as "plugging in." Imagine that the ground underneath your mat is like an electric current, and you want to plug your entire hand into that outlet so that you can get the energy to hold this pose. But if you pick up your hand and look at it (go ahead and do it right now; I'll wait), you'll see that your hand isn't perfectly flat; the palm sinks in a little. Now put your hand back down on the mat.

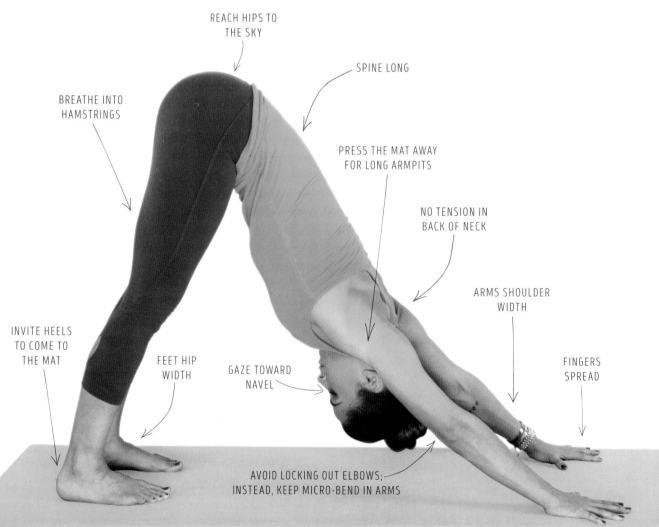

REACH HIPS TO THE SKY

SPINE LONG

BREATHE INTO HAMSTRINGS

PRESS THE MAT AWAY FOR LONG ARMPITS

NO TENSION IN BACK OF NECK

ARMS SHOULDER WIDTH

INVITE HEELS TO COME TO THE MAT

FEET HIP WIDTH

GAZE TOWARD NAVEL

FINGERS SPREAD

AVOID LOCKING OUT ELBOWS; INSTEAD, KEEP MICRO-BEND IN ARMS

Plug in every part of your hand with the exception of your palm. Grip into the mat like a rock climber and really notice each and every part of your hand being plugged into the mat. Then focus on the space underneath the center of your palm. Imagine that space is a suction cup that is sucking up energy from the ground underneath your mat. So you have two opposing lines of energy—the plugging-in, downward energy that goes into the mat and the line of energy pulling up through the center of your hand.

From here, lift your hips to the sky, intending to straighten your legs. If your legs don't straighten, who cares? It just means that your hamstrings are tight, and it's not a big deal. With practice, they'll straighten over time. Until then, keep pushing the mat away with your hands, reaching your hips to the sky, and inviting your heels to come down to the ground. Don't be discouraged if your heels don't reach the ground; just keep the intention there so that there is always a bit of tension in your hamstrings as they work to lengthen.

Now let your head go so that there is no tension in your neck. Gaze toward your navel and push the mat away even more so that your armpits are long. Breathe fully and deeply in this position for three to seven breaths before releasing.

✓ DO THIS   ✗ NOT THIS

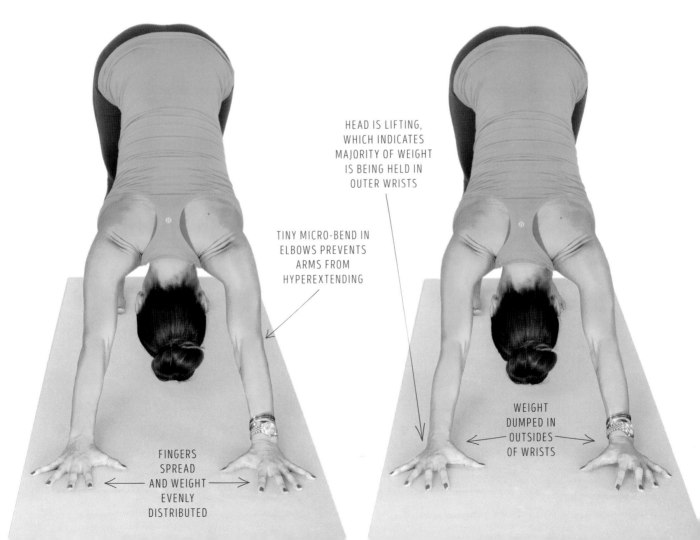

HEAD IS LIFTING, WHICH INDICATES MAJORITY OF WEIGHT IS BEING HELD IN OUTER WRISTS

TINY MICRO-BEND IN ELBOWS PREVENTS ARMS FROM HYPEREXTENDING

FINGERS SPREAD AND WEIGHT EVENLY DISTRIBUTED

WEIGHT DUMPED IN OUTSIDES OF WRISTS

STEPPING FORWARD FROM DOWNWARD DOG

Stepping forward from downward-facing dog (page 100) can be a frustrating thing for beginners. When people try to bring a foot forward, it often seems to get stuck and just doesn't make it to the front of the mat. Or sometimes a beginner can bring the foot forward, but the foot drops like a cement block at the front of the mat. Now, this isn't exactly wrong per se, but it's much better to bring your foot to the front of the mat with intention and control, because it means that you're using your strength and flexibility to get from point A to point B.

The best part of being a beginner is that every day is an opportunity to grow, and sometimes just one little explanation of something makes a huge difference. I often find that to be the case for stepping to the front of the mat. Here's what to do if you're struggling with this movement:

Begin in downward dog. Lift one leg as high as you can. As you do this, come up onto the toes of the other foot. Spread the lifted leg's toes (which helps engage the muscles throughout your leg) and come forward,

✓ DO THIS

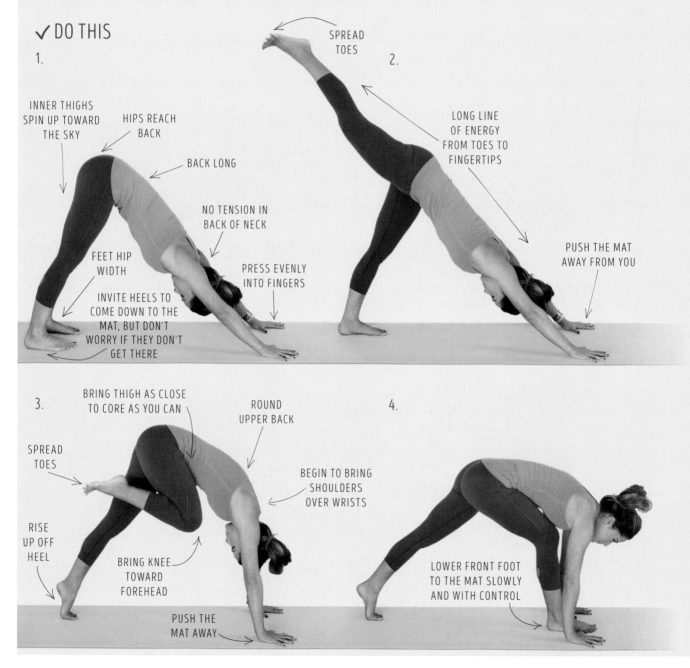

1.

INNER THIGHS SPIN UP TOWARD THE SKY

HIPS REACH BACK

BACK LONG

NO TENSION IN BACK OF NECK

FEET HIP WIDTH

PRESS EVENLY INTO FINGERS

INVITE HEELS TO COME DOWN TO THE MAT, BUT DON'T WORRY IF THEY DON'T GET THERE

2.

SPREAD TOES

LONG LINE OF ENERGY FROM TOES TO FINGERTIPS

PUSH THE MAT AWAY FROM YOU

3.

SPREAD TOES

RISE UP OFF HEEL

BRING THIGH AS CLOSE TO CORE AS YOU CAN

ROUND UPPER BACK

BEGIN TO BRING SHOULDERS OVER WRISTS

BRING KNEE TOWARD FOREHEAD

PUSH THE MAT AWAY

4.

LOWER FRONT FOOT TO THE MAT SLOWLY AND WITH CONTROL

pulling your knee into your chest as your shoulders come over your wrists.

Round your upper back as you do this. The idea here is to get as much room as you can between the floor and your chest so that you can easily place the lifted leg's foot down with control. Push the mat away from you as you find more space between your chest and the mat, then gently place your foot down. The trick is to push the mat away while using core strength to pull the lifted leg's knee into your chest.

The most common mistake I see students make when stepping to the front of the mat is that they don't actively push the mat away with their hands to create space for the leg to fit through. When there isn't enough space, the leg gets stuck. To fix this problem, you need to do two things:

1. Actively press into the mat with your hands until you feel that you've rounded your upper back.

2. Use core and hip flexor strength to pull your knee tightly into your chest as you come forward.

✕ NOT THIS

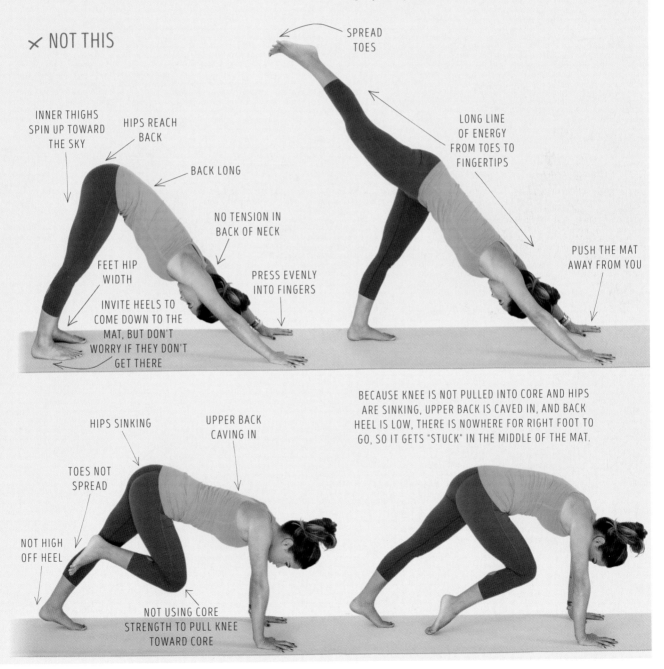

INNER THIGHS SPIN UP TOWARD THE SKY

HIPS REACH BACK

BACK LONG

NO TENSION IN BACK OF NECK

FEET HIP WIDTH

PRESS EVENLY INTO FINGERS

INVITE HEELS TO COME DOWN TO THE MAT, BUT DON'T WORRY IF THEY DON'T GET THERE

SPREAD TOES

LONG LINE OF ENERGY FROM TOES TO FINGERTIPS

PUSH THE MAT AWAY FROM YOU

HIPS SINKING

UPPER BACK CAVING IN

TOES NOT SPREAD

NOT HIGH OFF HEEL

NOT USING CORE STRENGTH TO PULL KNEE TOWARD CORE

BECAUSE KNEE IS NOT PULLED INTO CORE AND HIPS ARE SINKING, UPPER BACK IS CAVED IN, AND BACK HEEL IS LOW, THERE IS NOWHERE FOR RIGHT FOOT TO GO, SO IT GETS "STUCK" IN THE MIDDLE OF THE MAT.

If you tried the above fix and still weren't successful, it may be that your hips are tight—which is the normal result of things like desk jobs and binge-watching Netflix, but ultimately nothing to worry about. They'll open up as you develop your practice. Until then, you can use yoga blocks to help get you that extra space between the floor and your chest as you step forward.

MODIFIED VERSION

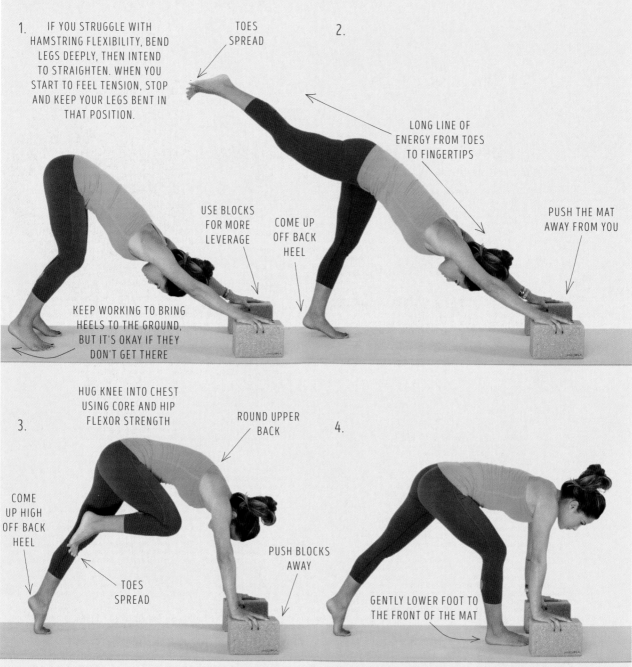

1. IF YOU STRUGGLE WITH HAMSTRING FLEXIBILITY, BEND LEGS DEEPLY, THEN INTEND TO STRAIGHTEN. WHEN YOU START TO FEEL TENSION, STOP AND KEEP YOUR LEGS BENT IN THAT POSITION.

TOES SPREAD

2.

LONG LINE OF ENERGY FROM TOES TO FINGERTIPS

PUSH THE MAT AWAY FROM YOU

USE BLOCKS FOR MORE LEVERAGE

COME UP OFF BACK HEEL

KEEP WORKING TO BRING HEELS TO THE GROUND, BUT IT'S OKAY IF THEY DON'T GET THERE

HUG KNEE INTO CHEST USING CORE AND HIP FLEXOR STRENGTH

ROUND UPPER BACK

3.

4.

COME UP HIGH OFF BACK HEEL

TOES SPREAD

PUSH BLOCKS AWAY

GENTLY LOWER FOOT TO THE FRONT OF THE MAT

VRKSASANA tree pose

The way we perform certain poses says a lot about what's going on with us. Tree pose is one of them. If you're stressed to the max and you've got a lot on your mind, I'm willing to bet that you won't be able to take more than a breath or two in tree pose before tumbling out of it. That's what I love about yoga: it forces you to take a hard look at what you're dealing with and make change in order to see results in your practice. Look at it as an opportunity to the chill the heck out.

To begin, stand with your feet together. Find a spot in front of you that's at eye level and not moving. This is your drishti, or focal point. Focus your gaze on that spot and relax the space between your eyebrows. Then lift your left toes, spread them, and set them down for a stable foundation in this balancing pose. On your next inhale, shift your weight to your left leg, feeling your weight evenly distributed across all four corners of your foot. Lift your right leg and place the right foot on the outside of your left calf muscle or left thigh. Avoid placing the foot against your knee joint, which compromises your knee.

From here, bring your hands to your hips and broaden your collarbones. Relax your shoulders away from your ears. You have the choice to stay like this or to bring your arms up overhead, out to the sides, or to reverse prayer position (page 195). It's entirely up to you. You can even close your eyes for an added challenge. There are lots of places to take the pose and test your balance. Do what feels best, and take three to seven breaths before switching sides.

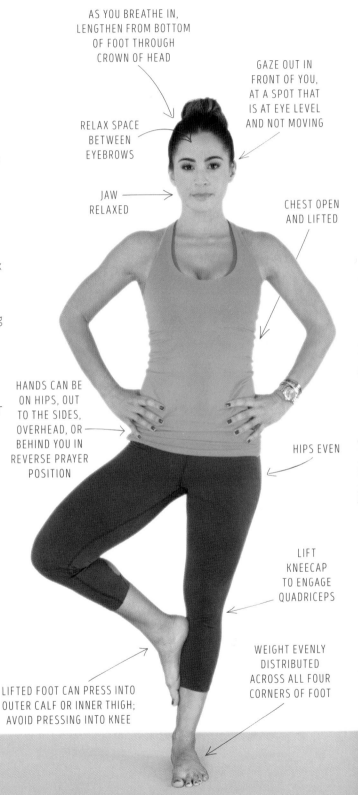

AS YOU BREATHE IN, LENGTHEN FROM BOTTOM OF FOOT THROUGH CROWN OF HEAD

GAZE OUT IN FRONT OF YOU, AT A SPOT THAT IS AT EYE LEVEL AND NOT MOVING

RELAX SPACE BETWEEN EYEBROWS

JAW RELAXED

CHEST OPEN AND LIFTED

HANDS CAN BE ON HIPS, OUT TO THE SIDES, OVERHEAD, OR BEHIND YOU IN REVERSE PRAYER POSITION

HIPS EVEN

LIFT KNEECAP TO ENGAGE QUADRICEPS

WEIGHT EVENLY DISTRIBUTED ACROSS ALL FOUR CORNERS OF FOOT

LIFTED FOOT CAN PRESS INTO OUTER CALF OR INNER THIGH; AVOID PRESSING INTO KNEE

TADASANA mountain pose

This pose doesn't look like much more than just standing there, but as a beginner I really struggled with it because it requires such good posture, and it was such an effort for me to hold my shoulders back and engage my lower core. Mountain pose is the start and end to every vinyasa, so I recommend getting very familiar with it. Don't knock it 'til you try it!

Begin standing with your feet together and your big toe mounds touching. Feel your weight evenly distributed across all four corners of both feet. Find a spot in front of you that's at eye level and not moving and focus your gaze on this spot with soft eyes.

Roll your shoulders back and let your arms hang heavy, with your hands naturally positioned slightly in front of your body. Tuck your tailbone slightly and engage your lower core by drawing your navel in and then up. Engage your quads, then tilt your chin until you feel it is parallel to the ground. Breathe in and lengthen through your entire body. Exhale and relax your shoulders away from your ears. Breathe fully and deeply for as long as it feels good.

GAZE OUT IN FRONT OF YOU, AT A SPOT THAT IS EYE LEVEL AND NOT MOVING

LIFT CHIN SLIGHTLY UNTIL IT'S PARALLEL WITH THE FLOOR

RELAX SHOULDERS AWAY FROM EARS

CHEST OPEN AND LIFTED

DRAW NAVEL IN AND UP

MICRO-TUCK TAILBONE FOR NEUTRAL HIPS

LET ARMS BE HEAVY AND HANDS HANG NATURALLY IN FRONT OF THE BODY

LIFT KNEECAPS TO ENGAGE QUADS

FEET TOGETHER WITH BIG TOE MOUNDS TOUCHING

UTTANASANA standing forward fold

Forward fold is a beast of a pose. It doesn't really look like much, but it requires so much openness in the backs of the hips and the hamstrings that, in my opinion, it's not really a beginner pose. But I'm putting it here because you'll see it time and again as a beginner, so I'm sparing you the agony of waiting until way down the road to learn how to do it properly. My best advice, especially if you are tight in the hamstrings and hips, is to follow the modified version until you develop more flexibility.

Begin in mountain pose (opposite). As you exhale, hinge at your hips and melt your belly over your thighs. This is important. This is the goal of the pose, if you will. If you can't reach your belly to your thighs without rounding your low back, simply bend your knees to modify. Bring your hands flat on the ground with your fingertips in line with your toes. If your hands won't lie flat on the ground, simply bend your knees more. Let your head hang heavy without any tension in your neck, and feel your weight evenly distributed across all four corners of both feet. Visualize your hip joints being stacked over your ankles.

If you're able to straighten your legs and keep your low back long, double-check that your hamstrings aren't hyperextending. To do this, lift your kneecaps to engage your quads or micro-bend your knees. Breathe fully and deeply for three to seven breaths before moving on.

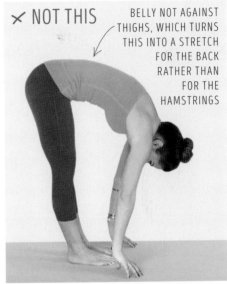

✗ NOT THIS — BELLY NOT AGAINST THIGHS, WHICH TURNS THIS INTO A STRETCH FOR THE BACK RATHER THAN FOR THE HAMSTRINGS

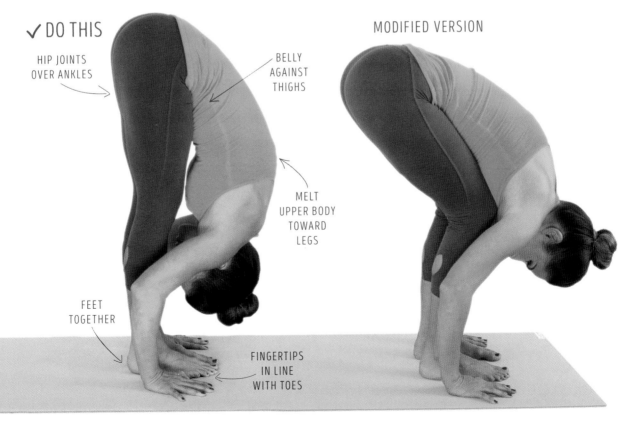

✓ DO THIS

HIP JOINTS OVER ANKLES

BELLY AGAINST THIGHS

MELT UPPER BODY TOWARD LEGS

FEET TOGETHER

FINGERTIPS IN LINE WITH TOES

MODIFIED VERSION

ARDHA UTTANASANA halfway lift

To be honest, I'd like to put this pose in the advanced chapter because it's quite challenging, but because it appears multiple times in a vinyasa, I thought I would bang it out here. I encourage you to be really mindful about this pose, because if you do it with improper alignment, you're liable to strain your back or hyperextend your legs. When done properly in its full or modified version, it's a fantastic pose for tight hamstrings and hips.

Begin in standing forward fold (page 107). As you inhale, ripple up through your spine to elongate your back and take your gaze about three feet out in front of you. Bring your fingertips in line with your toes and straighten your arms.

The most important thing is that your back is straight. Do not—I repeat, do *not*—round your back. If your back wants to round, it means that your hips and hamstrings are really tight. Set your back straight (see what I did there?) by bending your knees. Aim to reach your belly toward your thighs. This visualization brings your low back nice and long, which means that your hamstrings and hips will feel a *fan-freaking-tastic* stretch.

If your legs will straighten and your back is nice and long, too, just double-check that your hamstrings aren't hyperextending. To do this, visualize your hip joints stacked over your ankles, then either lift your kneecaps or micro-bend your knees to help protect your hamstrings. This pose generally comes in the middle of a vinyasa and is done for just one inhale before moving on. However, if you're doing it in a hatha class or you are working on your hamstring flexibility and want to spend more time in the pose, you're welcome to breathe for three to five breaths (or even longer!) before moving on.

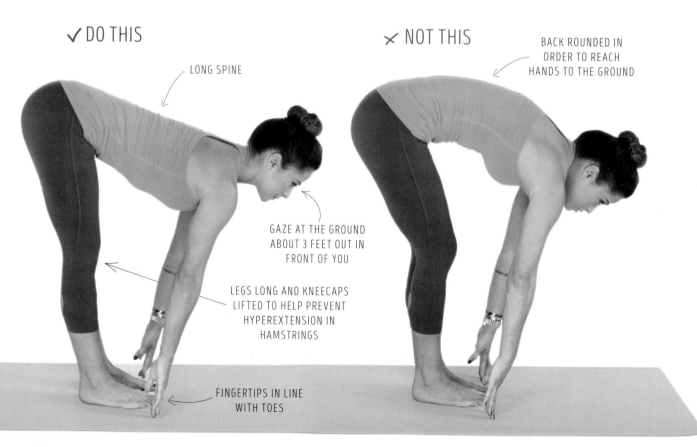

✓ DO THIS

LONG SPINE

GAZE AT THE GROUND
ABOUT 3 FEET OUT IN
FRONT OF YOU

LEGS LONG AND KNEECAPS
LIFTED TO HELP PREVENT
HYPEREXTENSION IN
HAMSTRINGS

FINGERTIPS IN LINE
WITH TOES

✗ NOT THIS

BACK ROUNDED IN
ORDER TO REACH
HANDS TO THE GROUND

UTTHITA CHATURANGA plank pose

When I first started practicing yoga, having to hold plank pose in class felt like a cruel and unusual punishment. It was torture for me. But you know what they say? The poses you dislike are the ones you need the most. What a weird saying. But, as it turns out, it's true, because guess what? With practice (and lots of cursing), I built up the strength to hold the pose for many, many breaths, and it no longer makes me want to roll up my mat and walk out of class.

Start on all fours with your knees hip width apart. Bring your wrists, elbows, and shoulders in one line and spread your fingers. Plug into the mat just as you did for downward-facing dog, then extend your legs, keeping your toes curled and your feet hip width. You're now in the basic plank position, but it's crucial to fine-tune it.

Push the mat away until you feel a little bit of rounding between your shoulder blades. Lift your hips slightly and make your legs so strong that if someone walked by and pressed on your hamstrings, they wouldn't budge. Press out of the bottoms of your feet, imagining that there is one long line of energy traveling from the crown of your head all the way through the bottoms of your feet. Activate your core strength, then check in with your hands. Avoid collapsing your weight into the outside edges of your palms. Dumping your weight here will stress your wrists and may cause injury. Instead, evenly distribute your weight across all four corners of your palms, pressing especially hard into the bases of your thumbs and index fingers. Breathe fully and deeply for as long as you can before moving on.

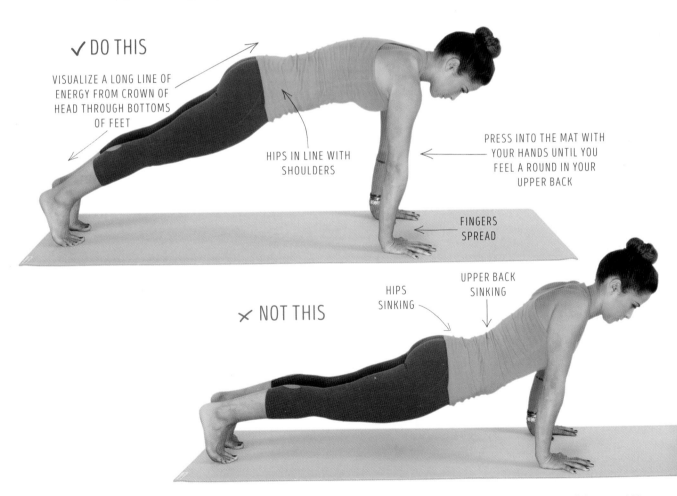

✓ DO THIS

VISUALIZE A LONG LINE OF ENERGY FROM CROWN OF HEAD THROUGH BOTTOMS OF FEET

HIPS IN LINE WITH SHOULDERS

PRESS INTO THE MAT WITH YOUR HANDS UNTIL YOU FEEL A ROUND IN YOUR UPPER BACK

FINGERS SPREAD

✗ NOT THIS

HIPS SINKING

UPPER BACK SINKING

CHATURANGA DANDASANA low plank pose

Here I am putting yet another pose that I consider to be advanced in the beginner chapter. How embarrassing! It's for your own good, though, because if I didn't and you went to a yoga class, you'd probably have to do this pose at least fifteen times, and you'd be mad that I didn't go over it. And I can't have you angry with me. But yeah, this pose? Performing it correctly requires so much strength. Please, for the sake of your shoulders, pay attention.

Begin in plank pose (page 109). Having a slight round in your upper back is crucial, so double-check that it's there. Then, as you exhale, use your toes to send your upper body as far forward as you can go. Notice how arched my feet are in the photo compared to the "what not to do" photo. It's important to use your toes to send yourself forward; if you don't, your hands won't be in the right position, and lowering down that way could compromise your shoulders.

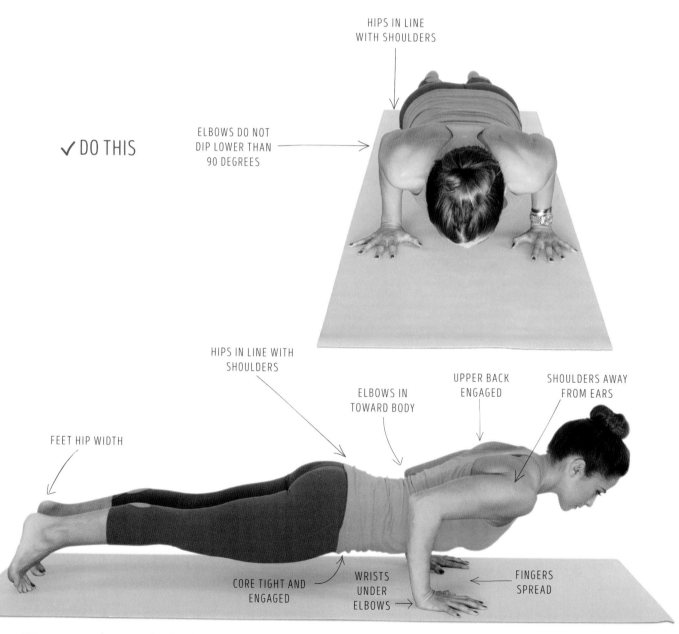

✓ DO THIS

HIPS IN LINE
WITH SHOULDERS

ELBOWS DO NOT
DIP LOWER THAN
90 DEGREES

HIPS IN LINE WITH
SHOULDERS

ELBOWS IN
TOWARD BODY

UPPER BACK
ENGAGED

SHOULDERS AWAY
FROM EARS

FEET HIP WIDTH

CORE TIGHT AND
ENGAGED

WRISTS
UNDER
ELBOWS

FINGERS
SPREAD

Now that you've come as far forward as you can, maintain that little round in your upper back and slowly lower down to a 90-degree bend in your elbows. Do not lower any more than that, because it could cause injury to your shoulders over time. Also, do not allow your elbows to open up to the sides. That happens when you've dumped your weight into the outside edges of your palms, which can be extremely painful for your wrists and may cause wrist injuries over time. When you're at 90 degrees with your elbows straight back behind you, keep your chest nice and broad, your core nice and strong, your knees engaged, and your legs strong. Keep your hips in line with your body. The tendency is either to let them sink or to lift them too high, but they should never be higher or lower than your chest. As this pose generally appears briefly yet repeatedly during vinyasa classes, you likely won't stay in the pose for very long. As you inhale, you'll probably come into either high lunge (page 112) or cobra pose (page 129). Alternatively, if you're looking to build strength and endurance, you could breathe in chaturanga for three to five breaths (or more).

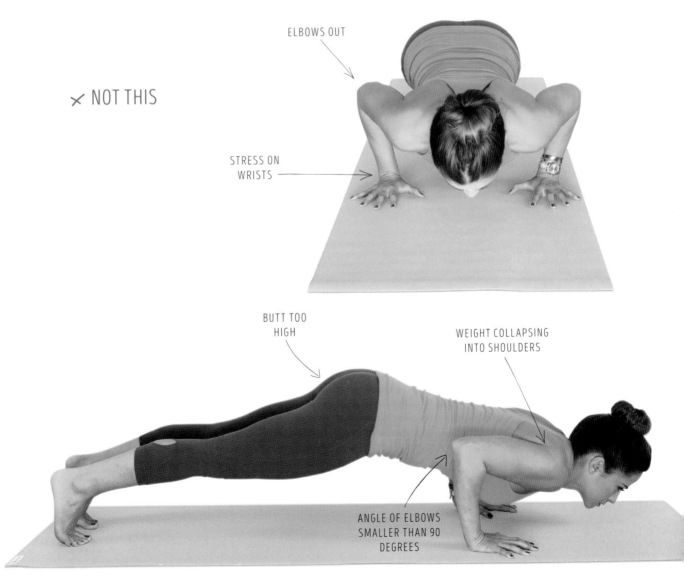

ELBOWS OUT

✕ NOT THIS

STRESS ON WRISTS

BUTT TOO HIGH

WEIGHT COLLAPSING INTO SHOULDERS

ANGLE OF ELBOWS SMALLER THAN 90 DEGREES

UTTHITA ASHWA SANCHALANASANA high lunge

High lunge feels incredible for the hip flexors, gently wakes up the leg muscles, and stretches the side body, making it one of my favorite poses to do first thing in the morning.

Begin by taking a big step forward with your right foot. Lift your left heel off the mat and look back to ensure that your toes are still facing forward. Press out of the bottom of your left foot so that your leg is long and strong. Bring your hands to your hips to ensure that your pelvis is even, then look down at your right knee. Your knee should be directly over or slightly behind your right ankle. Allowing it to come out in front of your ankle compromises your knee and may cause injury over time. As you inhale, lengthen through your torso so that your upper body is perpendicular to the mat. Tilt your chin until you feel that it's parallel to the ground and gaze out in front of you at a spot that is at eye level and not moving. On your next inhale, lift your arms overhead, and as you exhale, relax your shoulders away from your ears. If holding your arms overhead is too much for you, you can bring your hands to your heart in prayer position or bring your hands to your hips. Breathe fully and deeply for three to seven breaths before switching sides.

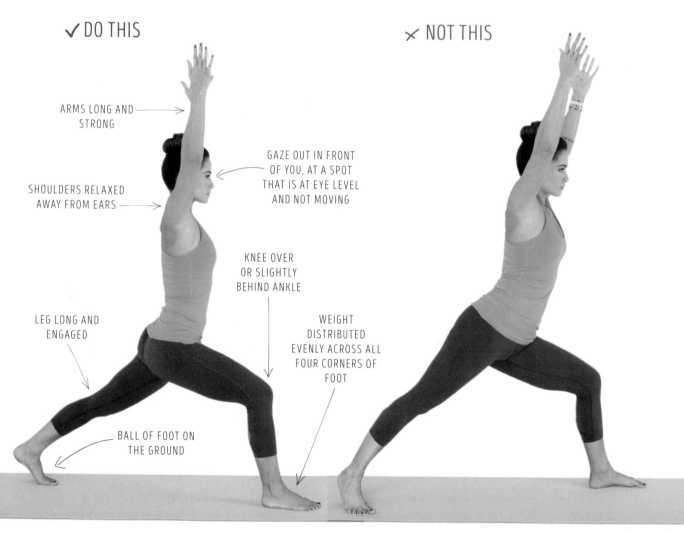

✓ DO THIS   ✗ NOT THIS

ARMS LONG AND STRONG

GAZE OUT IN FRONT OF YOU, AT A SPOT THAT IS AT EYE LEVEL AND NOT MOVING

SHOULDERS RELAXED AWAY FROM EARS

KNEE OVER OR SLIGHTLY BEHIND ANKLE

LEG LONG AND ENGAGED

WEIGHT DISTRIBUTED EVENLY ACROSS ALL FOUR CORNERS OF FOOT

BALL OF FOOT ON THE GROUND

VIRABHADRASANA 1 warrior 1

As a beginner, warrior 1 used to drive me bonkers because holding your arms up for a long time? That shiz is hard. The good news is that you can always modify the pose by taking your hands to prayer position at your chest, but I didn't know that at the time, so I was in agony. This is a great strength-building pose—it's excellent for shoulders and legs. It looks quite similar to high lunge—the difference being that your back foot is firmly planted on the ground at a 45-degree angle, whereas in high lunge just the ball of your foot is on the ground, facing forward.

Begin by taking a big step forward with your right foot and bend your right knee so that the knee is over or slightly behind your ankle. Do not allow your knee to come in front of your ankle, which will stress your knee. Turn your left foot out slightly so that the toes are pointed about 45 degrees to the left. Continue to press through the outer edge of your left foot—do not allow that part of the foot to lift. Your hips should be facing forward and your pelvis should be even. You can bring your hands to your hips to check that your pelvis is neutral. On your next inhale, bring your arms overhead with your palms facing one another.

As you exhale, relax your shoulders away from your ears and imagine that you are holding a watermelon between your arms. Maintaining this tension will help keep your arms long and strong. Be mindful not to hyperextend in the elbows. Micro-bend your elbows if you need to. Spread your fingers and breathe for three to seven breaths before doing the same thing on the other side.

If you need to modify this pose, bring your hands to prayer position at your chest.

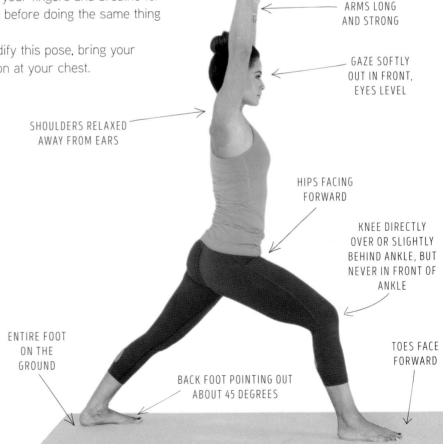

PALMS FACING
ONE ANOTHER

ARMS LONG
AND STRONG

GAZE SOFTLY
OUT IN FRONT,
EYES LEVEL

SHOULDERS RELAXED
AWAY FROM EARS

HIPS FACING
FORWARD

KNEE DIRECTLY
OVER OR SLIGHTLY
BEHIND ANKLE, BUT
NEVER IN FRONT OF
ANKLE

ENTIRE FOOT
ON THE
GROUND

BACK FOOT POINTING OUT
ABOUT 45 DEGREES

TOES FACE
FORWARD

VIRABHADRASANA 2 warrior 2

This pose doesn't look like much, but it's killer for the arms and legs when you hold it for breath after breath in class. The key is to breathe, breathe, breathe and try not to think. You'll be moving on before you know it.

Begin by taking a big step forward with your left foot. Turn your right foot 90 degrees to the right so that your hips are open and facing the long edge of your mat. Then open up your arms so that they're parallel to the ground, your left arm forward and right arm back, with your palms facing down. Spread your fingers and gaze over your left middle finger. Make your arms long and strong so that if someone tried to push them down, they wouldn't go anywhere.

✓ DO THIS

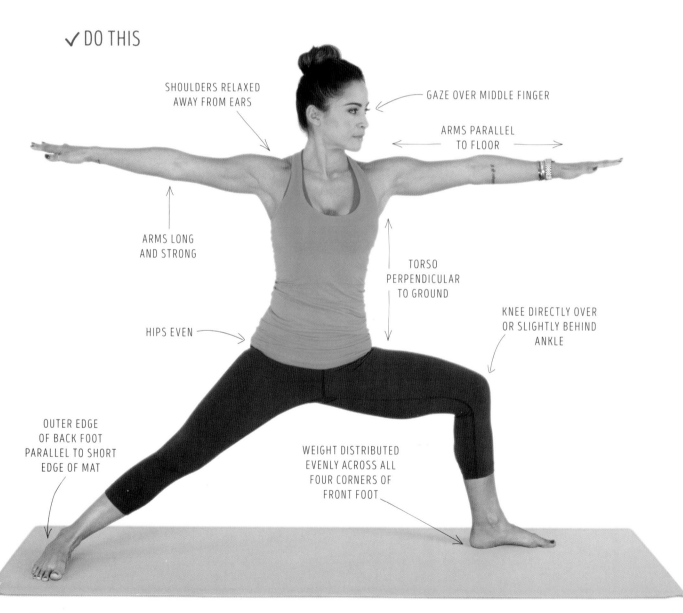

SHOULDERS RELAXED
AWAY FROM EARS

GAZE OVER MIDDLE FINGER

ARMS PARALLEL
TO FLOOR

ARMS LONG
AND STRONG

TORSO
PERPENDICULAR
TO GROUND

KNEE DIRECTLY OVER
OR SLIGHTLY BEHIND
ANKLE

HIPS EVEN

OUTER EDGE
OF BACK FOOT
PARALLEL TO SHORT
EDGE OF MAT

WEIGHT DISTRIBUTED
EVENLY ACROSS ALL
FOUR CORNERS OF
FRONT FOOT

Bend your left leg deeply so that your left knee is stacked over or slightly behind your left ankle. Avoid allowing your knee to come past your ankle, which compromises your knee and may cause injury over time.

Bring your hands to your hips for a second to feel that your pelvis is even and not tilted forward. Then bring your arms back into position. Draw your belly button in and up to activate your core and breathe fully and deeply. Press into the outside edge of your right foot, as it sometimes tends to lift. Take three to seven breaths before switching sides.

✗ NOT THIS

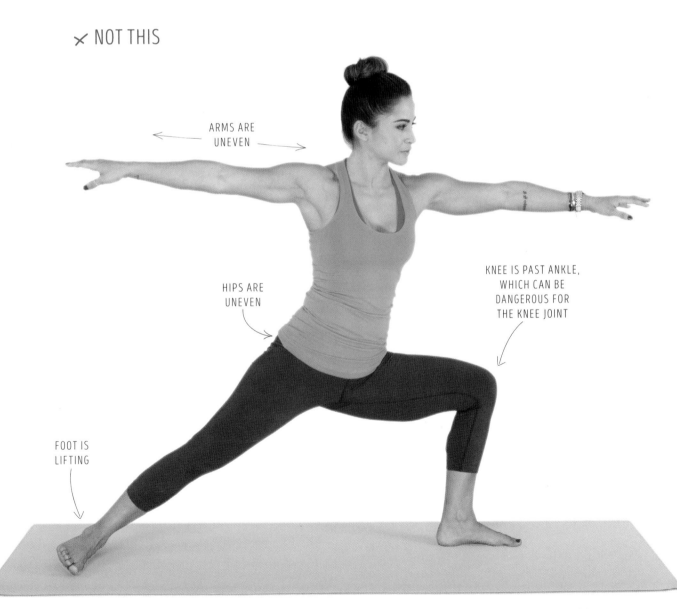

ARMS ARE
UNEVEN

KNEE IS PAST ANKLE,
WHICH CAN BE
DANGEROUS FOR
THE KNEE JOINT

HIPS ARE
UNEVEN

FOOT IS
LIFTING

VIPARITA VIRABHADRASANA reverse warrior

If you experience the afternoon slump as regularly as the sun rises, you're going to want to start incorporating this pose into your days. The nice side-body stretch helps get the blood flowing and wakes up a tired body.

Begin in warrior 2 (page 114) with your left leg forward. As you inhale, rotate your arms so that your left arm reaches up to the sky and your right hand rests on your right thigh. Sink low in your hips and reach high with your left arm as you look up toward your left hand. Rotate your hand so that the palm faces behind you. Breathe length through your left side body, imagining that you can breathe space into the left side of your rib cage.

Avoid collapsing in your right side body. Instead, use core strength for good posture to stay light and elongated through your spine. Relax your left shoulder away from your ear and breathe for three to seven breaths before switching sides.

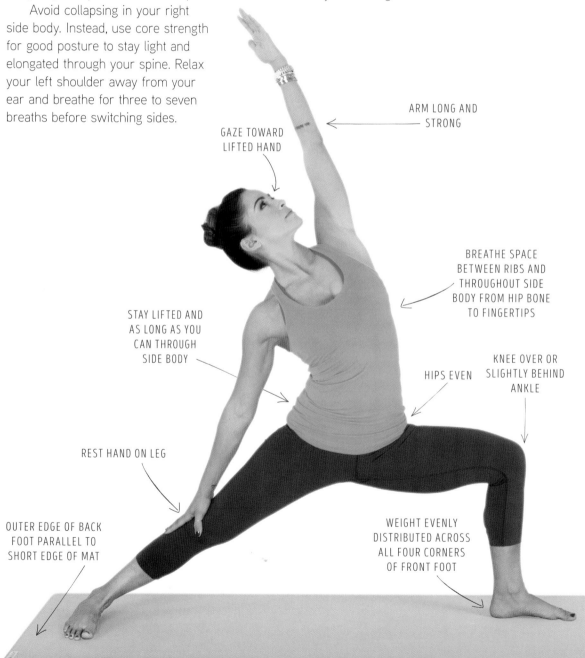

GAZE TOWARD
LIFTED HAND

ARM LONG AND
STRONG

BREATHE SPACE
BETWEEN RIBS AND
THROUGHOUT SIDE
BODY FROM HIP BONE
TO FINGERTIPS

STAY LIFTED AND
AS LONG AS YOU
CAN THROUGH
SIDE BODY

HIPS EVEN

KNEE OVER OR
SLIGHTLY BEHIND
ANKLE

REST HAND ON LEG

OUTER EDGE OF BACK
FOOT PARALLEL TO
SHORT EDGE OF MAT

WEIGHT EVENLY
DISTRIBUTED ACROSS
ALL FOUR CORNERS
OF FRONT FOOT

ANJANEYASANA low lunge

If low-back pain or sciatica has you constantly riding the struggle bus, you'll definitely want to start incorporating this pose morning, noon, and night. Gentle yet effective, it helps open up the hip flexors, which, when tight, can aggravate low-back issues, including sciatica.

Begin in high lunge (page 112) with your left leg forward. Take a deep breath in. As you exhale, lower your right knee to the ground, keeping the toes curled under. Inhale and lift your arms overhead if they aren't there already, and as you exhale, slowly press your hips forward until you feel a good stretch in your right hip flexor. On your next inhale, lift from your chest to create a mini backbend and breathe into your entire front body. Be mindful not to compress your low back, and instead breathe length into your spine and stay light and lifted through your chest. If it feels okay for your neck, look up. Inhale and breathe length through your entire body. Exhale your shoulders away from your ears. Breathe for three to seven breaths before switching sides.

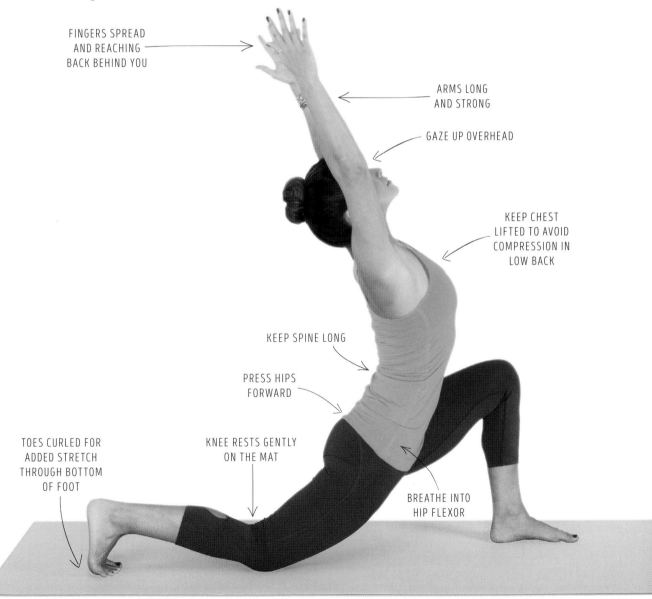

FINGERS SPREAD AND REACHING BACK BEHIND YOU

ARMS LONG AND STRONG

GAZE UP OVERHEAD

KEEP CHEST LIFTED TO AVOID COMPRESSION IN LOW BACK

KEEP SPINE LONG

PRESS HIPS FORWARD

TOES CURLED FOR ADDED STRETCH THROUGH BOTTOM OF FOOT

KNEE RESTS GENTLY ON THE MAT

BREATHE INTO HIP FLEXOR

modified UTTHITA HASTA PADANGUSTHASANA
standing hand-to-knee pose A and B

In Sanskrit, this pose literally translates to "extended hand-to-big-toe pose," but since this is the beginner chapter, I'm assuming that flexibility may be an issue for you. So I'm teaching a modified version of the pose here, which has you grab your knee rather than your toe to account for tight hamstrings. If you're worried about having to modify, relax. Everyone has to start somewhere. You'll still get a good stretch through your hip and inner thigh, and it'll still test your balance, so no worries there.

Begin in mountain pose (page 106). Lift your toes, spread them, and set them down for a stable foundation as you begin the balancing pose. Then find your drishti. For this pose, look for a spot out in front of you that is at eye level and not moving, and focus your gaze on that spot.

A)

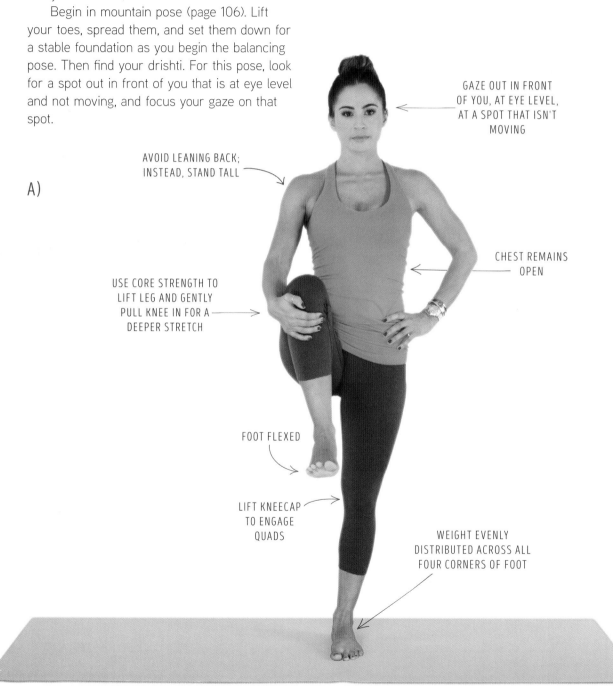

GAZE OUT IN FRONT OF YOU, AT EYE LEVEL, AT A SPOT THAT ISN'T MOVING

AVOID LEANING BACK; INSTEAD, STAND TALL

CHEST REMAINS OPEN

USE CORE STRENGTH TO LIFT LEG AND GENTLY PULL KNEE IN FOR A DEEPER STRETCH

FOOT FLEXED

LIFT KNEECAP TO ENGAGE QUADS

WEIGHT EVENLY DISTRIBUTED ACROSS ALL FOUR CORNERS OF FOOT

As you inhale, shift your weight onto your left foot as you use your core and hip flexor strength to lift your right leg. Gently wrap your right hand around the top of your right shin, flex your right foot, and bring your left hand to your left hip. Do not lean back. Instead, use your core strength and sense of balance to remain tall. Activate your core by bringing your navel in toward your spine and up toward your heart. Broaden your collarbones and relax your shoulders away from your ears. Breathe deeply for three to seven breaths here in part A before opening your right knee to the right. As you do this, slowly shift your gaze over your left shoulder.

This will definitely test your balance! If you wobble or fall over, who cares? Just get back into the pose slowly and try again. Breathe for three to seven breaths in part B before inhaling and bringing your knee back out in front of you. Slowly release and take the pose to the other side.

B)

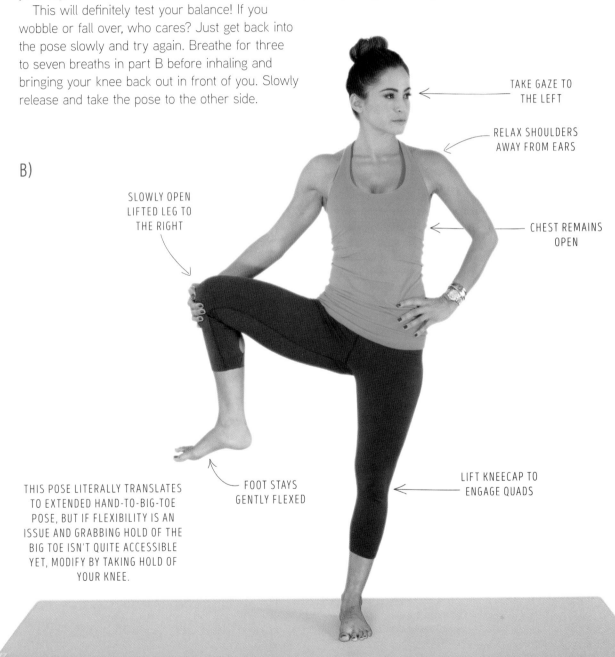

TAKE GAZE TO THE LEFT

RELAX SHOULDERS AWAY FROM EARS

SLOWLY OPEN LIFTED LEG TO THE RIGHT

CHEST REMAINS OPEN

FOOT STAYS GENTLY FLEXED

LIFT KNEECAP TO ENGAGE QUADS

THIS POSE LITERALLY TRANSLATES TO EXTENDED HAND-TO-BIG-TOE POSE, BUT IF FLEXIBILITY IS AN ISSUE AND GRABBING HOLD OF THE BIG TOE ISN'T QUITE ACCESSIBLE YET, MODIFY BY TAKING HOLD OF YOUR KNEE.

PRASARITA PADOTTANASANA A wide-leg forward fold A

If you've ever been to a torturous Bikram yoga class, you know that forward folds come about two-thirds of the way through the class and signify that the end is in sight. For that reason, whenever I do this pose in my personal practice, it always makes me smile and simultaneously feel grateful that I'm not in Bikram, sloshing around in my own sweat. Not that there's anything wrong with that; it just makes me question my sanity sometimes.

Anyway, to do this awesome hip opener, start by facing the wide edge of your mat and taking a wide stance. Lift your kneecaps to engage your quads. Turn your toes inward so that you are slightly pigeon-toed and bring your hands to your hips. As you inhale, press your hips forward, lean back, and lift your heart. As you exhale, hinge from your hips and bring your hands down to the ground with your fingertips in line with your toes. Look straight down between your hands and bring your elbows straight back behind you. Then shift your weight forward to bring your hips in line with your ankles. Breathe fully and deeply through the backs of your legs for three to seven breaths. When you're ready to release, bend your knees deeply, bring your hands to your hips, and round your back to come up vertebra by vertebra.

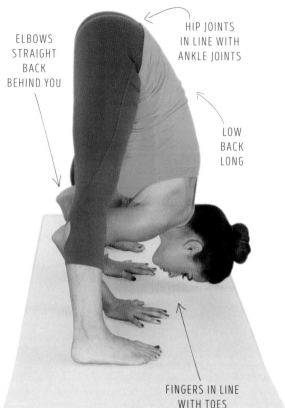

ELBOWS STRAIGHT BACK BEHIND YOU

HIP JOINTS IN LINE WITH ANKLE JOINTS

LOW BACK LONG

FINGERS IN LINE WITH TOES

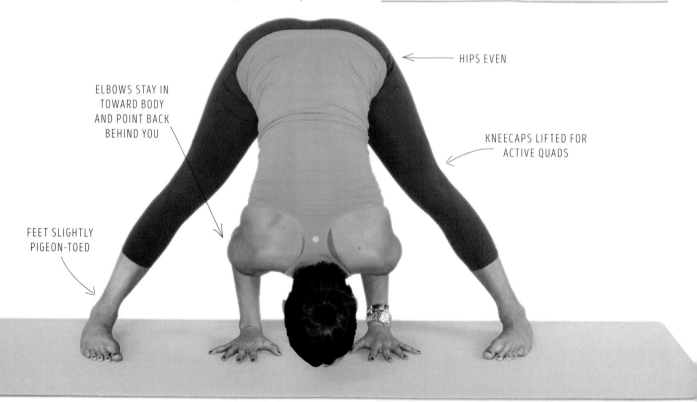

HIPS EVEN

ELBOWS STAY IN TOWARD BODY AND POINT BACK BEHIND YOU

KNEECAPS LIFTED FOR ACTIVE QUADS

FEET SLIGHTLY PIGEON-TOED

PRASARITA PADOTTANASANA B wide-leg forward fold B

This is the next phase of this awesome hip-opening sequence, and as you move deeper, you may feel a glorious release…or like your hamstrings might rip! Stay mindful and breathe, imagining that with each breath you're able to comb through the tangles of tension.

Start by facing the wide edge of your mat and taking a wide stance. Lift your kneecaps to engage your quads. Turn your toes inward so that you are slightly pigeon-toed and bring your hands to your hips. As you inhale, press your hips forward, lean back, and lift your heart. As you exhale, hinge from your hips and fold forward. Look straight down at your mat and keep your collarbones broad. Then shift your weight forward to bring your hips in line with your ankles. Breathe fully and deeply through the backs of your legs for three to seven breaths. When you're ready to release, bend your knees deeply and round your back to come up vertebra by vertebra.

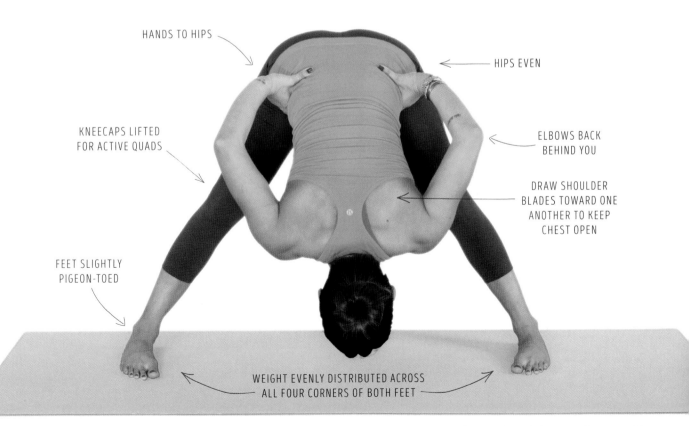

HANDS TO HIPS

HIPS EVEN

KNEECAPS LIFTED
FOR ACTIVE QUADS

ELBOWS BACK
BEHIND YOU

DRAW SHOULDER
BLADES TOWARD ONE
ANOTHER TO KEEP
CHEST OPEN

FEET SLIGHTLY
PIGEON-TOED

WEIGHT EVENLY DISTRIBUTED ACROSS
ALL FOUR CORNERS OF BOTH FEET

PRASARITA PADOTTANASANA C wide-leg forward fold C

This is an excellent pose for people who are dealing with tight chests. I always recommend it for athletes and anyone who spends the majority of the day hunched over a computer.

Start by facing the wide edge of your mat and taking a wide stance. Lift your kneecaps to engage your quads. Turn your toes inward so that you are slightly pigeon-toed and bring your hands behind your back, interlacing the fingers and pressing your palms together. Now, if you're an athlete or extremely tight through your chest, this position might not be accessible to you yet. In that case, modify by grabbing opposite elbows or as close to your elbows as you can.

As you inhale, press your hips forward, lean back, and lift your heart. As you exhale, hinge from your hips and fold forward, keeping your arms glued to your back. Look straight down at the mat, and when you can't fold forward any farther, lift your arms. If your fingers are interlaced, press your palms together as you bring your arms forward. This is important because pressing the palms together activates the muscles through your arms and helps protect your shoulders. If you've been doing the modified version and grabbing your elbows or forearms, lift your arms as much as you comfortably can. Then shift your weight forward to bring your hips in line with your ankles. Breathe fully and deeply through the backs of your legs for three to seven breaths. When you're ready to release, slowly bring your arms to your back. When your arms are glued to your back, bend your knees deeply and round your back to come up vertebra by vertebra.

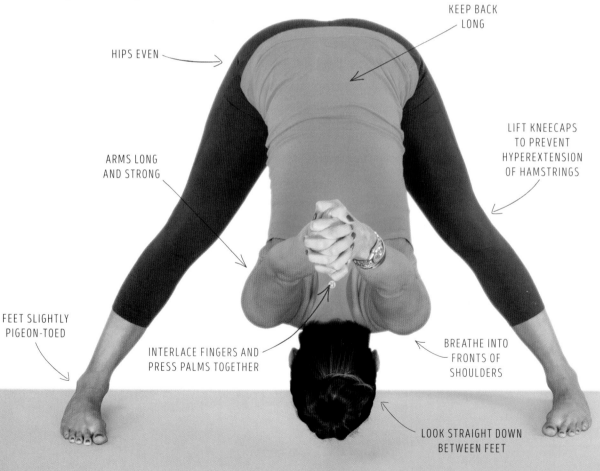

HIPS EVEN

KEEP BACK LONG

LIFT KNEECAPS TO PREVENT HYPEREXTENSION OF HAMSTRINGS

ARMS LONG AND STRONG

FEET SLIGHTLY PIGEON-TOED

INTERLACE FINGERS AND PRESS PALMS TOGETHER

BREATHE INTO FRONTS OF SHOULDERS

LOOK STRAIGHT DOWN BETWEEN FEET

PRASARITA PADOTTANASANA D wide-leg forward fold D

For the last pose in this series, you'll come into a deep hamstring-opening stretch. It's definitely a pose you'll want to incorporate if tight hips and hamstrings are trouble spots.

Start by facing the wide edge of your mat and taking a wide stance. Lift your kneecaps to engage your quads. Turn your toes inward so that you are slightly pigeon-toed and bring your hands to your hips. As you inhale, press your hips forward, lean back, and lift your heart. As you exhale, hinge from your hips and gently wrap your peace fingers around your big toes. Look straight down between your hands and bring your elbows straight out to the sides. Then shift your weight forward to bring your hips in line with your ankles. Breathe fully and deeply through the backs of your legs for three to seven breaths. When you're ready to release, bend your knees deeply, bring your hands to your hips, and round your back to come up vertebra by vertebra.

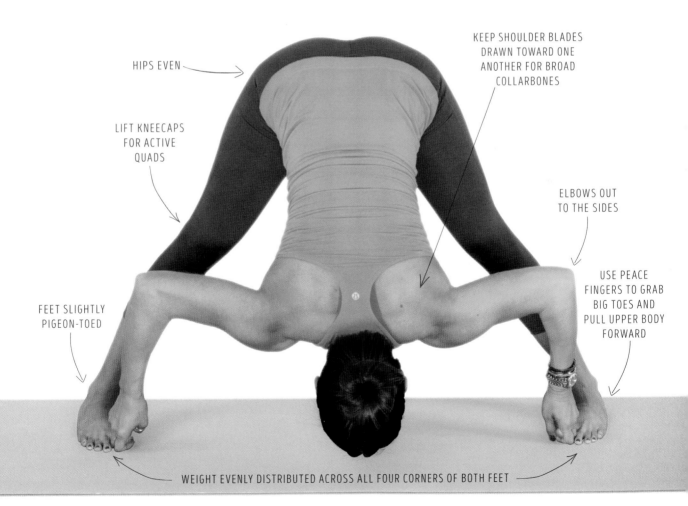

HIPS EVEN

KEEP SHOULDER BLADES DRAWN TOWARD ONE ANOTHER FOR BROAD COLLARBONES

LIFT KNEECAPS FOR ACTIVE QUADS

ELBOWS OUT TO THE SIDES

FEET SLIGHTLY PIGEON-TOED

USE PEACE FINGERS TO GRAB BIG TOES AND PULL UPPER BODY FORWARD

WEIGHT EVENLY DISTRIBUTED ACROSS ALL FOUR CORNERS OF BOTH FEET

UTTANASANA variation rag doll pose

This pose is a crowd-pleaser, so if you're a new yoga teacher and you're constantly scratching your head wondering what you can do to please the masses, throw in this bad boy. You're welcome. It's likely that it's such a class favorite because it gently opens up the hamstrings, which are notoriously tight for, like, everyone.

Begin standing with your feet a little wider than hip width apart. Lift your toes, spread them, and set them down for a stable foundation. On your next inhale, lengthen through your entire body. As you exhale, hinge from your hips and fold forward, letting your arms hang heavy. Grab opposite elbows and bend your knees until you feel your stomach against your thighs. Once your stomach is lying over your thighs, intend to straighten through your legs as you keep your low back long, visualizing your hip joints stacked over your ankles. As you inhale, breathe length through your hamstrings. As you exhale, melt your upper body over your thighs and feel your upper body being pulled down by gravity. Stay in this pose for as long as you like—five breaths, five minutes, or more—before releasing.

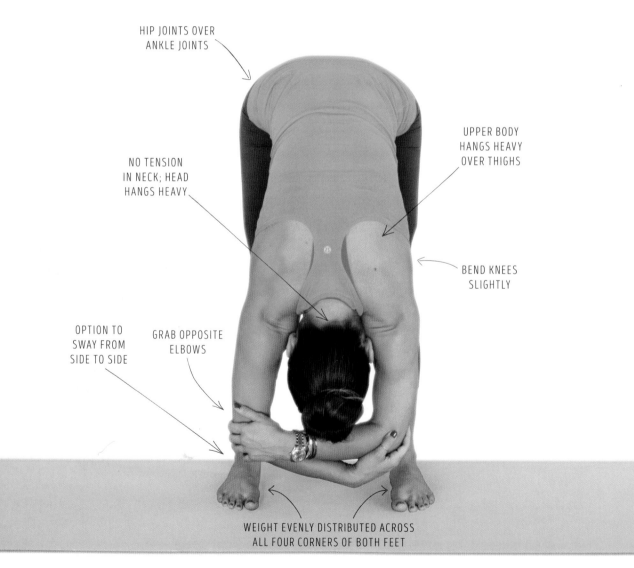

HIP JOINTS OVER
ANKLE JOINTS

UPPER BODY
HANGS HEAVY
OVER THIGHS

NO TENSION
IN NECK; HEAD
HANGS HEAVY

BEND KNEES
SLIGHTLY

OPTION TO
SWAY FROM
SIDE TO SIDE

GRAB OPPOSITE
ELBOWS

WEIGHT EVENLY DISTRIBUTED ACROSS
ALL FOUR CORNERS OF BOTH FEET

UTKATASANA chair pose

This pose cracks me up because so many people feel such intense emotion around it. I have a very good guy friend who can bench-press a million and a half pounds, but seven deep breaths in chair pose makes him want to crawl into a hole and wither away. Another friend of mine, a former ballerina, says that this pose makes her "stabby." So, if you're feeling inexplicable rage while in chair pose, just know that you're not alone. Breathe through it, and with lots of practice the rage should melt away.

Begin in mountain pose (page 106). Lift your toes, spread them, and set them down for a stable foundation. On your next inhale, lengthen through your body. As you exhale, squeeze your legs together and sink your hips as if you're about to sit down in a chair. From here, lift your arms. Now, you have a few options with your arms. Beginners can bring the hands together in prayer position. If you need more of a challenge, lift your arms overhead. Your arms can be by your ears with the palms facing one another or parallel to the ground with the palms facing down—it's totally up to you.

Once you're in your expression of the pose, tune in to your alignment. Keep the majority of your weight in your heels. When you glance down, you should be able to see your big toes. If your knees are blocking the view of your pigglies, your weight distribution is too far forward in your feet (which may stress your knees), so redistribute your weight into your heels. Next, check for length in your spine. Avoid swaying your low back. Instead, slightly tuck your tailbone for a neutral spine. Breathe for three to seven breaths in this pose before releasing.

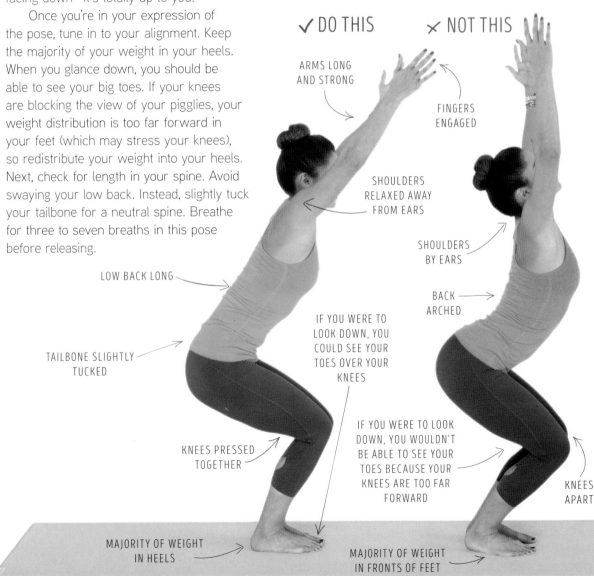

✓ DO THIS   ✗ NOT THIS

ARMS LONG AND STRONG

FINGERS ENGAGED

SHOULDERS RELAXED AWAY FROM EARS

SHOULDERS BY EARS

LOW BACK LONG

BACK ARCHED

TAILBONE SLIGHTLY TUCKED

IF YOU WERE TO LOOK DOWN, YOU COULD SEE YOUR TOES OVER YOUR KNEES

IF YOU WERE TO LOOK DOWN, YOU WOULDN'T BE ABLE TO SEE YOUR TOES BECAUSE YOUR KNEES ARE TOO FAR FORWARD

KNEES PRESSED TOGETHER

KNEES APART

MAJORITY OF WEIGHT IN HEELS

MAJORITY OF WEIGHT IN FRONTS OF FEET

UTKATASANA variation chair twist

This pose is both detoxifying and strengthening, and it's liable to have you huffing and puffing if your teacher throws it into the middle of a hot yoga class and leaves you breathing there for five or so breaths! My advice? Just stick with it and try to keep your cool.

Begin in mountain pose (page 106). As you inhale, lift your arms overhead. As you exhale, squeeze your legs together and sit your hips back as if you're about to sit down in a chair. Keep a neutral spine and avoid arching your back. As you inhale, bring your hands together in prayer position at your heart. As you exhale, gently tip your torso slightly forward and initiate a twist to the right from your navel. Hook the outside of your left arm onto the outside of your right knee. Keep squeezing your knees together to keep your left knee from coming forward. You have the option of keeping your hands in prayer position or opening them wide, with the left arm pointed down toward the ground and the right arm pointed up toward the sky with the palms away from you. Breathe for three to seven breaths in whichever expression of the pose you choose before bringing your hands back to prayer position and returning to center.

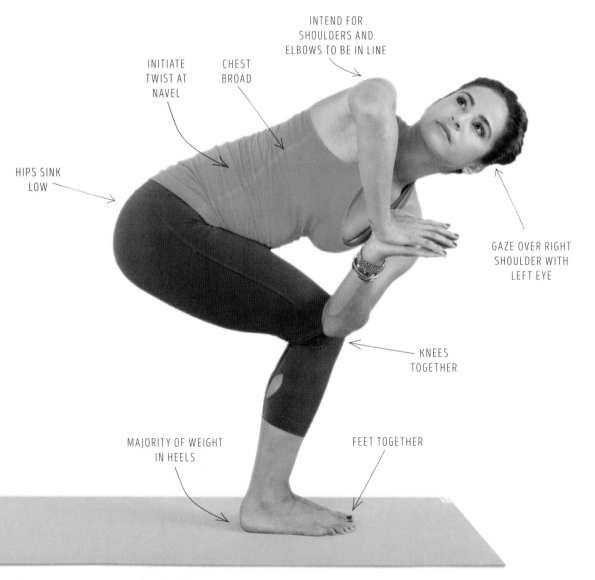

INTEND FOR
SHOULDERS AND
ELBOWS TO BE IN LINE

INITIATE
TWIST AT
NAVEL

CHEST
BROAD

HIPS SINK
LOW

GAZE OVER RIGHT
SHOULDER WITH
LEFT EYE

KNEES
TOGETHER

MAJORITY OF WEIGHT
IN HEELS

FEET TOGETHER

ARDHA PURVOTTANASANA reverse table pose

This pose is excellent for people with tight shoulders and chests.

    Begin by sitting on your mat with your legs straight out in front of you and your feet hip width apart. Take a deep breath in. As you exhale, slide your hands back about eight inches behind you, with your fingers spread and pointed toward your body. Then bring your feet halfway in to your pelvis, keeping them hip width apart, and press into your feet and hands evenly to lift your hips off the mat. Bring your hips up so that they're in line with your shoulders and knees. If it feels okay for your neck, you can let your head go back. Breathe into the fronts of your shoulders. Be mindful that your knees stay hip width apart and do not splay out to the sides. Breathe fully and deeply for three to seven breaths before exhaling your hips back down to the mat.

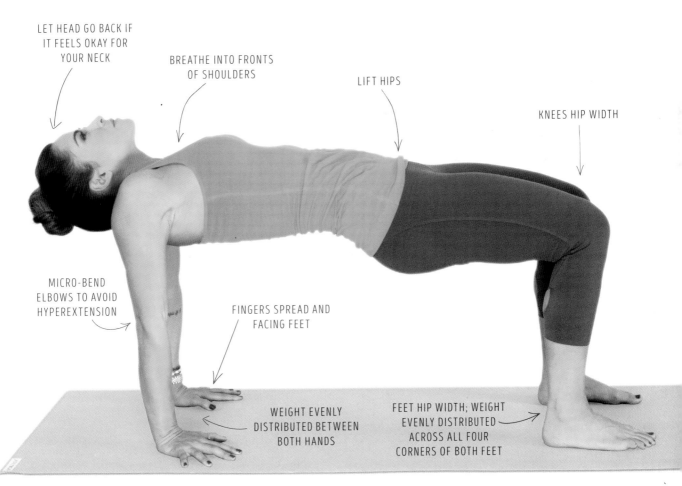

LET HEAD GO BACK IF IT FEELS OKAY FOR YOUR NECK

BREATHE INTO FRONTS OF SHOULDERS

LIFT HIPS

KNEES HIP WIDTH

MICRO-BEND ELBOWS TO AVOID HYPEREXTENSION

FINGERS SPREAD AND FACING FEET

WEIGHT EVENLY DISTRIBUTED BETWEEN BOTH HANDS

FEET HIP WIDTH; WEIGHT EVENLY DISTRIBUTED ACROSS ALL FOUR CORNERS OF BOTH FEET

PADAHASTASANA gorilla pose

This pose reminds me of being a little kid. If you can do it with a straight face, then gold star for you. Silly as you may feel in gorilla pose, it's a wonderful way to open up tight hips and simultaneously get a little hand massage. What's better than that?

Begin by standing on your mat with your feet hip width apart. Inhale and get as tall as you can. As you exhale, bend your knees slightly and hinge at the waist as you come into a forward fold. Bend your knees deeper so that you can easily slide your hands underneath your feet with your palms facing up. The most common mistake I see is people not sliding the hands far enough under the feet. You want to be sure that your toes are touching your wrists. Once your hands are sufficiently under your feet, let your head hang heavy and begin to straighten your legs, visualizing your hip joints lining up over your ankles. Take a deep breath, then begin to rock slightly back and forth, using the pressure of your feet to give your hands a little massage. Breathe fully and deeply, letting your arms and entire upper body be very heavy. When you're ready to release, remove your hands from under your feet, bend your knees deeply, and come up vertebra by vertebra until you're standing tall.

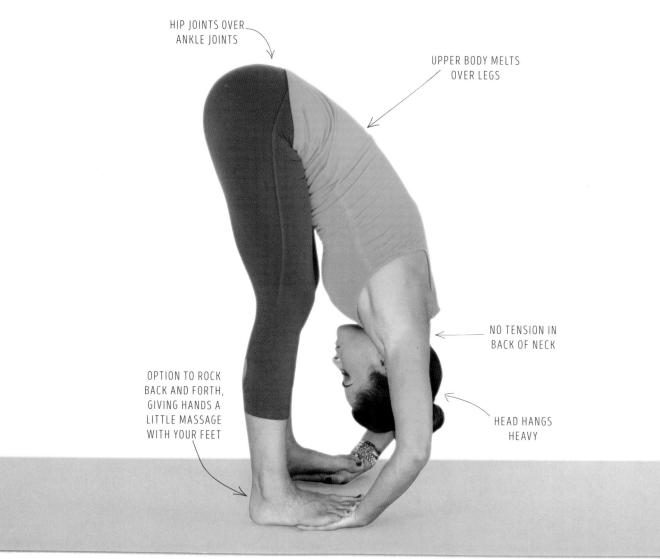

HIP JOINTS OVER
ANKLE JOINTS

UPPER BODY MELTS
OVER LEGS

NO TENSION IN
BACK OF NECK

OPTION TO ROCK
BACK AND FORTH,
GIVING HANDS A
LITTLE MASSAGE
WITH YOUR FEET

HEAD HANGS
HEAVY

BHUJANGASANA cobra pose

This pose is an effective way for beginners to develop back and upper-body strength. If you struggle with upward dog (page 198), cobra pose is a good substitute in the middle of your vinyasas.

Begin by lying on your stomach. Bring your hands underneath your shoulders with your fingers spread and your elbows drawn back and slightly in toward your body. Press the tops of your feet into the mat and, as you inhale, begin to straighten your arms to use your back-body strength to peel your chest off the mat. Tuck your tailbone slightly and press through your pubis into the mat. If your pelvis starts to lift up off the mat, you've gone too far. You want to keep your pubis connected to the mat. Relax your shoulders away from your ears and firm your shoulder blades down your back, lifting through your chest. Visualize length through your spine, imagining that your body is making a sideways J-shape rather than a sideways L-shape. Breathe fully for three to seven breaths before slowly coming down.

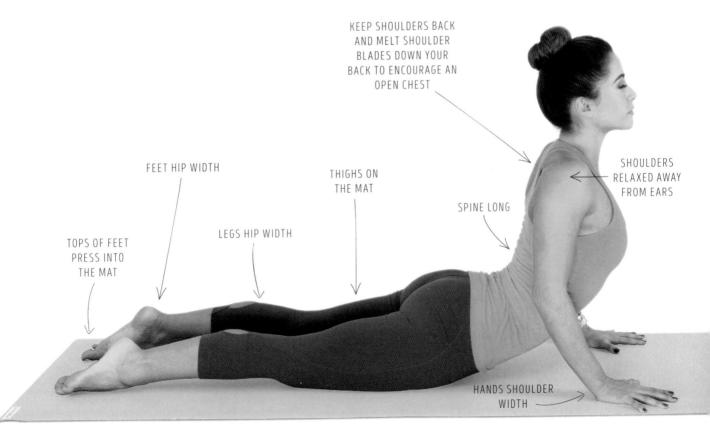

KEEP SHOULDERS BACK AND MELT SHOULDER BLADES DOWN YOUR BACK TO ENCOURAGE AN OPEN CHEST

SHOULDERS RELAXED AWAY FROM EARS

FEET HIP WIDTH

THIGHS ON THE MAT

SPINE LONG

TOPS OF FEET PRESS INTO THE MAT

LEGS HIP WIDTH

HANDS SHOULDER WIDTH

ANANDA BALASANA happy baby pose

If you've ever been to one of my yoga classes, you know that the vibe is pretty relaxed. I never want it to feel stuffy or like students can't ask questions, so I try to keep it lighthearted and approach teaching with humor and ease. During one class I said, "Okay, now draw your knees in toward your armpits as you come into happy baby pose." And another student chimed in, "Or, as my boyfriend calls it, 'Happy boyfriend pose!'"

The entire class just about died from laughter. Totally inappropriate and totally hysterical. And now you're going to think it every time you get into the pose and probably suffer a laugh attack. #sorrynotsorry

Begin by lying on your back with your knees bent. Press your low back to the mat and engage your core. As you exhale, use your core strength to lift your legs, inviting your knees in toward your armpits. Grab hold of the outside edges of your feet if you can. If they aren't accessible to you yet, grab hold of your ankles or anywhere on your lower shins. Use your biceps strength to pull your legs in even more. Then tuck your chin slightly so that the back of your neck is long. Lengthen through your tailbone and breathe.

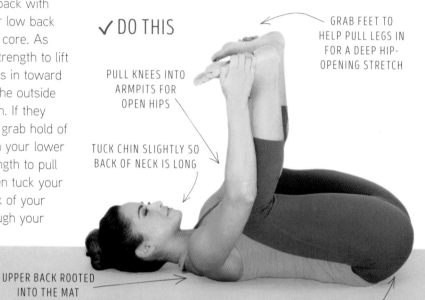

✓ DO THIS

GRAB FEET TO HELP PULL LEGS IN FOR A DEEP HIP-OPENING STRETCH

PULL KNEES INTO ARMPITS FOR OPEN HIPS

TUCK CHIN SLIGHTLY SO BACK OF NECK IS LONG

UPPER BACK ROOTED INTO THE MAT

REACH TAILBONE TOWARD THE MAT

One common mistake I see is people with the top of their head on the mat. Tuck your chin so that this doesn't happen. I also see people grabbing the right part of the foot, but at the expense of lifting their upper body off the mat, which means that their flexibility isn't quite developed enough. A better option is to place a yoga strap around the center of each foot (or do it one at a time with the opposite leg extended) or to grab hold of your ankles or anywhere on your lower shins.

Take three to seven deep breaths before gently releasing.

✗ NOT THIS

GRABBING THE RIGHT PLACE BUT AT THE EXPENSE OF LIFTING THE UPPER BODY WHICH MEANS THE FLEXIBILITY ISN'T QUITE DEVELOPED ENOUGH SO IT'D BE BETTER TO USE A YOGA STRAP OR GRAB AT THE ANKLES OR CALVES

TOP OF HEAD ON THE MAT

UPPER BACK LIFTED

SUPTA GOMUKHASANA reclined cow face pose

Attention, runners, athletes, people who work at desks, people with long commutes, and—okay, everyone with tight hips! You're going to want to add this pose to your daily practice to help open up those hips. It's fantastic because it targets the outer hips and provides nearly instant relief for tightness.

Begin by lying on your back with your legs bent. Tuck your chin slightly so that the back of your neck is long. Inhale and press your low back into the mat. As you exhale, use your core strength to lift your legs. Cross your left thigh over your right thigh and scissor the shins so that they're about parallel with the ground. Lift your arms and grab hold of the outside edges of your feet. Take a deep breath in and, as you exhale, gently use your biceps strength to bring your legs in toward your body. You should feel a very deep stretch through the outer edge of your left hip. Breathe fully and deeply, visualizing the tension being released with each breath. When you're ready, switch sides.

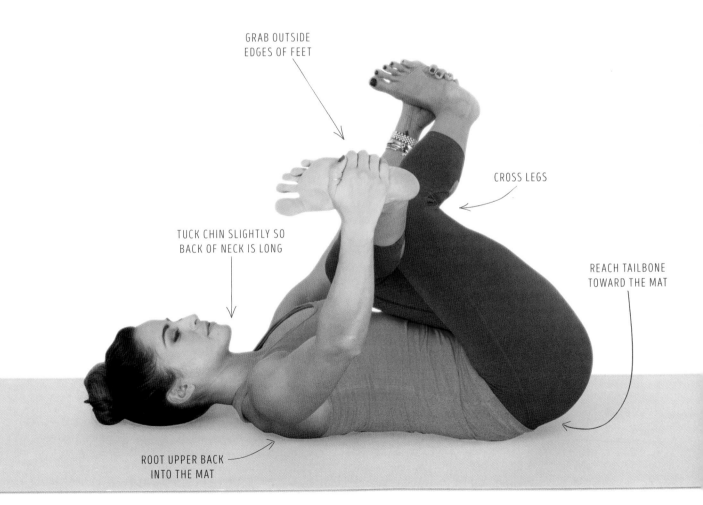

GRAB OUTSIDE
EDGES OF FEET

CROSS LEGS

TUCK CHIN SLIGHTLY SO
BACK OF NECK IS LONG

REACH TAILBONE
TOWARD THE MAT

ROOT UPPER BACK
INTO THE MAT

SETU BANDHA SARVANGASANA bridge pose

This posture offers a nice, gentle stretch for the chest, shoulders, and hip flexors. It's also the prerequisite for wheel pose (page 236), a deep backbend, so if you're looking to get your backbend on, this is a good starting point.

Begin by lying on your back with your legs bent and your feet on the mat. Bring your heels close to your pelvis with your feet hip width apart. Lift your toes, spread them, and set them down for a stable foundation. Press evenly into your feet to lift your hips. Avoid squeezing your bum; instead, press through your heels and feel your hamstrings engage. Gently rock from side to side until you can interlace your fingers underneath you and press into your arms. You may need to rock until the sides of your arms are on the mat so that you can lift your chest as well. Do not allow your knees to open up. Place a block between your legs if your knees are splaying out to the sides. Micro-tuck your tailbone so that you have a very long spine, and breathe into your shoulders and through your chest. Without turning your head, breathe fully and deeply for three to seven breaths before releasing your hands and lowering your hips to the ground.

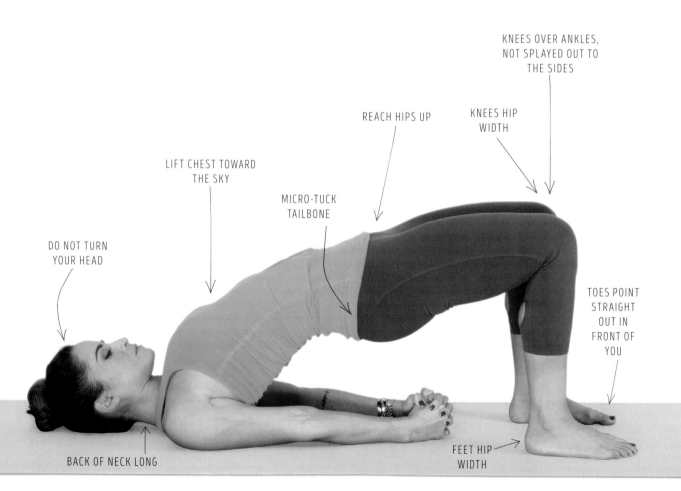

KNEES OVER ANKLES, NOT SPLAYED OUT TO THE SIDES

REACH HIPS UP

KNEES HIP WIDTH

LIFT CHEST TOWARD THE SKY

MICRO-TUCK TAILBONE

DO NOT TURN YOUR HEAD

TOES POINT STRAIGHT OUT IN FRONT OF YOU

BACK OF NECK LONG

FEET HIP WIDTH

SALAMBA BHUJANGASANA sphinx pose

Sphinx pose is a nice way to wake up the back muscles and offers a gentle stretch through the torso. Like bridge and cobra, it is a good beginner pose for backbends.

Begin on your stomach with your legs hip width apart. Bring your elbows underneath your shoulders with your forearms out in front of you, palms facing down. Press into the tops of your feet and then press into your forearms to peel your chest off the mat. As you press into your forearms, see if you can push into your hands as well to create the sensation that you're trying to pull yourself forward on your mat. This will help you lengthen through your entire spine. Focus your gaze about three feet out in front of you on the ground. Relax your shoulders away from your ears and melt your shoulder blades down your back. Breathe length through your chest and spine and visualize your body making a very gradual sideways J-shape rather than a sideways L-shape. This helps prevent compression in the low back. Breathe fully and deeply for three to seven breaths before releasing your chest to the ground.

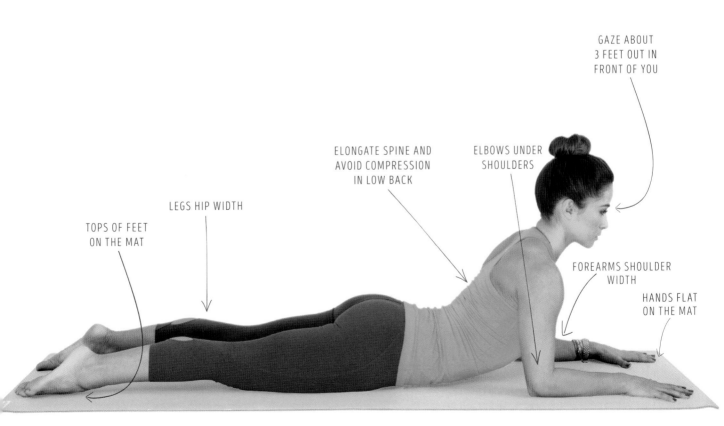

GAZE ABOUT
3 FEET OUT IN
FRONT OF YOU

ELONGATE SPINE AND
AVOID COMPRESSION
IN LOW BACK

ELBOWS UNDER
SHOULDERS

LEGS HIP WIDTH

TOPS OF FEET
ON THE MAT

FOREARMS SHOULDER
WIDTH

HANDS FLAT
ON THE MAT

PARIVRTTA JANU SIRSASANA revolved head-to-knee pose

The previous poses were gentle openers for the chest, back, and front body. With this pose, we're moving into the side body—the spaces between the ribs. Opening up that notoriously tight area is like opening up the gates of heaven, all blue skies and singing birds. Sounds great, right? Let's get to it.

Begin seated on your mat with your legs spread a little wider than 90 degrees. As you inhale, bend your right leg and place your right foot against your left inner thigh, as close to your pelvis as you can. Then lengthen through your spine and lift your arms overhead. As you exhale, lean to the left and place your left arm against the inside of your left calf muscle with your palm facing up. Then wrap your fingers around the arch of your foot. If your hand doesn't reach, wrap a yoga strap around the center of your foot and grab it as close to your foot as you can. From here, inhale and rotate your chest so that the right side of your rib cage is facing up. Lift your right arm overhead and grab hold of the top of your foot. If it doesn't reach, wrap another yoga strap around the back of your heel and grab it as close to your foot as you can. Turn your gaze up underneath your right arm if it feels okay for your neck and breathe into any tension you feel in your side body. Tune in to your hips and ensure that both hips are evenly on the ground—do not allow your right hip to come up. With each breath, comb through any tightness you feel from the top of your right hip bone all the way up through your right armpit. Take three to seven deep breaths in this position before gently releasing and switching to the other side.

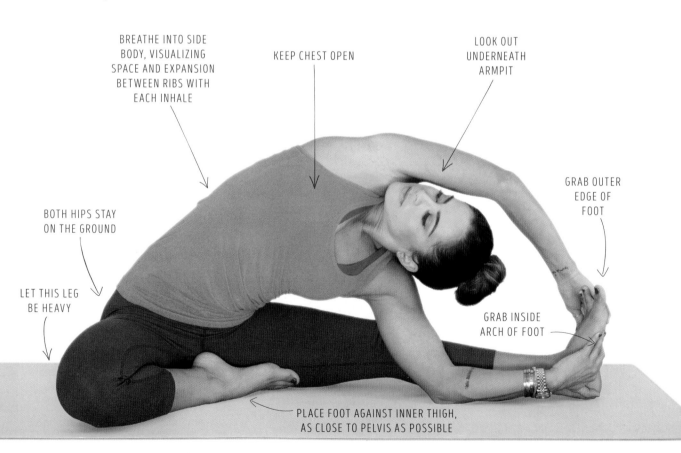

BREATHE INTO SIDE BODY, VISUALIZING SPACE AND EXPANSION BETWEEN RIBS WITH EACH INHALE

KEEP CHEST OPEN

LOOK OUT UNDERNEATH ARMPIT

GRAB OUTER EDGE OF FOOT

BOTH HIPS STAY ON THE GROUND

LET THIS LEG BE HEAVY

GRAB INSIDE ARCH OF FOOT

PLACE FOOT AGAINST INNER THIGH, AS CLOSE TO PELVIS AS POSSIBLE

SUPTA BADDHA KONASANA reclined bound angle pose

If you're looking for an alternative to savasana at the end of your practice, this pose is a great option. It's so relaxing and wonderful for opening up the inner thighs. Most often, though, you'll see this pose toward the end of your hatha or vinyasa yoga class just before you come into savasana.

Begin by lying on your back with your legs bent and your feet together on the mat. Slowly open up your knees so that the bottoms of your feet are touching and the knife-edges of your feet are on the mat. If you are extremely tight in your hips and find that you can't relax your knees, place a block or thick rolled blanket underneath each knee for support.

You have a few options for your hands. You can bring them to your sides with your palms facing up or bring them to your stomach, as shown. Alternatively, you can open your arms very wide as if you were going in for a big hug or bring your arms overhead if you have an open chest. Essentially, do whatever feels best for you.

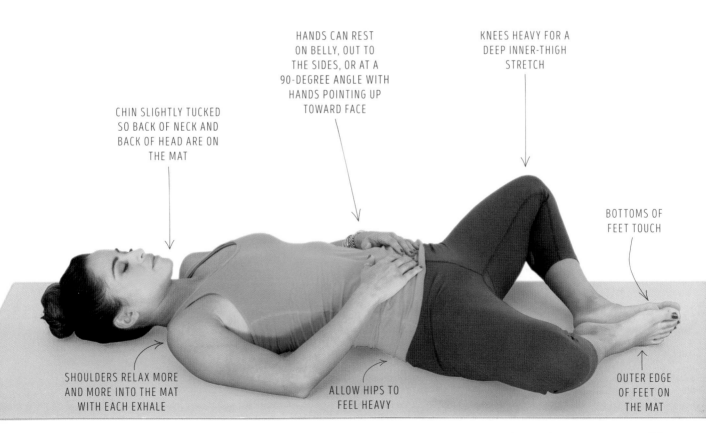

HANDS CAN REST
ON BELLY, OUT TO
THE SIDES, OR AT A
90-DEGREE ANGLE WITH
HANDS POINTING UP
TOWARD FACE

KNEES HEAVY FOR A
DEEP INNER-THIGH
STRETCH

CHIN SLIGHTLY TUCKED
SO BACK OF NECK AND
BACK OF HEAD ARE ON
THE MAT

BOTTOMS OF
FEET TOUCH

SHOULDERS RELAX MORE
AND MORE INTO THE MAT
WITH EACH EXHALE

ALLOW HIPS TO
FEEL HEAVY

OUTER EDGE
OF FEET ON
THE MAT

SAVASANA corpse pose

Savasana is meant to be the ultimate relaxing pose, and for most people it is. But for some people—particularly those who have low-back issues or are quite overweight—it can be painful. If you find that savasana aggravates your low back, you can place a rolled blanket underneath your knees to alleviate the pressure. If you're significantly overweight, you may find that your head tilts too far back to be comfortable. In that case, slide a folded blanket underneath your head so that your head is at the same height as the top of your spine.

Begin in a supine position and spread your legs mat width apart. Take your arms out to the sides with your palms facing up. Let your feet splay out to the sides. Close your eyes and let your eyes sink into the sockets. Scan your body from your head to your toes and, as you move from part to part, allow each part to totally relax. This pose should feel effortless. Take full, deep breaths for as long as you like before slowly wiggling your fingers and toes and rolling over onto your right side. Yoga instructors often have you roll to the right after savasana because the heart is on the left side, so rolling to the right applies less pressure and therefore allows you to remain in a calm state.

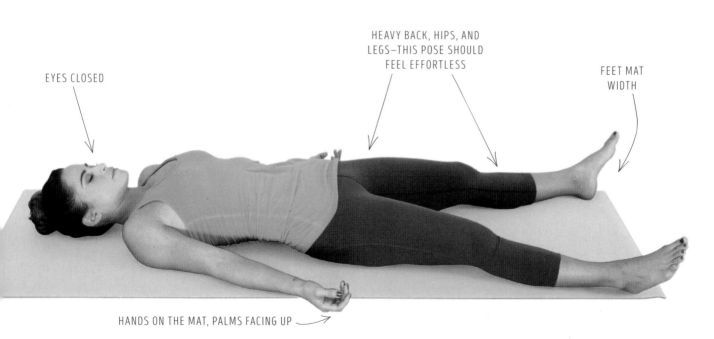

HEAVY BACK, HIPS, AND LEGS—THIS POSE SHOULD FEEL EFFORTLESS

EYES CLOSED

FEET MAT WIDTH

HANDS ON THE MAT, PALMS FACING UP

You can practice yoga poses individually, or you can do them in sequences. The following beginner sequences are comprised of poses covered in this chapter. They're a nice way to get accustomed to linking poses together as you develop your personal practice. Use them as a guide, and feel free to weave in any other poses you've learned that seem like natural next steps from what's offered. Remember, as long as your alignment is on point, you don't have to worry about much else. Play, explore, and don't take it too seriously.

sequence 1

1. MOUNTAIN POSE
(page 106)

2. STANDING FORWARD FOLD (page 107)

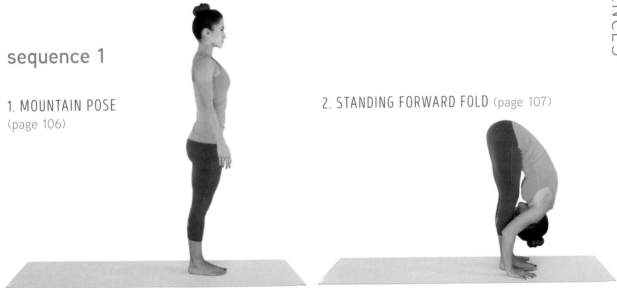

3. HALFWAY LIFT (page 108)

4. STANDING FORWARD FOLD

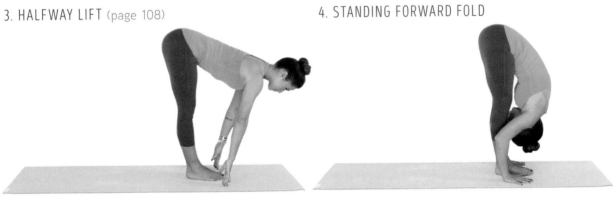

5. PLANK (page 109)

6. CAT/COW POSE (page 83)
A)

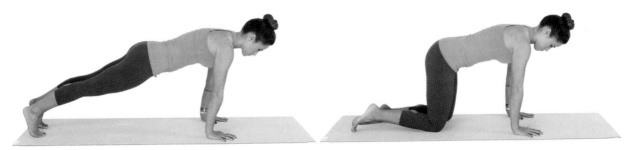

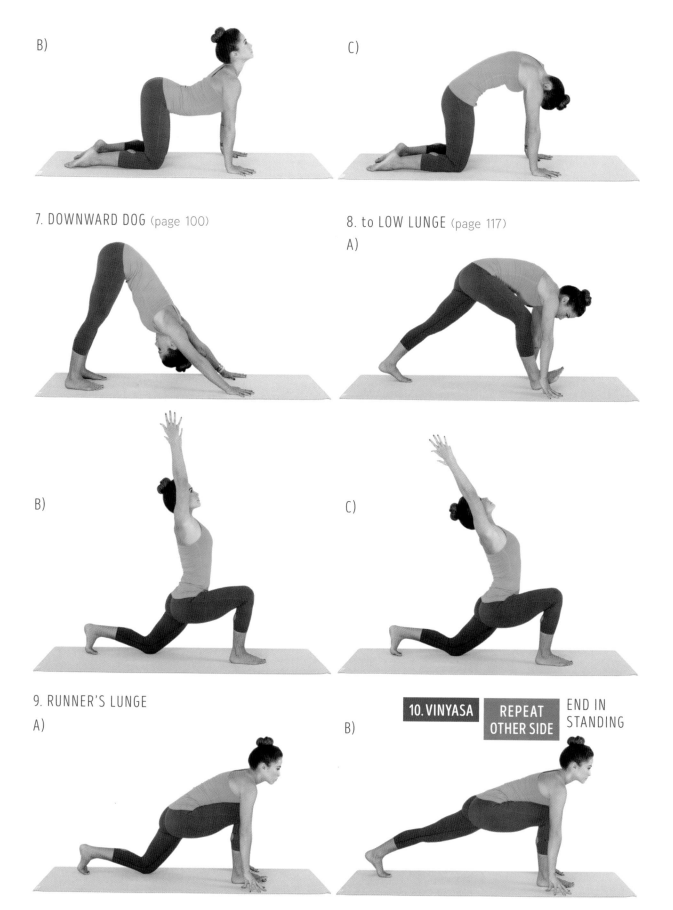

B)

C)

7. DOWNWARD DOG (page 100)

8. to LOW LUNGE (page 117)

A)

B)

C)

9. RUNNER'S LUNGE

A)

10. VINYASA | **REPEAT OTHER SIDE** | END IN STANDING

B)

sequence 2

1. EASY POSE
(page 90)

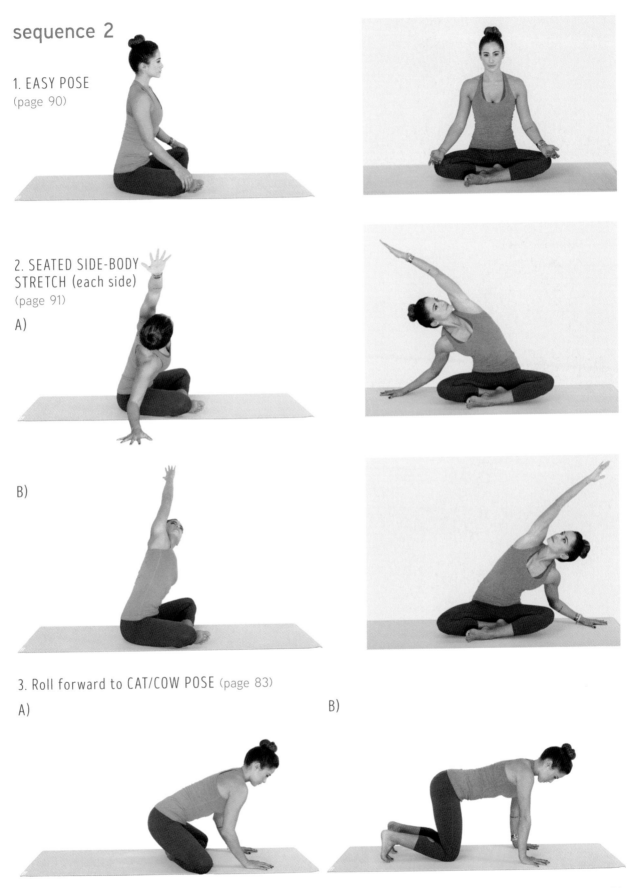

2. SEATED SIDE-BODY STRETCH (each side)
(page 91)

A)

B)

3. Roll forward to CAT/COW POSE (page 83)

A)

B)

C) 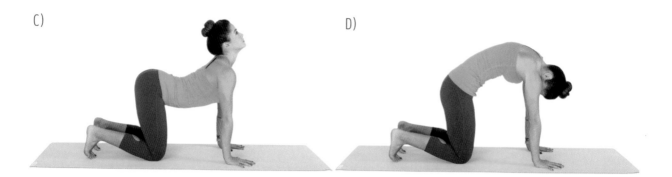 D)

4. DOWNWARD DOG (page 100)

5. WARRIOR 1
(page 113)

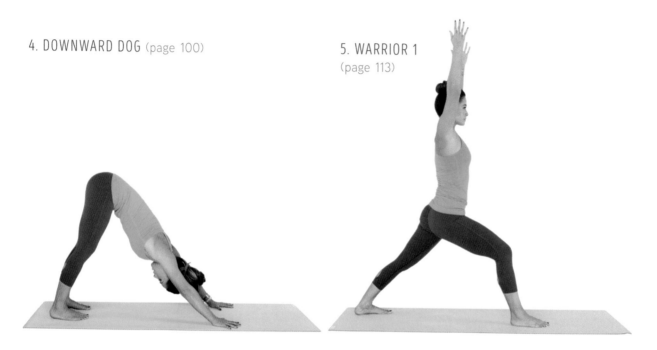

6. GORILLA POSE (page 128)

7. TREE POSE (page 105)

8. VINYASA

REPEAT OTHER SIDE

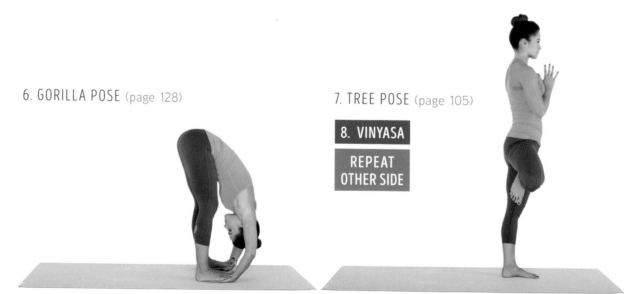

9. DOWNWARD DOG (page 100) to seated

A)

B)

C)

D)

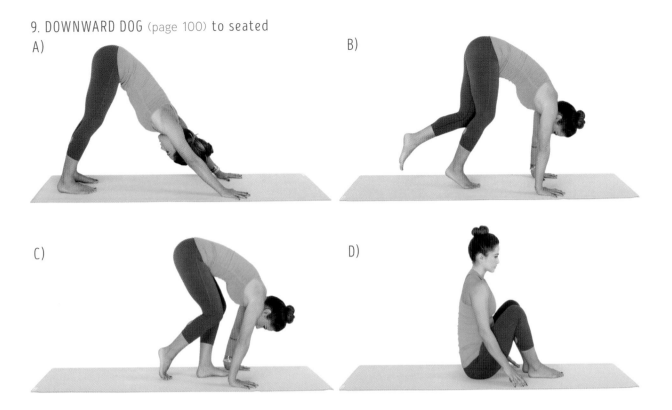

10. BRIDGE POSE (page 132)

11. CORPSE POSE (page 136)

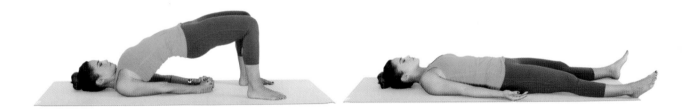

sequence 3

1. COBBLER'S POSE (page 88)

2. FIRE LOG POSE
(page 87)

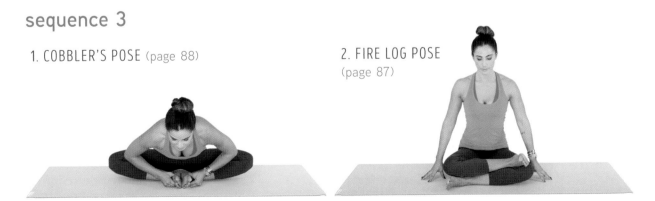

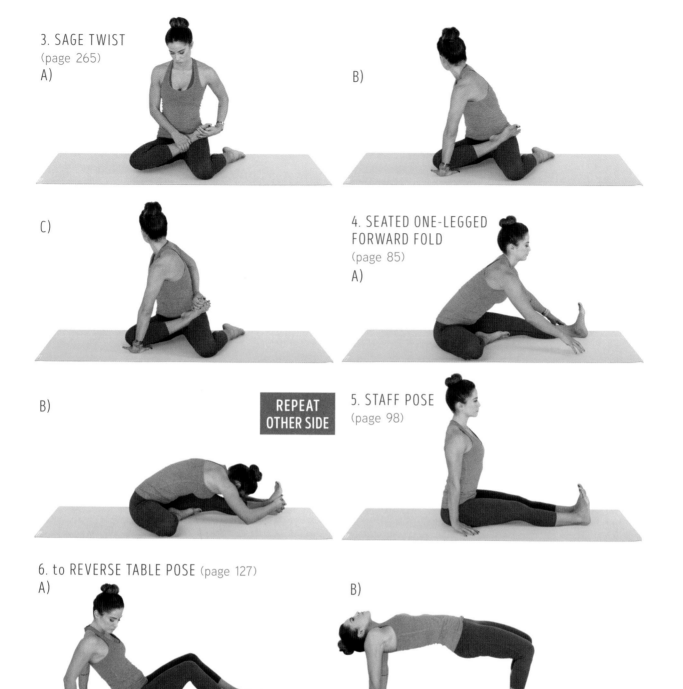

3. SAGE TWIST
(page 265)
A)

B)

C)

4. SEATED ONE-LEGGED FORWARD FOLD
(page 85)
A)

B)

REPEAT OTHER SIDE

5. STAFF POSE
(page 98)

6. to REVERSE TABLE POSE (page 127)
A)

B)

7. CORPSE POSE (page 136)

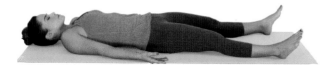

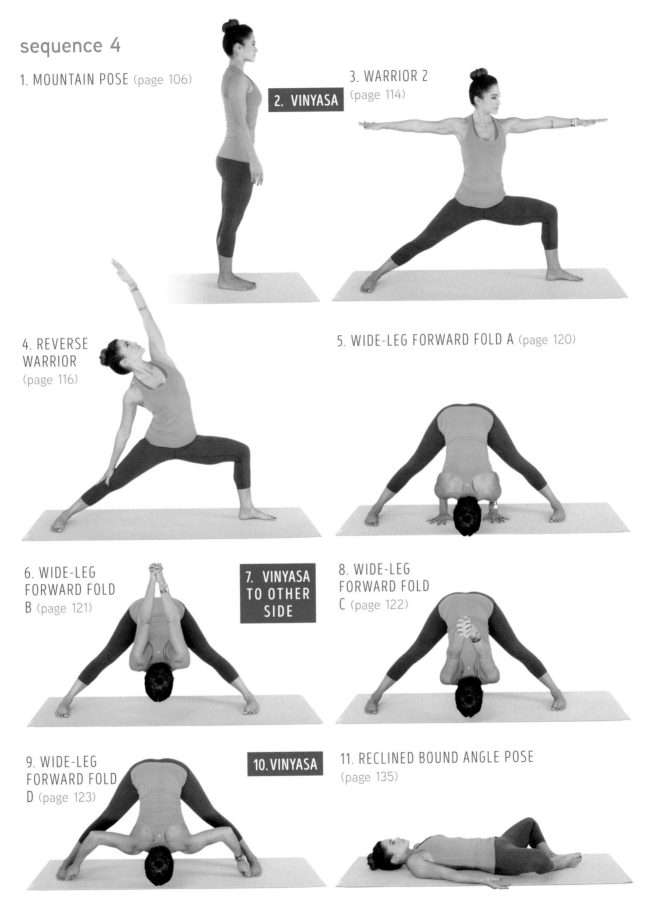

sequence 4

1. MOUNTAIN POSE (page 106)

2. VINYASA

3. WARRIOR 2 (page 114)

4. REVERSE WARRIOR (page 116)

5. WIDE-LEG FORWARD FOLD A (page 120)

6. WIDE-LEG FORWARD FOLD B (page 121)

7. VINYASA TO OTHER SIDE

8. WIDE-LEG FORWARD FOLD C (page 122)

9. WIDE-LEG FORWARD FOLD D (page 123)

10. VINYASA

11. RECLINED BOUND ANGLE POSE (page 135)

sequence 5

1. CHAIR POSE (page 125)

2. CHAIR TWIST (page 126)
A)

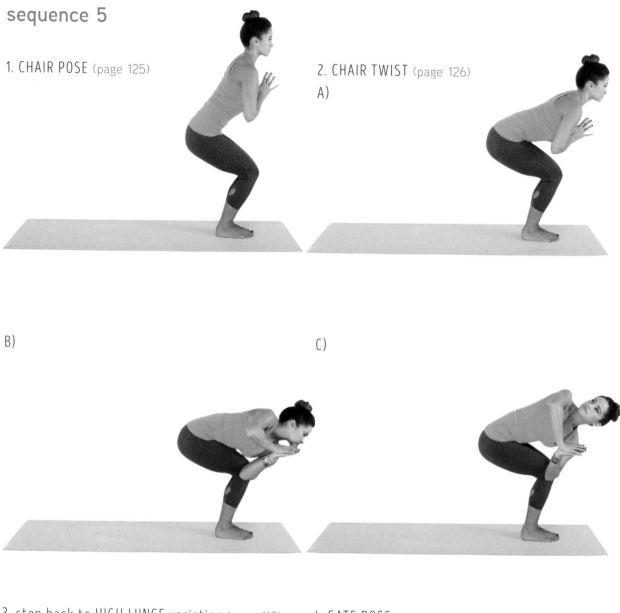

B)

C)

3. step back to HIGH LUNGE variation (page 112)

4. GATE POSE (page 84)
A)

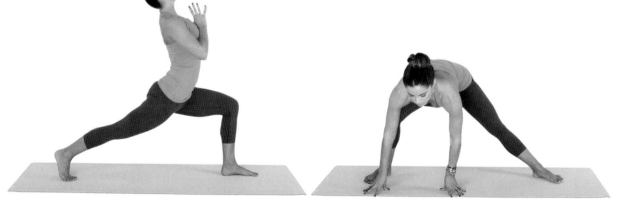

B)

C)

5. VINYASA

REPEAT OTHER SIDE

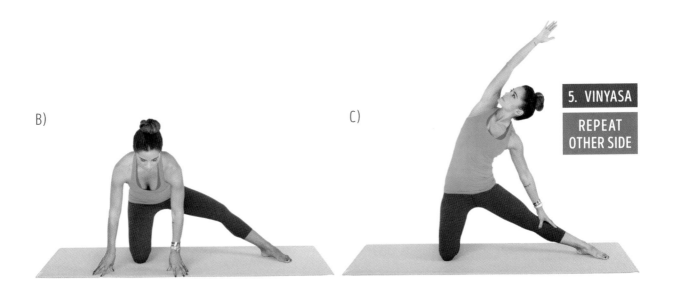

6. DOWNWARD DOG (page 100)

7. CHILD'S POSE (page 93)

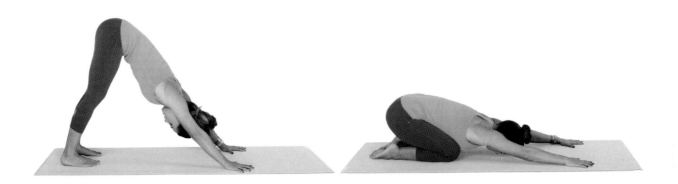

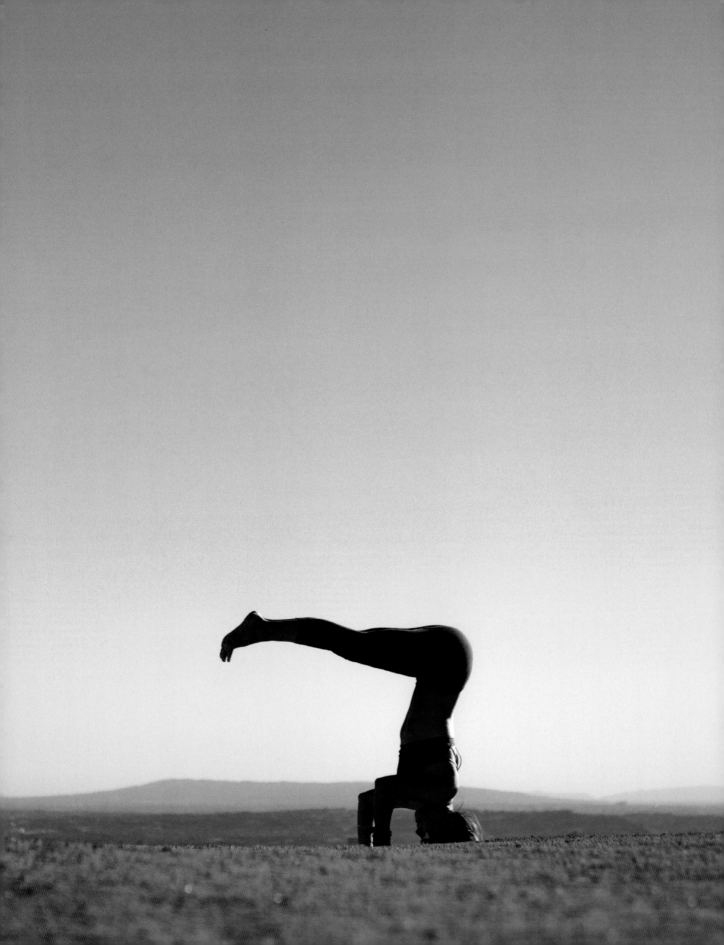

a taste of independence in Thailand

March 2012

The flight from Munich to Bangkok is pretty much an eight-hour-long panic attack for me. After nearly a year on heavy-duty antibiotics, I'm physically well enough to travel and the majority of my Lyme disease symptoms have disappeared or diminished, but I'm far from the picture of health.

My joints ache and feel brittle. They audibly click first thing in the morning, and I have to move slowly and carefully when I get out of bed so as not to startle the joints in my feet, which send searing, electric pain through my body if I move too quickly or put too much pressure on them before they're sufficiently warmed up. A weird new symptom has popped up— my stomach gurgles all the time—but it doesn't seem like a big deal, so I mostly ignore it. I've lost a lot of weight and am extremely thin despite eating all the time, but again, I don't think much of it.

Despite my lack of picture-perfect health, I've crossed off a bucket list item. No, make that two bucket list items. I'm traveling to Thailand, and I've committed to attending a yoga teacher training program. Travel more *and* take a yoga teacher training program? Check and check. The sheer pride I feel for crossing both of them off my list could move me to tears, but to be honest, this whole ordeal has had me crying for the last few years, and I'm sick of crying, happy tears or not.

Right now I need to deal with the problem at hand: how the hell I'm going to get to sleep if I have to listen to the newlyweds in the hotel room next door having sex all night.

It dawns on me that little else makes me feel as uncomfortable as having to listen to another couple go at it all night and then seeing them at breakfast a few hours later. I feel like a total creep, but there's nothing I can do, because this boutique hotel that I've chosen here in northern Thailand doesn't have TVs or radios. So I just lie there, staring at the ceiling and wondering how I got to this point in my life.

I am jet-lagged and my stomach hurts, and I can't tell if the pain is from the jet lag or from the discomfort of having to listen to the moans and bed creaks for the last thirty minutes.

Suddenly I remember that I have my headphones. I leap out of bed, grab them from my carry-on, slip them into my ears, and drift off to sleep on the hardest bed I've ever lain on (it's a Thai thing).

I swear, every little thing I do feels like a milestone these days. I wake up feeling exceedingly proud of myself. I lie in bed for a second, the crisp white sheets cool against my skin, with a smile so big it almost hurts my face. This is not just any old day. I am waking up in *Thailand*. I am on the other side of the world—the opposite side of the one where I lay in bed, frozen in this exact same position, unable even to lift my arms over my head due to joint pain.

I smile bigger. Now it's one of those stupid-looking, way-too-big smiles with far too much gum showing to be cute, but I have no one to impress and everything to smile about. I stretch my arms overhead.

I stretch my arms overhead!

My arms!

Overhead!

This, too, is a milestone.

I laugh at the simultaneous absurdity and beauty of it all. I fought to get myself out of the hole that Lyme disease had dragged me into and the deeper hole that the medication had pulled me into, and now here I am, literally living out one of my dreams.

I glance at my watch. 5 a.m.

Thank you, jet lag, I think. I am wide awake and ready to rock and roll. I get up and dress conservatively in a black maxi skirt, tank top, and oversized, sheer T-shirt. I have four days here before I report to another venue for yoga teacher training, and I've got stuff to do.

I eat breakfast and notice with relief that I seem to be early enough not to have to encounter the newlyweds, who are probably sleeping off last night's efforts. I dish up a bowl of the freshest fruit I've ever had, along with eggs and pancakes. I'm a hungry girl with a full day ahead of me. I sit down to eat and audibly moan when I taste the pineapple. How is it that pineapple could be so delicious? As my teeth sink into the juicy, stringy piece, I close my eyes, trying to burn this moment into my memory forever.

I swallow and begin a mental list of everything I love about Thailand.

Reason #1 why I love Thailand: this pineapple.

The first order of business is to secure a yoga mat. The waifish, delicate Thai girl who works at the hotel cocks her head to the side when I try to ask her where I can buy one.

I take a deep breath and suppress a smile because I realize that I'm going to need to get creative with how I explain myself, given that she does not speak English and I don't know much more Thai than "hello," "thank you," and "goodbye." I welcome the challenge.

When I was in high school, my mom came home one day and announced that we would be hosting Japanese exchange students for a week. The two girls didn't know any English, and we didn't know any Japanese. This made for interesting interactions. Each person in my family had a different approach to communication. My brother and dad mostly smiled at them but stayed silent. My mom spoke slow, very loud English. And I used props. "Do you want some SPAGHETTI?" I'd ask, holding the package of pasta in my hand and pointing. Fortunately, everyone had a great attitude, and we laughed off our miscommunications and tried our best to understand each other. Sometimes we succeeded by miming.

I look at the Thai girl and pretend that I'm playing a game of charades.

"Uh, okay," I say. I start showing her some yoga moves.

She cocks her head even further to the side and squints at me like she's trying to guess what I'm doing. Then I squat down on the ground, draw a giant imaginary rectangle with my index finger, and take an exaggerated step onto my imaginary mat.

"You know, so no OUCH!" I say, jumping back as if I'd just stepped on glass, as if that's going to help. Then I roll up my imaginary mat and hold it in my arms.

"So…?" I look at her hopefully, hold out my arms, and shrug my shoulders. I take out my credit card. "So *I buy*," I say, waving the card, "the *mat*," I finish, bouncing my imaginary yoga mat in my arms.

Suddenly she says, "Ahhhhh!!!!!"

Relief washes over both of us, and we laugh at my sub-par acting skills. She performs a similar game of charades accompanied by a Thai translation. I gather that she isn't sure I'll have luck finding a yoga mat, but there is a giant market down the road, and it's worth a look. If not, there's a mall farther down the road. To this day, I have no idea how in the world we came to this understanding, but that's the beauty of traveling—magic like this just happens.

"*Kop khun kah,*" I say with one hand on my heart, because I figure that gesture is a universal "thank you" in the very probable case that my Thai sucks.

Reason #2 why I love Thailand: charades.

She grins from ear to ear, puts her hands in Namaste, and bows her head. I set out walking for the market with her hand-drawn map.

My heart soars. Not only did I essentially have a conversation with someone with whom I do not share a common language, but I figured out what to do! A few months ago, I couldn't even concentrate on someone speaking *English*, and now look at me! Kicking ass and taking names, doing ninja moves in the middle of the courtyard at my tiny hotel in Thailand(!!) and figuring shit out. Go, me!

NAMASLAY COMMANDMENT #9:
DEFY YOUR LIMITS.

As I walk down the road, my confidence starts to wane as I become very aware of just how much I stick out.

In Europe, where Greg and I have lived for the past few hockey seasons, we have learned how to dress in order to blend in. You don't wear baseball caps. You don't wear college sweatshirts. The only sweatpants that you wear in public are the super tailored kind commonly referred to as "joggers." Greg may or may not have purchased (and worn) capris made for men. I usually pay a little more attention to what I wear, and when I do, I am sometimes mistaken for Spanish and sometimes for Italian.

In Thailand, it's not as easy to blend in. For one, um, I'm not Thai. My Lebanese-Ecuadorian skin is sort of olive, but it's a distinctly different shade than the warm brown skin of the Thai people. My eyes are almond-shaped and hooded, and my hair is not the jet-black beautiful mane that everyone else sports here. And in case that weren't enough, even at barely over five feet tall, I am taller than most of the people I walk by.

And I have to walk by *a lot* of people.

This morning, they are mostly men, sitting outside garages, electronics stores, pawn shops, and gas stations.

I walk as I've learned to walk when I'm traveling alone: head held high, eyes forward, face calm but determined, as if I know exactly where I'm going. No eye contact. With each step I take, though, my confidence wanes. I inwardly cringe and prepare for the usual thing that happens when a woman walks by a group of men: the dreaded cat-calling.

I am a pretty calm person, but nothing makes me rage the way being cat-called makes me rage. It's a poisonous rage that I have a very hard time controlling, starting deep within and bubbling up with each whistle, hoot, and kissy sound. When it happens, I want to run up to the men and shake the shit out of them and say, "Don't you have a mother? A sister? Any woman you care about in your life? Why are you doing this?! Why are you dead set on making me feel so uncomfortable that I want to jump out of my skin?!"

Now, I've never actually done that, but I fantasize about it every time I am cat-called. I'll never do it because it's dangerous, and I especially will not do it in Thailand when I am traveling alone. I cannot act a fool here and land myself in a Thai prison because first of all, my parents hate to travel, and second of all, Thai prison.

But as I walk by man after man after man, the strangest thing happens: nothing. There are groups of men perched on buckets in front of shops that are still closed. There are groups of men sitting on the ground talking. There are groups of men leaning against dilapidated buildings and eating out of takeout cartons. And they don't even glance my way. They don't look up from their morning papers, their food, or their friends. They don't care about me at all, and at this moment, it's the best feeling in the world.

Reason #3 why I love Thailand: as a solo female traveler, I feel safe.

About a half mile and three turns away, I decide that I should check the map. I don't want to look like I'm lost, so I discreetly open my bag and glance at the map. Shit. I'm definitely lost. My heart flutters and a wave of panic washes over me. I tell myself that it's the jet lag and follow my gut instinct to keep going straight.

Suddenly I see an old man wheeling a basket piled high with fish. His face is calm yet determined. He is walking with purpose. I cannot for the life of me come up with one reason why one man would need so many fish so early in the morning other than the fact that he's going to sell them at the market.

Follow that man! my inner child yells out, and I smile because now I'm playing a game called Get Un-lost. (It's a working title; don't judge me.)

Feeling a little like a detective, I try to follow the man without looking like I'm following him, which is hard to do when you two are the only ones walking down the middle of the street. But it's all good, because pretty soon I start to hear sounds. Market sounds.

A Thai market sounds a lot like you'd imagine—people negotiating in Thai, and the whack, whack, whack of butchers chopping, and shrieks of laughter from children chasing each other through the aisles, and mothers consoling crying babies. There are easily over a thousand booths packed into this one market, with row after row of people and flowers and trinkets and clothing and musical instruments. I walk by splashing buckets of live eels, and snails and crabs, and mysterious sea creatures that I could not identify if my life depended on it. At first, my eyes are like saucers. It's incredible! I did it! Another milestone! I successfully found my way to the market that I only learned about through a game of charades with one of the hotel employees who speaks Thai. I. Am. Awesome.

But then I start to feel hot. A little overwhelmed. The all-too-familiar wave of anxiety splashes over me and I feel uneasy, despite my best efforts to push the feeling aside.

The market is sensory overload. I start to feel claustrophobic in aisles overcrowded with shoppers, but I push on. There are lanterns and yarn and brightly colored scarves. There is rice and potatoes and scallions and weird-shaped fruits that I cannot name. There is smoked fish and sausages and patties of mystery meat. There are towels and radios and books and makeup. There are old shoes and paintings and handmade soaps. There are pirated DVDs and handmade jewelry and Buddha statues. This place has *everything*.

Everything, it seems, except for a yoga mat.

When I can't take the claustrophobia anymore, I flag down a tuk tuk driver to take me to the mall. It's only 9:30 a.m., but the sun beats down violently as we putter down the street. My loose cotton maxi skirt feels like a wool blanket, and I'm holding out hope that the mall is air-conditioned. As we drive, we pass whole families piled onto dirt bikes and mopeds. I watch incredulously as a father drives with a toddler behind him, the mother behind the toddler, and an infant perched precariously over the handlebars. No one wears helmets as they bounce down the roads. I am in awe. The traffic is unbelievable and there are people everywhere, but things just seem to function in a sort of organized chaos. These parents have everything to worry about with their children, the loves of their lives, bouncing along, but everyone seems cool, calm, and collected. It is a good lesson for me.

We finally arrive at the mall, and as I step into the building, the air-conditioning slaps me across the face. I feel like I've just stepped into an ice-cold shower, and I could twirl and dance a jig of happiness, but making a scene is frowned upon in Thailand.

The mall has a department store in which I locate a purple yoga mat.

The mat is nothing special—it's the same type of cheapo mat that you'd find at your local big box store—but yoga mats have always been somewhat sacred to me. During college, my mat was the one place I could go where the debilitating anxiety wouldn't creep up on me. I step onto every mat on which I practice with reverence and appreciation for the space and safety it provides. I'm so excited about this ordinary yoga mat, about the fact that this is the one on which I will spend the next six weeks developing the foundation I need to be the great teacher I know I can be. As I pay, I am filled with pride that I was able to get myself to a Thai market and get a tuk tuk driver to take me to the mall, where I successfully found a mat. Now I can take a tuk tuk back to the hotel and relax.

I find my way outside. It is even more sweltering now, at 10:30 a.m., but my driver is all smiles when I show him the business card of the hotel, on which the name and address are written in Thai. We negotiate using charades, in which I am apparently fluent, and after agreeing to a price, he flashes his biggest smile and gets in the front seat.

Reason #4 why I love Thailand: it lives up to its name: the land of smiles.

****

Three weeks later, I am halfway through yoga teacher training and I feel raw. The training has been the most intense thing that I've ever done mentally, physically, and dare I say spiritually?

The yoga practice is like a mirror that forces you to look inside and see what's going on internally. It forces you to examine everything you do and everything you are. The intensity of this training has cut me open and exposed my insecurities, my self-doubts, my constant inner battles. It has stripped me of my masks, my layers of armor, my Tough Girl exterior. It has reopened old wounds that feel as painful as they did when they first happened. I feel naked and vulnerable. I experience excruciating waves of sadness and anxiety and emotional release.

Sifting through all that *stuff* is like organizing fifty shoe boxes of old photos—sticky with who knows what, fuzzy and out of focus—but it also leaves me feeling good. Feeling a tremendous sense of accomplishment. The entire process makes me nostalgic and happy and frustrated and exhausted and proud.

So, despite my fear of the unknown, I soldier on. I fan the flames of hope that I feel growing within me. These are the best days of my life because I am going through something so transformational. Every single day, I feel like I'm learning something new about myself. Every single day, I feel like I've peeled back another layer—like an onion—to get to the best, most delicious part of myself. This is sacred time to work on me. And while you could argue that for the last year or so, all I'd done was work on myself, this is different. That is focusing on me so I can get back to even kilter. This is focusing on me so that I can let go of all the baggage that I've been carrying around and reveal the person I am at my core—a strong, determined woman with a heart of gold and a desire to help other people.

And then one day it all comes together.

It's a sweltering afternoon, easily over 110 degrees, and the twenty or so of us yoga teacher trainees are in the shala. Our shala is like a giant open tree house. The yoga platform sits in the middle of the biggest tree I've ever seen. The floor is well over twenty feet wide and just as deep. There is a thatched roof, and although there are no walls, a few gauzy white curtains help keep out the mosquitoes once the sun starts to set. With eyes glazed over we stare at our teacher, who, equally fatigued and sluggish from the long day in the heat, is explaining the intricacies of tree pose.

"You want to watch out for the student putting the foot on the knee joint. That's a common mistake, and it puts a lot of stress on the joint," she explains. We are too tired to really compute what she's saying.

Now, I'm a teacher at heart. When we were kids I used to make my brother play a very originally titled game called School. Being four years older, I, naturally, was the teacher. I taught him important lessons like how to balance a checkbook (we used Mom's expired checkbooks, which felt fancy and legitimate) and how to write in cursive (which to this day he does not do, so I sometimes wonder if I failed him).

In first grade, when my fellow classmates didn't understand concepts, I was always the first to jump in and explain it another way.

In third grade, my art teacher told us to draw a fish. Everyone else drew a standard goldfish—you know, with a triangle for the tail and a long oval for the body. I drew a lionfish, which is this crazy-looking poisonous fish with up to eighteen brown-and-white-striped dorsal fins and a funny face that looks like it's frowning because of its big old sad eyes. I was so psyched about that fish because I'd seen it the night before on the Discovery Channel. I showed my teacher my somewhat abstract drawing, filled with pride because I knew that it was different from everyone else's.

This particular teacher was one of those who never left her desk. In fact, I don't think I ever even saw her stand up. When I brought her my fish, she exclaimed, "That's not a fish! Go to the library and get a book on fish, and then come back and draw one."

My heart sank. It felt like she had stepped on me, squashing my bubbling enthusiasm with her dismissal of my silly little fish. But even then, as a third grader, I knew that what she'd said wasn't right. I relayed the story to my mom that night, and the next day she withdrew me from public school and enrolled me in a Rudolf Steiner school in the Berkshires, where the Waldorf pedagogy is rooted in creative play and artistic expression and the words "standardized testing" mean nothing.

It was a weird place, but as I've learned, all the best things in life are weird, and in that school I developed an even greater love of teaching and learning. I remember how we created our own textbooks and learned about fractions by drawing tree branches. My family could only afford to send me to Steiner school for a little over a year, but the education I received there was priceless.

The Waldorf approach served me well years later, when I became a Spanish teacher at a school that specialized in TPR Storytelling, which is a method of teaching foreign languages based on the idea that students learn best through reading and telling stories.

Teaching is my thing. No, it's my *thang*. I totally nerd out on it. Anytime I take a yoga class, I evaluate the instruction—not to compare teachers, but just for fun. What can I learn from this teacher? What did she do that I can implement? What didn't I like about what she did? Did the teacher have a good read on the class? Did he or she offer modifications or adjustments? Did the teacher have a sequence that made sense for the body? Did the class start and end on time? These things were important to me as a student, and I always mentally took notes and vowed to implement the things I liked that will work for me and my teaching style.

I firmly believe that everyone I meet knows something that I don't. Everyone is a teacher. Therefore, I am a teacher to everyone I meet, so I do my best to share what I know with others without threatening what they know. That way, we both can continue to learn and grow, because here's something else I am crazy for: learning.

I love to learn. I am forever a student.

Sorry, I went off on a tangent there, but it's important because as I'm sitting in that yoga shala in Thailand on the hottest day of our training, more than seven hours into our schedule for the day, I think to myself, *Jeez, it would be so much more useful if we had a visual for these tree pose points she's trying to make.*

And instantly I can picture it in my head: a photo of a person in tree pose, cut out and pasted against a white background, with lines drawn all over the photo to indicate proper alignment, breath, and foundation.

Being a blog lover and knowing that there aren't any yoga blogs out there that I love, I decide right then and there that I will create a yoga blog that features these types of cutouts. The blog will be rooted in real talk—no mumbo jumbo I'm-greater-than-thou guru stuff. This will be a modern blog that everyday people can dive into without feeling like they don't belong to the club. None of that exclusivity shit; this blog will be for everyone.

Reason #5 why I love Thailand: it's the place where I dreamed up my destiny.

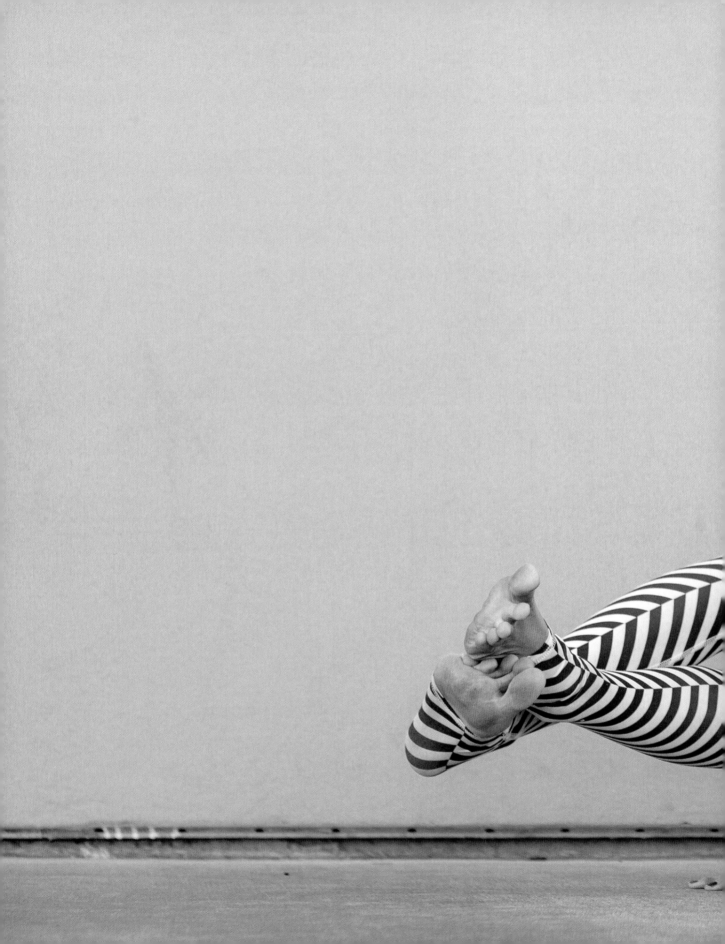

CHAPTER 4:

the intermediate practice

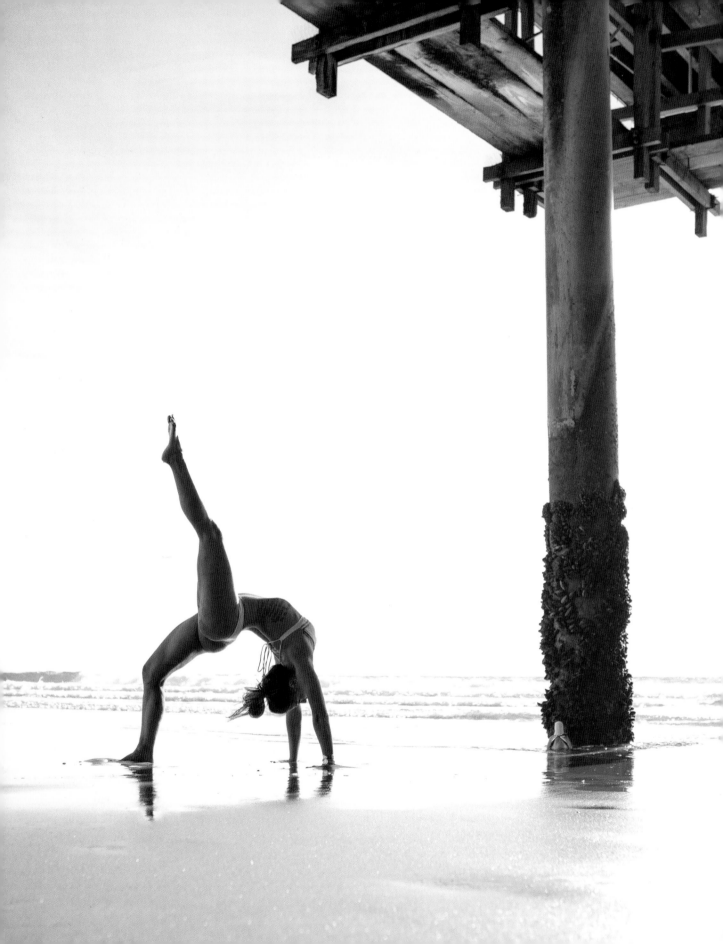

the space between

2015

I'm in my apartment in the Czech Republic. We have an east-facing window and the morning light streams in, drenching the living room in warmth.

I've been practicing yoga for over a decade, practicing daily for the last five years or so, and I feel good. No, I feel great. My practice is thriving, and the trick, I've learned, is to surrender. I've let go of having expectations for myself. I've thrown out the idea that by now I should know how to do *X, Y,* or *Z* pose.

I know yoga isn't about that. *You* know yoga isn't about that. But let's be real: sometimes it's nice to be able to do your dream pose.

Anyway, I'm at that weird stage in the practice where I'm no longer a beginner, but I'm not quite advanced, either. I'm in between, and it's my favorite place to be because I really love the struggle.

I *really* love the struggle.

That's an unlikely thing to say, but let me explain.

The struggle is where it all goes down. It's the blood, sweat, and tears of the making of a masterpiece. It's the grind, the dance, the meditation in motion that builds up my strength and exposes my layers. It challenges the negative committee inside my head and tells it to sit down and STFU.

You might step back from whatever it is you're dealing with and think that there's no way you can make it through. You might even try to look for an alternate route, but when you do, you'll quickly realize that there is no shortcut. You can't avoid the struggle. It's there, as sure as the jitters on your first day of school, as sure as the thrill of your first solo drive after being granted your license, as sure as the pounding of your heart as you go in for the first kiss of your longtime crush. And you have to choose to keep fighting through, to keep giving it all you've got. To let yourself be cut open and exposed. To cry and kick and scream and release everything you've been holding onto for so many years. To choose to push through day after day. To get back up after being knocked down time and again. Because one day you will conquer, thrive, and soar, and it will all be worth it. This is true for the yoga practice, and it is true for life.

In my yoga practice, I sweat as I move. My arms shake underneath me. My legs, which have developed the tiniest teardrop quads, quiver. My breathing intensifies. The work is physically hard for me.

But the mental aspect? That's harder.

The mental aspect requires sifting through years of wearing masks—masks of indifference, of irritation, of various shades of my ego. It's peeling back layer after layer that I put up to block out the world and protect myself, to stay safe. It's going through old habits, years of negative self-talk, and the belief that I'm not good enough, that I can't.

I can't.

Psh. What a waste of breath. Because here's the thing I've learned.

Actually? I *can.* I can do *anything.*

I have lived through family tragedy that's shaken me to my core. I have lived through a mystery illness that a number of doctors couldn't figure out. I have beaten that disease by taking medication and by following my own intuition, and subsequently I've traveled all over the world, alone, and completed a rigorous yoga teacher training program that consisted of fifteen hours a day of training, so actually? This little headstand action? No, I might not be able to do it, like, *right now,* but you can bet that I will work and sweat and grind and show myself that just like everything else in my life, I *can.*

I can do *anything* I put my mind to and work toward.

And so can you.

We, my friend, are powerful beyond measure. When we get out of our own way, we can do anything.

So when I'm on the mat, I breathe, and I move, and I think absolutely nothing, guided by unshakable faith in my abilities and motivated by the fact that so far, no matter how bad the day, I have survived and mostly thrived. Guided by love in my heart and determination running through my veins, I know that I can do, be, and have anything I work toward.

Right now I'm working on supported headstand. My arms are in place, my head is down on the mat, and I curl my toes and lift my hips. My legs are straight and I breathe in, feeling the breath comb through the slight tension I feel in my hamstrings. The breath untangles the tension, and I walk my feet forward, feeling the stretch in the backs of my hips. On my next inhale, I give the tiniest hint of a hop and spread my toes like they're wings, and suddenly my legs are lifting up, slowly reaching toward the sky as I push into my forearms, using the strength of my back muscles and my core. I could cry I am so proud of myself, so in awe, so loving these precious moments of in-between—the space between the starting position and the full expression of the pose.

These in-between moments—the moments between the day we are born and the day we die, the dash between our birth and death years on our tombstones, all the temporary stages—are life. It's our choice how we spend this in-between time. It's our move to make it count. It's our decision to give it all we've got. So I move through the moment and surrender to whatever happens. No expectations, no deadlines, no thoughts at all—just doing my best to lift, lift, lift my legs all the way up and enjoy every shake that my body responds with, every drop of sweat that trickles down my arms, and every breath that fuels me through this simple yet glorious experience.

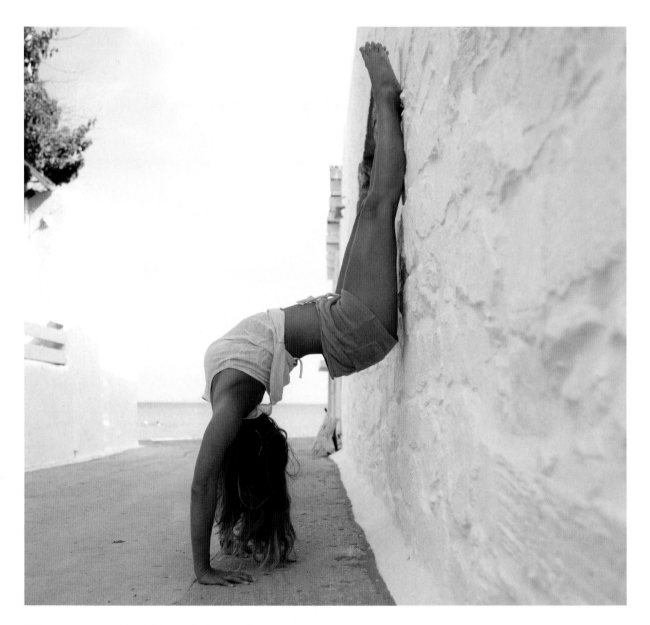

On one hand, being an intermediate yoga student is like being a sophomore in college. You're still somewhat new to collegiate stuff, but you've got the basics down. You know a solid amount, yet there's still so much more to learn.

On the other hand, if you start creeping down to negative town, being an intermediate yoga student can be somewhat frustrating. You're definitely not a beginner, but you're most certainly not pressing up into handstands. As you continue to build strength and prepare for more advanced poses, the practice can feel very repetitive, and it's not unheard of for people to become frustrated by the seeming absence of progress.

My advice is to remember this: we inhabit our bodies day in and day out, and therefore we don't recognize the micro-growth that we experience daily. So I encourage you to stick with it and aim for a well-rounded practice. Balance out your drive to achieve those crazy pretzel poses by adding in some much-needed yin and restorative yoga. Stay hyper-aware of which types of yoga you avoid and which parts of the yoga practice (like pranayama or meditation) you tend not to do enough of. When you are honest about who you are and what you do and you strive to make changes for a well-rounded yoga experience, you will see breakthroughs.

NAVASANA boat pose

I have a feeling that boat pose got its name from the fact that it's easy to fall back and "rock the boat," if you will. The key is developing hip flexor and core strength. The bad news is that the lactic acid–burning feeling that you experience while developing hip flexor and core strength feels about as good as a sunburn, but the good news is that in my experience, that strength develops quite quickly (much like a sunburn, in fact!). Add navasana to your practice regularly and you'll be amazed by how much strength you gain.

Begin seated on your mat with both legs straight out in front of you. Pull the flesh from underneath your sitting bones so that they are firmly rooted into the mat. Then bend your knees, bringing the feet together on the ground. As you inhale, elongate your spine and broaden your collarbones so that your chest is open. Then extend your arms so that they are parallel to the floor, keeping them plugged into your torso. From here, gently lean back until you are balancing on your sitting bones and lift your shins until they're parallel to the ground.

MODIFIED VERSION

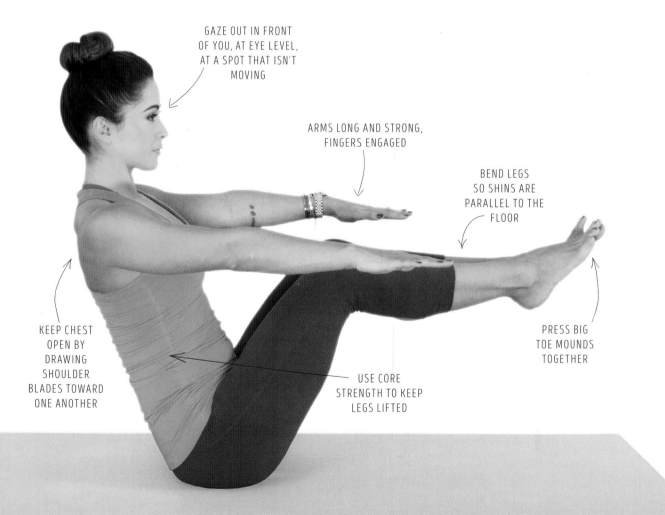

GAZE OUT IN FRONT OF YOU, AT EYE LEVEL, AT A SPOT THAT ISN'T MOVING

ARMS LONG AND STRONG, FINGERS ENGAGED

BEND LEGS SO SHINS ARE PARALLEL TO THE FLOOR

KEEP CHEST OPEN BY DRAWING SHOULDER BLADES TOWARD ONE ANOTHER

USE CORE STRENGTH TO KEEP LEGS LIFTED

PRESS BIG TOE MOUNDS TOGETHER

If you want to take it a step further, you can press out of the bottoms of your feet to extend your legs, keeping your big toe mounds touching. Spread your toes and breathe.

Keeping your chest lifted and your arms long and strong, breathe fully and deeply. If you want to take it another step further, you can do alternate toe taps to the rhythm of your breath or rotate your torso, initiating the twist at your navel. Aim for at least three breaths, but you can stay in this pose for as many breaths as you like before releasing.

FULL EXPRESSION

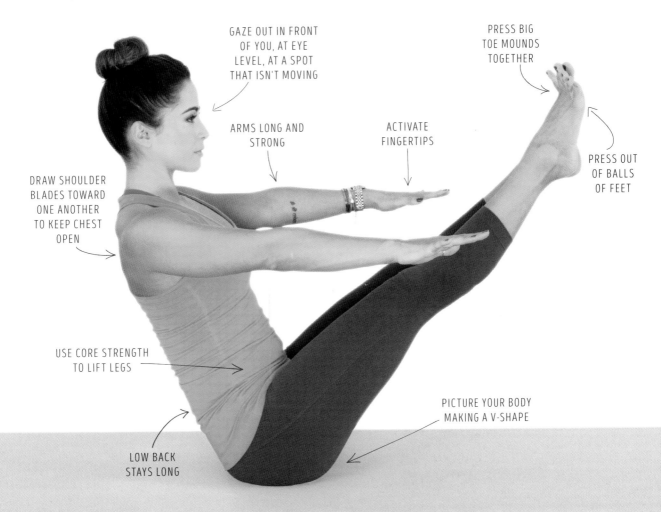

GAZE OUT IN FRONT OF YOU, AT EYE LEVEL, AT A SPOT THAT ISN'T MOVING

PRESS BIG TOE MOUNDS TOGETHER

ARMS LONG AND STRONG

ACTIVATE FINGERTIPS

PRESS OUT OF BALLS OF FEET

DRAW SHOULDER BLADES TOWARD ONE ANOTHER TO KEEP CHEST OPEN

USE CORE STRENGTH TO LIFT LEGS

PICTURE YOUR BODY MAKING A V-SHAPE

LOW BACK STAYS LONG

UPAVISTHA KONASANA A seated wide angle posture a

Upavistha konasana A is a seated angle posture that can be a little confusing to get into because the tendency is to spread the legs as wide as possible, as if you were doing a split. This pose isn't about doing a perfect split, so open your legs to about a 90-degree angle. From here, bring your hands to your hips to check that they are open enough for the pose. If they tilt slightly forward and your low back stays long, you are fine and can continue to open your legs wider until you feel like you're on your "edge."

If your hips tilt backward and your low back wants to round, however, you are pretty tight and should modify the pose by sitting on the edge of a folded blanket or yoga block. If you're modifying, stay in this position with your fingers on the ground behind you, encouraging your hips to tilt forward, and make sure to keep your legs engaged to protect your knees and hamstrings.

If you do not need to modify, you have a few options. The first is to bring your hands to the ground in front of you and gently push them into the mat to pull your upper body forward while maintaining length in your back and openness in your chest. This is key to keep the stretch in the hips.

The second option, if you're slightly more open, is to take your hands down toward your feet. If you can't wrap your peace fingers around your big toes, you can wrap a yoga strap around each foot and grab the strap as close to the foot as you can, or you can take hold of your shins or anywhere on your legs that's comfortable.

If you're ready for the full expression of the pose (as shown in the photo), wrap your peace fingers around your big toes on an inhale as you lengthen through your spine. Then, as you exhale, use your biceps strength to pull yourself forward, bringing your chin to the ground. Be mindful to keep your legs engaged to protect your knees and hamstrings, and be sure to stay long in your low back and open in your chest.

Wherever you are in the posture, breathe fully and deeply for three to seven breaths before releasing.

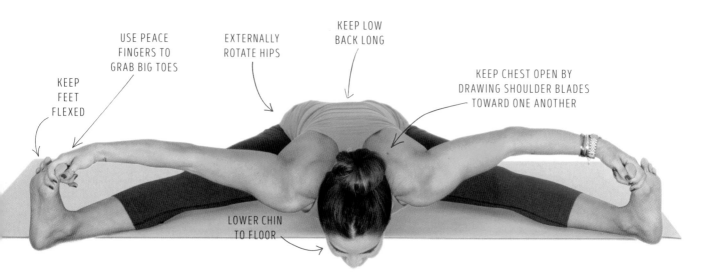

KEEP FEET FLEXED

USE PEACE FINGERS TO GRAB BIG TOES

EXTERNALLY ROTATE HIPS

KEEP LOW BACK LONG

KEEP CHEST OPEN BY DRAWING SHOULDER BLADES TOWARD ONE ANOTHER

LOWER CHIN TO FLOOR

UPAVISTHA KONASANA B seated wide angle posture b

The next form of the seated angle series is sort of a variation of boat pose (page 158).

Begin seated on your mat and gently pull the flesh from underneath your sitting bones so that your sitting bones are firmly rooted into the mat. Bend your knees and lean back, activating your core. Roll your shoulders back, reach down, and either take hold of the outside edges of your feet or wrap your peace fingers around your big toes. Slowly begin to lift your feet and press out of the bottoms of your feet to extend your legs. If the legs don't come fully straight, no worries. Just keep pressing out of the bottoms of your feet to encourage your hamstrings to open up. Focus on keeping your back long and your chest open. Take three to seven breaths in this position before gently releasing.

FULL EXPRESSION

MODIFIED VERSION

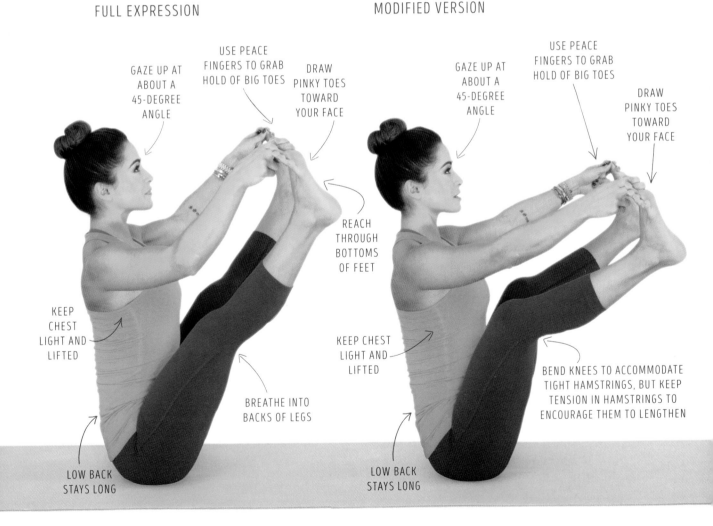

GAZE UP AT ABOUT A 45-DEGREE ANGLE

USE PEACE FINGERS TO GRAB HOLD OF BIG TOES

DRAW PINKY TOES TOWARD YOUR FACE

REACH THROUGH BOTTOMS OF FEET

KEEP CHEST LIGHT AND LIFTED

BREATHE INTO BACKS OF LEGS

LOW BACK STAYS LONG

GAZE UP AT ABOUT A 45-DEGREE ANGLE

USE PEACE FINGERS TO GRAB HOLD OF BIG TOES

DRAW PINKY TOES TOWARD YOUR FACE

KEEP CHEST LIGHT AND LIFTED

BEND KNEES TO ACCOMMODATE TIGHT HAMSTRINGS, BUT KEEP TENSION IN HAMSTRINGS TO ENCOURAGE THEM TO LENGTHEN

LOW BACK STAYS LONG

JANU SIRSASANA head-to-knee pose

This is a fantastic stretch for tight hamstrings. Many people find that opening up the hamstrings by doing forward folds like Janu sirsasana helps alleviate low-back pain, so it's definitely a pose that you'll want to incorporate if you deal with back pain.

Begin seated on your mat with both legs straight out in front of you. Pull the flesh from underneath your sitting bones so that your sitting bones are firmly rooted into the mat. Then bend your right leg, position your right heel against your pubis, and press the bottom of your foot against your left inner thigh. From here, square your body over your left leg and activate the left leg and foot. Inhale and lengthen through your spine, then exhale and come forward, keeping your back long and your chest open. If you can, wrap your hands around the bottom of your left foot. If you can't, no worries—just grab a yoga strap and pull yourself as close to your leg as you can while maintaining the integrity of the pose with your back elongated and your collarbones broad. Breathe for three to seven breaths before switching sides.

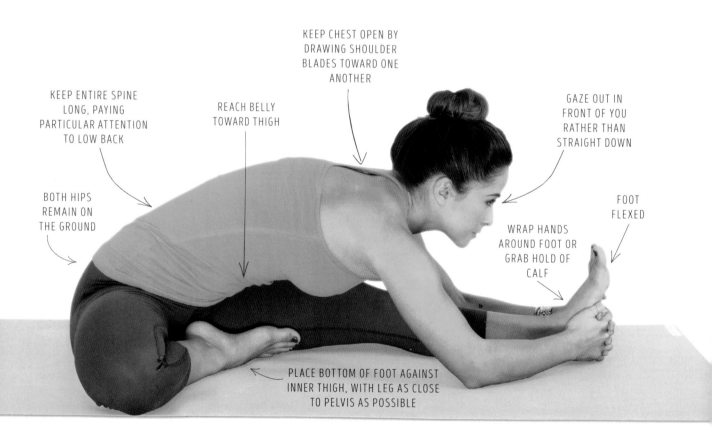

KEEP CHEST OPEN BY DRAWING SHOULDER BLADES TOWARD ONE ANOTHER

KEEP ENTIRE SPINE LONG, PAYING PARTICULAR ATTENTION TO LOW BACK

REACH BELLY TOWARD THIGH

GAZE OUT IN FRONT OF YOU RATHER THAN STRAIGHT DOWN

BOTH HIPS REMAIN ON THE GROUND

FOOT FLEXED

WRAP HANDS AROUND FOOT OR GRAB HOLD OF CALF

PLACE BOTTOM OF FOOT AGAINST INNER THIGH, WITH LEG AS CLOSE TO PELVIS AS POSSIBLE

TIRIANG MUKHA EKA PADA PASCHIMOTTANASANA
three limbs facing intense west stretch

The name of this pose is a mouthful, but it's not nearly as complicated as it sounds. If you're freaking out, calm down, my friend. It's all good in the 'hood.

Begin seated on your mat with both legs straight out in front of you. Gently pull the flesh from underneath your sitting bones so that your sitting bones are firmly rooted into the mat. Bend your right leg so that your right foot is in line with your right hip. With your right hand, move your right calf muscle to the right so that the back of your right leg can touch the mat with your knees hip width apart. On your next inhale, rise up through your spine, and as you exhale, reach your stomach toward your thighs as you come into a forward fold. Keep your low back long as you move your torso forward. When you can't come any farther, interlace your fingers around the bottom of your left foot or grab hold of your left leg wherever you can. Use your biceps strength to actively bring your stomach toward your thighs. The point is not to get your head to your knee, which will stretch your back, but to bring your stomach to your thighs, which will keep the focus on the hips. Keep your left foot gently flexed and take three to seven deep breaths before rising up and taking it to the other side.

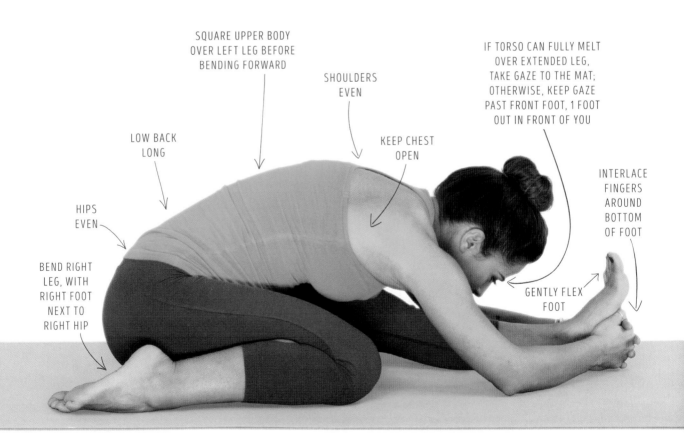

SQUARE UPPER BODY
OVER LEFT LEG BEFORE
BENDING FORWARD

SHOULDERS
EVEN

IF TORSO CAN FULLY MELT
OVER EXTENDED LEG,
TAKE GAZE TO THE MAT;
OTHERWISE, KEEP GAZE
PAST FRONT FOOT, 1 FOOT
OUT IN FRONT OF YOU

LOW BACK
LONG

KEEP CHEST
OPEN

INTERLACE
FINGERS
AROUND
BOTTOM
OF FOOT

HIPS
EVEN

BEND RIGHT
LEG, WITH
RIGHT FOOT
NEXT TO
RIGHT HIP

GENTLY FLEX
FOOT

EKA PADA RAJAKAPOTASANA (king pigeon pose) variation
mermaid pose

This pose is gorgeous and feels just as amazing. It requires a lot of openness in the chest, upper back, front body, hip flexors, and hips, and developing all that flexibility can take a while, but if you stick with it, the pose will come to you.

Begin in pigeon pose (page 97) with your left leg forward, right leg back, and hips facing forward. As you inhale, bend your right leg and place the foot in your right elbow crease, keeping your foot gently flexed to protect your ankle. On your next inhale, reach your left arm overhead and bend at the elbow until your hands clasp. Gently twist from your navel to look to the right and breathe here for three to seven breaths before taking it to the other side.

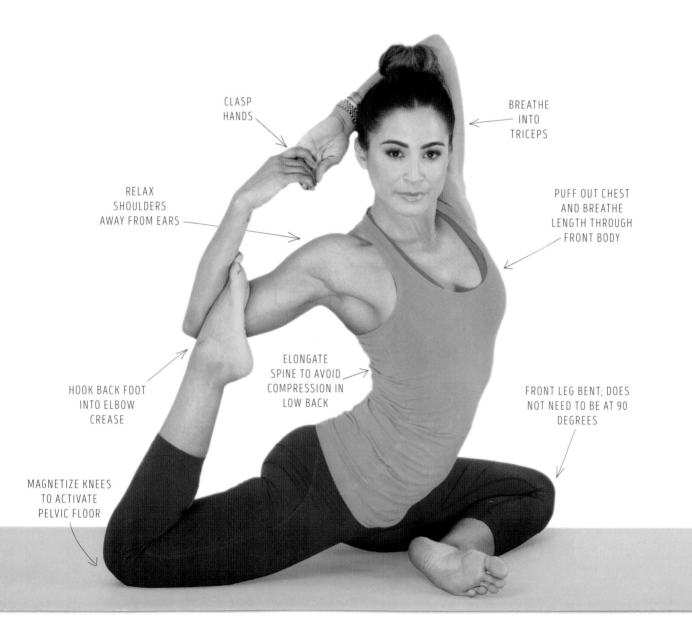

CLASP HANDS

BREATHE INTO TRICEPS

RELAX SHOULDERS AWAY FROM EARS

PUFF OUT CHEST AND BREATHE LENGTH THROUGH FRONT BODY

HOOK BACK FOOT INTO ELBOW CREASE

ELONGATE SPINE TO AVOID COMPRESSION IN LOW BACK

FRONT LEG BENT; DOES NOT NEED TO BE AT 90 DEGREES

MAGNETIZE KNEES TO ACTIVATE PELVIC FLOOR

SASANGASANA rabbit pose

This pose feels particularly wonderful for those who are sedentary for most of the day because it really opens up the low back.

Begin in child's pose (page 93) with your knees hip width apart. Cup your palms over your heels. On your next inhale, place the top of your head on the mat, as close to your knees as you can get it. Then lift your hips high, breathing length through your back. Take three to seven breaths before releasing the pose.

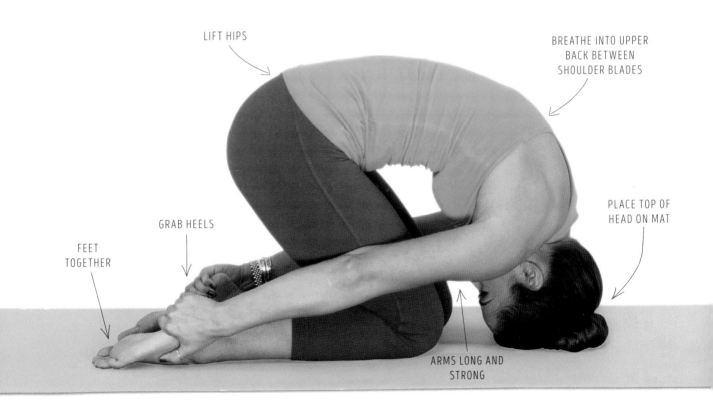

LIFT HIPS

BREATHE INTO UPPER
BACK BETWEEN
SHOULDER BLADES

PLACE TOP OF
HEAD ON MAT

GRAB HEELS

FEET
TOGETHER

ARMS LONG AND
STRONG

MARICHYASANA A pose dedicated to the sage marichi

To be honest, I didn't feel anything going on in this pose for the longest time. It was clear that I was supposed to come forward, but I just couldn't! I felt like I was stuck. It took a while for me to realize that this pose targets deep within the hip, and if you can't come forward, it simply means that you're tight. Keep practicing, and I promise that with time you'll be able to find some movement.

Begin seated on your mat with both legs straight out in front of you and your feet hip width apart. Gently flex your left foot. Then bend your right leg and place the right foot on the mat in line with the head of your right femur, as close to your pelvis as you can get it. This will likely feel awkward; just go with it. Intend to keep your right knee pointed straight up to the sky rather than let it splay out to the right. On your next inhale, lengthen through your spine as you sit up tall. As you exhale, hinge at the waist and fold forward with your arms parallel to the ground, fingers spread, thumbs pointing up to the sky, and right arm on the inside of your right leg. When you can't come any farther forward, turn your right thumb down toward the ground so that the right pinky is pointed up to the sky. Then bend your right arm and wrap it in front of your right shin as you reach behind you. Then reach your left arm behind you until your hands clasp. If they don't quite connect, use a yoga strap to make the connection. Intend to keep your shoulders even. Once you've made a connection either with or without the help of a strap, guide your head down toward your left leg. If you find that you're having a hard time getting any movement, it just means that your hips are tight; wherever you are, take three to seven deep breaths before releasing the pose and taking it to the other side.

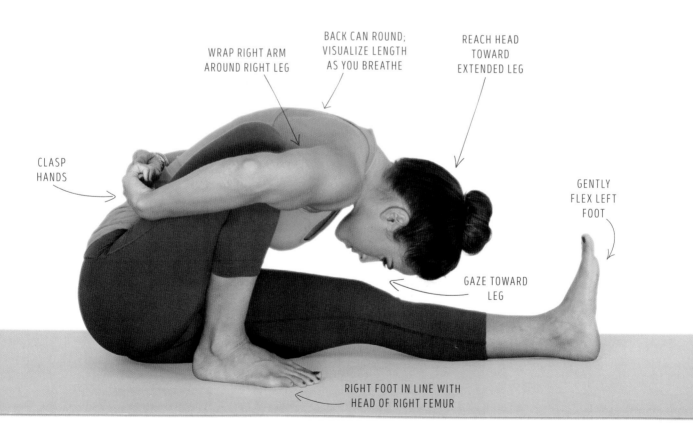

WRAP RIGHT ARM AROUND RIGHT LEG

BACK CAN ROUND; VISUALIZE LENGTH AS YOU BREATHE

REACH HEAD TOWARD EXTENDED LEG

CLASP HANDS

GENTLY FLEX LEFT FOOT

GAZE TOWARD LEG

RIGHT FOOT IN LINE WITH HEAD OF RIGHT FEMUR

MARICHYASANA C marichi's pose

This detoxifying twist is energizing for the body and a great way to open up the hips.

Begin seated on your mat with both legs straight out in front of you. Pull the flesh from underneath your sitting bones so that your sitting bones are firmly rooted into the mat. Then, as you inhale, bend your right leg and place the right foot on the mat in line with the head of your right femur, as close to your pelvis as you can get it. As you exhale, gently twist from your navel to the right and wrap your left arm around the outside of your right knee. Reach behind you with both hands until they clasp. If they don't, use a yoga strap to make the connection. As you continue to breathe, find length through your torso and chest as you look over your right shoulder with your left eye. Breathe for three to seven breaths in this pose before switching sides.

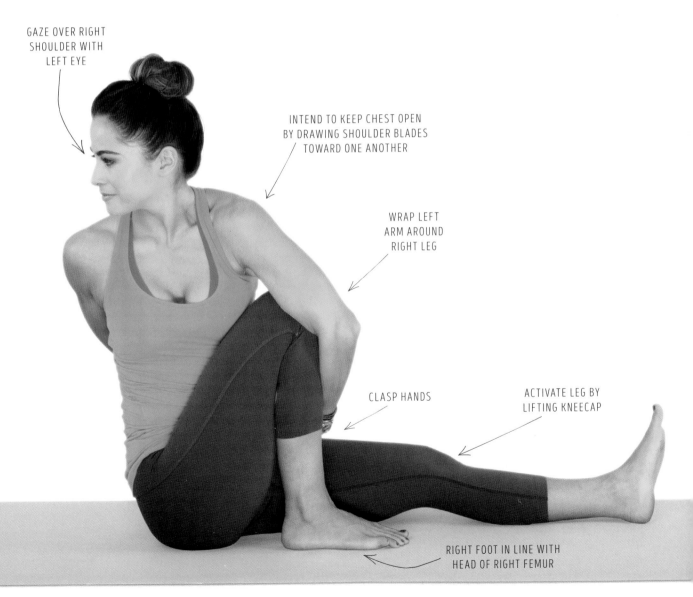

GAZE OVER RIGHT SHOULDER WITH LEFT EYE

INTEND TO KEEP CHEST OPEN BY DRAWING SHOULDER BLADES TOWARD ONE ANOTHER

WRAP LEFT ARM AROUND RIGHT LEG

CLASP HANDS

ACTIVATE LEG BY LIFTING KNEECAP

RIGHT FOOT IN LINE WITH HEAD OF RIGHT FEMUR

ARDHA BADDHA PADMA PASCHIMOTTANASANA
half-lotus seated forward fold

This pose is an excellent hip opener, but there's a lot going on with it, so if it seems intimidating, I get it. No worries; I'm here to help.

If you are new to the pose, begin seated on your mat with both legs straight out in front of you. Pull the flesh from underneath your sitting bones so that your sitting bones are firmly rooted into the mat. Then bend your left leg and bring your gently flexed foot into your right hip crease, where your leg meets your torso. Keep your left foot gently flexed to help prevent ankle sickling. Then wrap a yoga strap around your left foot and hold on to the other end of the strap with your left hand.

On your next inhale, lengthen through your spine. As you exhale, come forward, intending for your belly to meet your thighs (which ensures that you feel the stretch through the hamstring rather than in your back). Intend to keep your shoulders even as you come down (the left shoulder tends to want to lift), then grab hold of your right big toe with your right peace fingers. If your right hand isn't able to grab hold of the right foot, use another yoga strap. You should be feeling this pose through the back of your right leg, through the back of your left hip, and through your left shoulder and chest. Breathe for three to five breaths before switching sides.

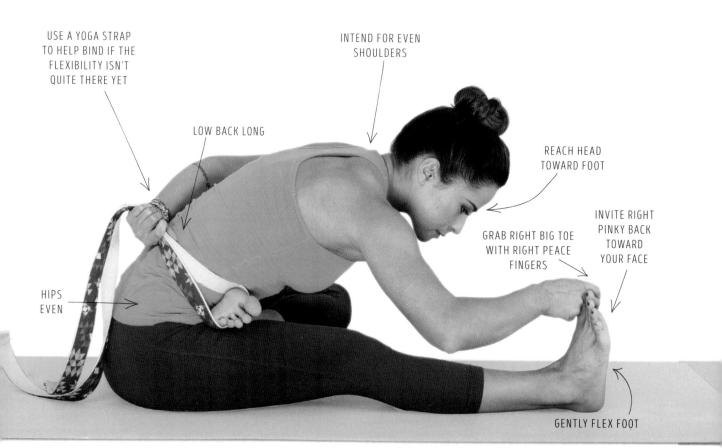

USE A YOGA STRAP TO HELP BIND IF THE FLEXIBILITY ISN'T QUITE THERE YET

INTEND FOR EVEN SHOULDERS

LOW BACK LONG

REACH HEAD TOWARD FOOT

INVITE RIGHT PINKY BACK TOWARD YOUR FACE

GRAB RIGHT BIG TOE WITH RIGHT PEACE FINGERS

HIPS EVEN

GENTLY FLEX FOOT

MODIFIED VERSION

If you're a bit more open, do the same thing, but without a yoga strap. With each breath, intend to feel a bit of movement through your body as you keep your shoulders even and your spine long. Breathe for three to seven breaths in the pose before switching sides.

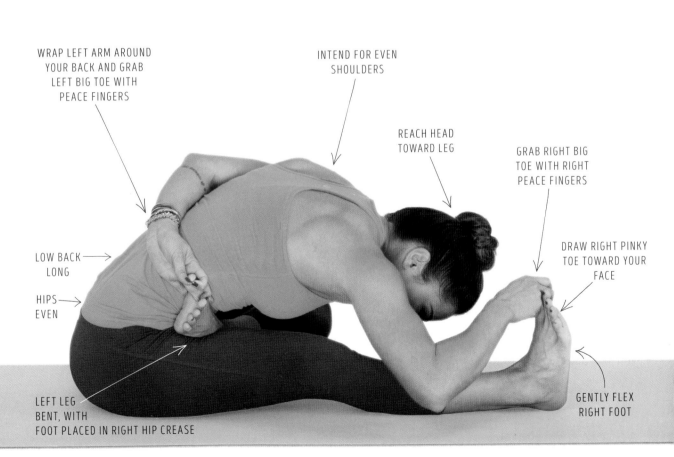

WRAP LEFT ARM AROUND YOUR BACK AND GRAB LEFT BIG TOE WITH PEACE FINGERS

INTEND FOR EVEN SHOULDERS

REACH HEAD TOWARD LEG

GRAB RIGHT BIG TOE WITH RIGHT PEACE FINGERS

DRAW RIGHT PINKY TOE TOWARD YOUR FACE

LOW BACK LONG

HIPS EVEN

LEFT LEG BENT, WITH FOOT PLACED IN RIGHT HIP CREASE

GENTLY FLEX RIGHT FOOT

GOMUKHASANA cow face pose

This pose is a game-changer for so many people. Want to improve your posture? Add this pose. Want to improve your snatch lift? Add this pose. Want to improve your running? Add this pose. Want to improve your relationship? Well, I can't help you there, but who knows, adding this pose to your practice might not be a bad idea!

Now, I have no clue why they call it cow face pose. I've scrutinized the shape for longer than I care to admit, and I don't see a cow face no matter which way I look at it. So let's just agree that it's a mystery and carry on.

To begin, sit tall with both legs straight out in front of you. Bend your knees and swing your right leg to the left so that the outside of your right knee is on the ground in front of you and bent at a 45-degree angle. Then swing your left leg in the opposite direction, positioning your left knee so that it is stacked on top of the right knee and bent at a 45-degree angle. Do not force your knees into place. If they don't stack perfectly, don't worry about it; it just means that you're tight through the hips. With time and consistent practice, it'll come. If your legs are comfortably in proper position, you can hinge at the hips and fold forward either with your arms in the full expression or with the aid of a strap. Only fold forward if your hips and knees feel okay.

Once your legs are in position, it's time to get your arms in their proper spots. Begin by lifting your left arm straight up overhead. Then bend at the elbow, letting your left hand come down past the base of your neck. From here, bring your right arm to your side and bend at the elbow, positioning your right hand up your spine. Reach until your hands clasp.

If your hands don't clasp, it just means that you're tight in the shoulders/triceps/armpit/chest area, and you can modify with a yoga strap. Whether or not you use a strap to help your hands connect, take three to seven deep breaths in the pose before switching sides.

MODIFIED VERSION

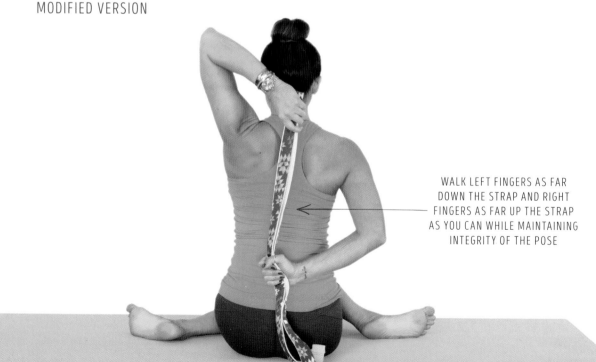

WALK LEFT FINGERS AS FAR DOWN THE STRAP AND RIGHT FINGERS AS FAR UP THE STRAP AS YOU CAN WHILE MAINTAINING INTEGRITY OF THE POSE

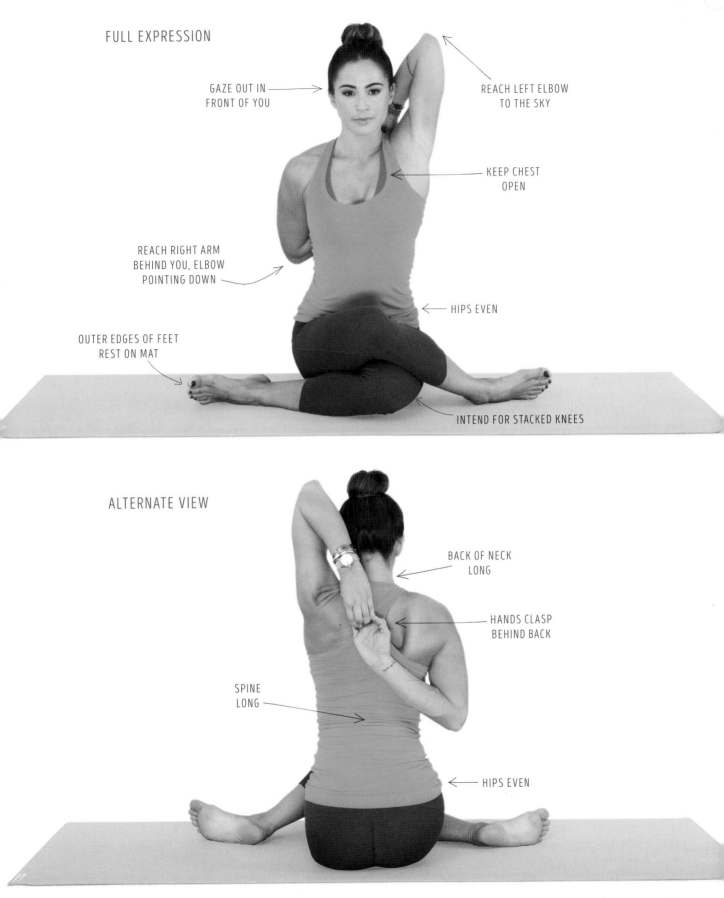

FULL EXPRESSION

GAZE OUT IN
FRONT OF YOU

REACH LEFT ELBOW
TO THE SKY

KEEP CHEST
OPEN

REACH RIGHT ARM
BEHIND YOU, ELBOW
POINTING DOWN

HIPS EVEN

OUTER EDGES OF FEET
REST ON MAT

INTEND FOR STACKED KNEES

ALTERNATE VIEW

BACK OF NECK
LONG

HANDS CLASP
BEHIND BACK

SPINE
LONG

HIPS EVEN

ARDHA MATSYENDRASANA half spinal twist

This delicious, detoxifying, energizing posture is always a class favorite. It targets the backs of the hips and the chest, and the twist offers the internal organs a gentle massage.

Begin seated on your mat with both legs straight out in front of you. Gently pull the flesh out from underneath your sitting bones so that your sitting bones are firmly rooted into the mat. Bend your right leg, placing your foot on the ground just outside your left thigh. Then bend your left leg and bring your left foot in line with your right hip, with the left knee out in front of you. If this places too much pressure on your knee, you can keep your left leg extended. Take a deep breath in and lengthen through your spine, sitting up nice and tall. As you exhale, initiate a twist at your navel and place your right fingertips on the mat behind you, in line with the base of your spine. On your next inhale, reach your left arm up to the sky, visualizing space being created between the ribs on the left side of your body. As you exhale, deepen your twist from the navel and hook your left elbow to the outside of your right knee. Keep drawing your shoulder blades toward one another so that your chest remains open. Inhale and sit up taller, then exhale and twist a bit more, looking out over your right shoulder with your left eye. Breathe fully and deeply here, trying to find a bit more movement with each breath, growing taller with each inhale and twisting from your navel with each exhale.

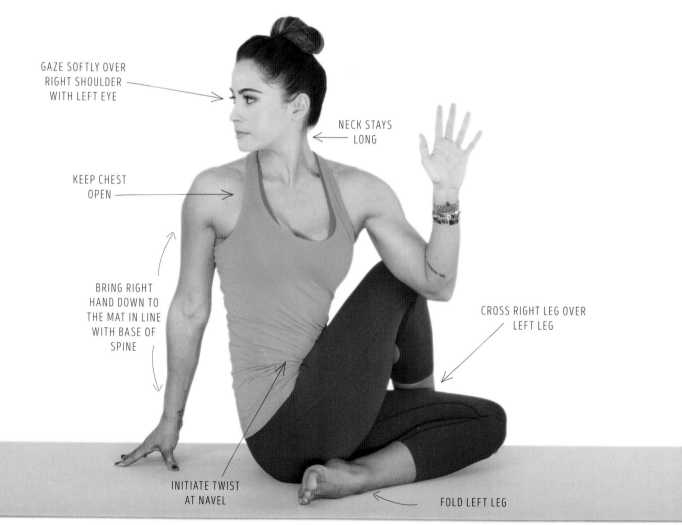

GAZE SOFTLY OVER RIGHT SHOULDER WITH LEFT EYE

NECK STAYS LONG

KEEP CHEST OPEN

BRING RIGHT HAND DOWN TO THE MAT IN LINE WITH BASE OF SPINE

CROSS RIGHT LEG OVER LEFT LEG

INITIATE TWIST AT NAVEL

FOLD LEFT LEG

If you'd like to take it a step further, you can thread your left hand through the hole created between your bent legs. Then reach back with your right hand until the hands clasp. If you aren't able to make contact, use a yoga strap to help you. This bind (the linking of your hands) will deepen the stretch through your chest.

Breathe fully and deeply for three to five breaths before slowly releasing the same way you went in and taking it to the other side.

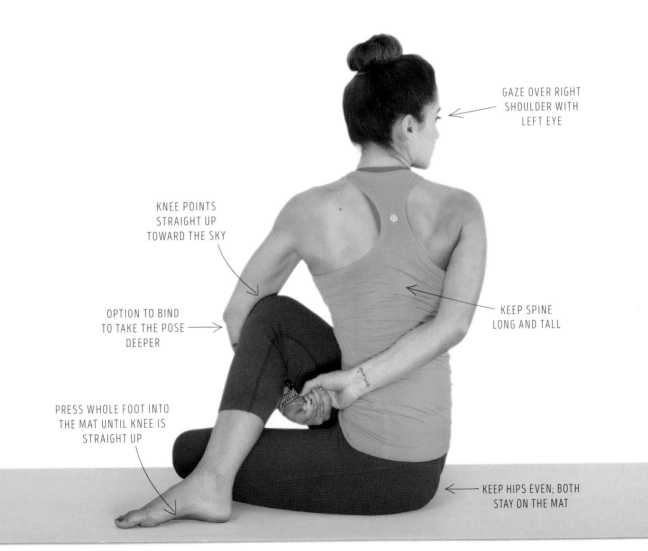

GAZE OVER RIGHT
SHOULDER WITH
LEFT EYE

KNEE POINTS
STRAIGHT UP
TOWARD THE SKY

OPTION TO BIND
TO TAKE THE POSE
DEEPER

KEEP SPINE
LONG AND TALL

PRESS WHOLE FOOT INTO
THE MAT UNTIL KNEE IS
STRAIGHT UP

KEEP HIPS EVEN; BOTH
STAY ON THE MAT

KROUNCHASANA heron pose

Full disclosure: Prior to shooting the photos for this book, I'd done this pose only a handful of times. I never came across it as a student in a class, probably due to how tricky it can be for the knees. If you struggle with knee issues, go gently and be mindful, or skip this one altogether.

If your knees are healthy, here's how to do it: Begin seated on your mat with both legs straight out in front of you. Then bend your left leg and place the top of your left foot on the mat next to your left hip. You may need to push the calf muscle to the left to make space for your left thigh. Sitting fully on both sitting bones, bend your right leg and place the right foot on the ground in front of you. Interlace your fingers around the bottom of your foot and then, as you inhale, lengthen through your spine and hamstring as you sit tall and extend your leg. Keep the toes active to encourage muscle activation throughout your right leg, and take three to seven deep breaths here before switching sides.

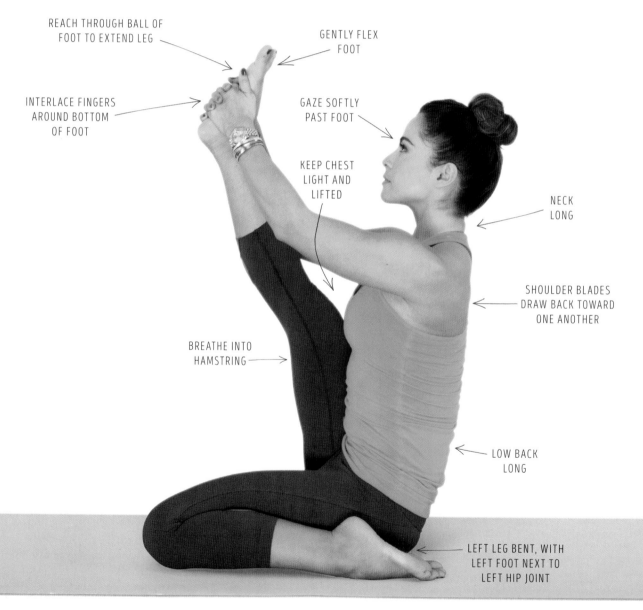

REACH THROUGH BALL OF
FOOT TO EXTEND LEG

GENTLY FLEX
FOOT

INTERLACE FINGERS
AROUND BOTTOM
OF FOOT

GAZE SOFTLY
PAST FOOT

KEEP CHEST
LIGHT AND
LIFTED

NECK
LONG

SHOULDER BLADES
DRAW BACK TOWARD
ONE ANOTHER

BREATHE INTO
HAMSTRING

LOW BACK
LONG

LEFT LEG BENT, WITH
LEFT FOOT NEXT TO
LEFT HIP JOINT

EKA PADA ADHO MUKHA SVANASANA three-legged dog

You'll see three-legged dog time and again if you participate in vinyasa classes, so it's a good idea to have the basics down. There are two ways to do this pose. The first is to open the top hip on the inhale. This allows your leg to come higher, and it's a good stretch for your hip flexor and a nice way to set up for wild thing pose (page 208). The second way has the hips even. Your leg likely won't come as high, but that's okay because you'll be getting a killer stretch in the bottom leg's hamstring. This is the variation that you'll want to work on if you're trying to focus on your hamstrings. Neither variation is wrong, and in my opinion it's a good idea to practice both since each one offers unique benefits.

Begin in downward-facing dog (page 100). On your next inhale, lift your right leg high and decide whether or not you'll open up the hip. (My hip is open in the photo.) Regardless of whether your hip is open, spread your toes. This encourages the leg muscles to stay engaged and helps develop flexibility. Take three to seven deep breaths in the pose before taking it to the other side.

TOES SPREAD

YOU HAVE OPTIONS WITH THE TOP LEG: 1) LET HIP OPEN SLIGHTLY AS YOU REACH THE LEG AS HIGH AS YOU CAN (SHOWN), OR 2) KEEP HIPS SQUARE AND TOES OF TOP FOOT POINTING DOWN TO THE MAT, WHICH KEEPS THE FOCUS ON THE BOTTOM LEG'S HAMSTRING

BREATHE INTO HAMSTRING

SPINE LONG

BACK OF NECK LONG

FINGERS SPREAD

PUSH THE MAT AWAY FROM YOU

ARDHA CHANDRASANA half moon pose

Okay, time for confessions of a yoga teacher: Half moon pose used to scare the hell out of me. Every time I did it, I'd fall backward, and without a way to really catch yourself, that's scary. So I avoided the pose for ages. That's basically the worst thing you can do with a pose you don't like. They always say that the pose you avoid is the one you need the most.

I'm not sure what happened, but I somehow became friends with half moon. I mean, I'm not about to invite her over for a sleepover, but I'm down to grab coffee once in a blue moon.

My point is, I come across a lot of people who don't like this pose (or others), and the best advice I can give is to kill it with kindness and make it your friend. Or acquaintance. Whatever.

To start, come into warrior 2 (page 114) with your left foot forward. As you inhale, send your torso forward and rotate your arms so that the left fingertips are on the ground and the right arm is pointing straight up to the sky. Keeping your right foot gently flexed, lift the right leg and press out of the bottom of your right foot. The trick is to keep your leg muscles engaged and the line of energy through your right leg a-buzzin'. Gaze softly at the ground toward the front of your mat as shown or, if you're up for more of a challenge, look to the side or straight up toward the sky.

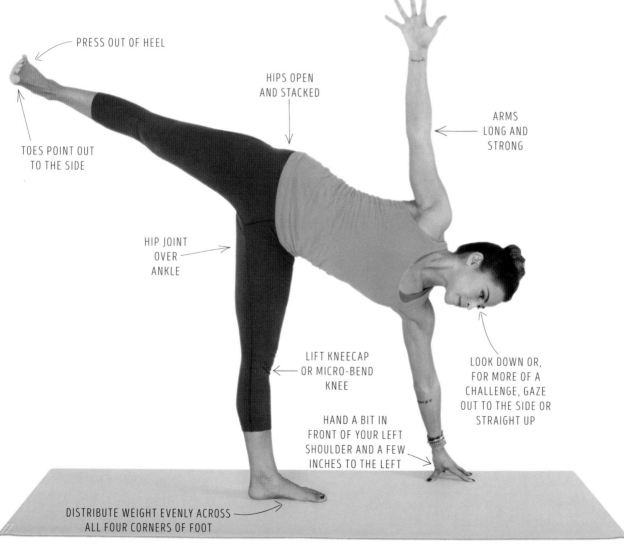

PRESS OUT OF HEEL

HIPS OPEN AND STACKED

ARMS LONG AND STRONG

TOES POINT OUT TO THE SIDE

HIP JOINT OVER ANKLE

LIFT KNEECAP OR MICRO-BEND KNEE

LOOK DOWN OR, FOR MORE OF A CHALLENGE, GAZE OUT TO THE SIDE OR STRAIGHT UP

HAND A BIT IN FRONT OF YOUR LEFT SHOULDER AND A FEW INCHES TO THE LEFT

DISTRIBUTE WEIGHT EVENLY ACROSS ALL FOUR CORNERS OF FOOT

MODIFIED VERSION

If this pose is too much for you because you're a bit tight, you can modify it by placing a yoga block on the ground in line with your left shoulder and resting your hand on the block. Breathe for three to seven breaths before moving on to the other side.

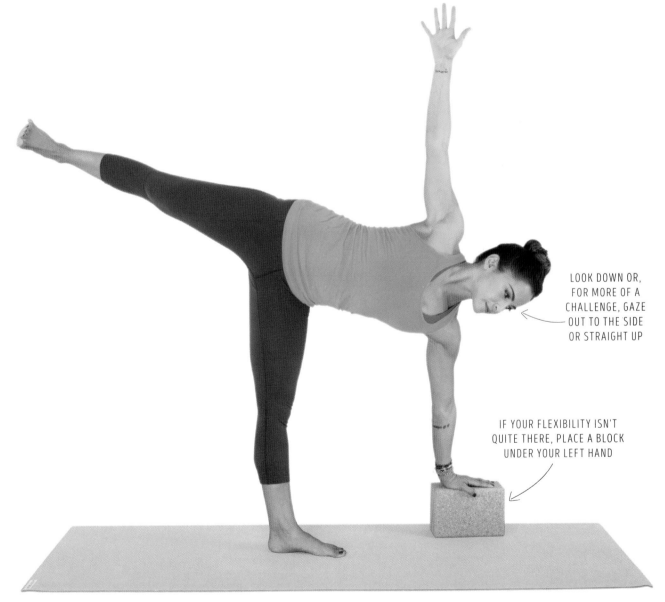

LOOK DOWN OR, FOR MORE OF A CHALLENGE, GAZE OUT TO THE SIDE OR STRAIGHT UP

IF YOUR FLEXIBILITY ISN'T QUITE THERE, PLACE A BLOCK UNDER YOUR LEFT HAND

CHAPASANA sugarcane pose

Chapasana is a kickass name, isn't it? That's really the only reason I was interested in giving this pose a go when I first practiced it. Hey, I'm only being honest! This is the next step in the progression once you've got a steady half moon pose.

Begin in half moon pose (page 176), then bend your top leg and grab hold of the foot with your hand. Be mindful to keep your toes spread and maintain that sensation of a lift through your entire body. Take three to seven deep breaths here before switching sides.

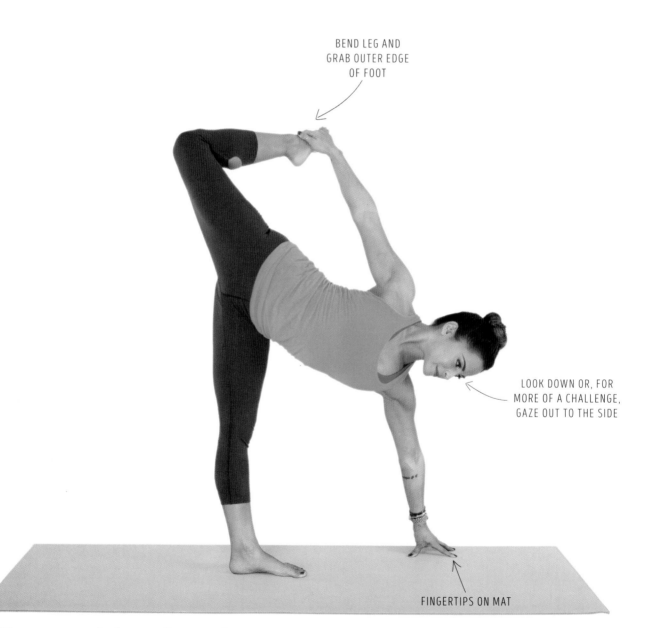

BEND LEG AND
GRAB OUTER EDGE
OF FOOT

LOOK DOWN OR, FOR
MORE OF A CHALLENGE,
GAZE OUT TO THE SIDE

FINGERTIPS ON MAT

NATARAJASANA dancer's pose

Dancer's pose has been a longtime favorite of mine. To me, it feels as beautiful as it looks because it opens up so many parts of the body—chest, hip flexors, hamstrings, back, the whole front body, and more. I love it.

Begin in mountain pose (page 106). Inhale, spread your toes, and set them down for a stable foundation in this balancing pose. Find a spot in front of you that's at eye level and not moving. Softly gaze at this focal point while you're in the pose.

Lift your left arm so that it's in line with your left ear. Bend your right elbow 90 degrees, with your forearm out to the right, your palm facing up, and your thumb pointing behind you.

Next, shift your weight onto your left foot and begin to lift your right foot back behind you. It's really important to grab the foot from the inside arch, so double-check that you've done so. On your next inhale, come forward with your chest as you lift your right leg as high as you can.

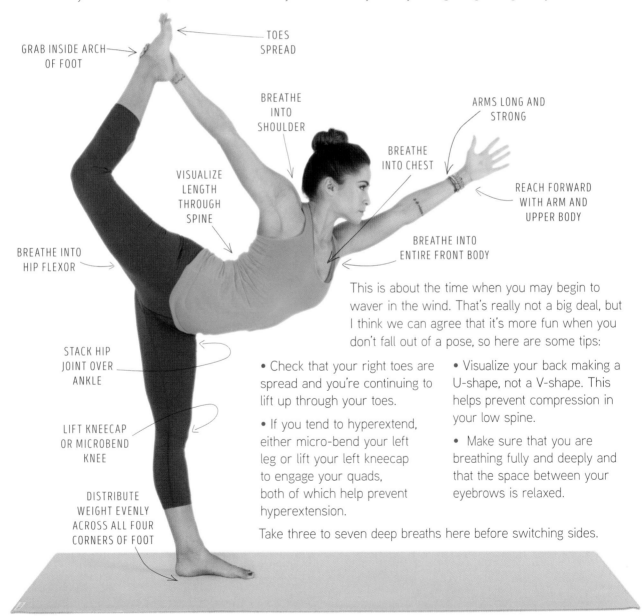

GRAB INSIDE ARCH OF FOOT

TOES SPREAD

BREATHE INTO SHOULDER

ARMS LONG AND STRONG

BREATHE INTO CHEST

VISUALIZE LENGTH THROUGH SPINE

REACH FORWARD WITH ARM AND UPPER BODY

BREATHE INTO HIP FLEXOR

BREATHE INTO ENTIRE FRONT BODY

STACK HIP JOINT OVER ANKLE

LIFT KNEECAP OR MICROBEND KNEE

DISTRIBUTE WEIGHT EVENLY ACROSS ALL FOUR CORNERS OF FOOT

This is about the time when you may begin to waver in the wind. That's really not a big deal, but I think we can agree that it's more fun when you don't fall out of a pose, so here are some tips:

• Check that your right toes are spread and you're continuing to lift up through your toes.

• If you tend to hyperextend, either micro-bend your left leg or lift your left kneecap to engage your quads, both of which help prevent hyperextension.

• Visualize your back making a U-shape, not a V-shape. This helps prevent compression in your low spine.

• Make sure that you are breathing fully and deeply and that the space between your eyebrows is relaxed.

Take three to seven deep breaths here before switching sides.

VIRABHADRASANA 1 (warrior 1) variations

Virabhadrasana is such a cool pose because there are so many places to go from here. Think of it like getting your first car (and how awesome was that—it took you from A to B and felt like freedom!) and then, just when you thought things couldn't get any better, being cast as a guest on *Pimp My Ride*. How sick is that?! We're talking custom monogrammed velvet seats and a subwoofer that shakes your whole body as you cruise (safely!) down the highway. Okay, so maybe *Pimp My Ride* isn't everyone's cup of tea, but you get what I'm saying—this is no longer an "okay, cool" pose, but a "holy smokes, this is taking me places!" pose. Basically, what I'm trying to say is that warrior 1 has endless options.

The legs stay the same as in regular warrior 1—hips facing forward, left foot facing forward, and right foot turned out about 45 degrees, fully on the ground. You have a deep bend in your front knee, and the knee is stacked above or slightly behind the ankle.

From here, you have total freedom. One thing you can do is to interlace your fingers behind your back (just for fun, interlace them in the way that feels weird) and then press your palms together. Hang out here or send your torso forward as shown and lift your arms to the sky for an incredible chest stretch.

Another option is to take goddess arms, with your arms out to the sides and bent about 90 degrees and the fingers spread as wide as you can. This is a nice way to open up the chest. Add a mini backbend for even more front-body opening.

A third option is to interlace your fingers around the back of your head and lean back for a little backbend. This feels awesome through the entire front body and is a good way to open up the upper back and chest.

Still not sick of learning about your options? You could do arms overhead by your ears. You could do cow face arms (see page 170). You could do eagle arms (see page 204). You could do "walk like an Egyptian" arms or the YMCA. I'm not even kidding. That's how great yoga is—there are no rules.

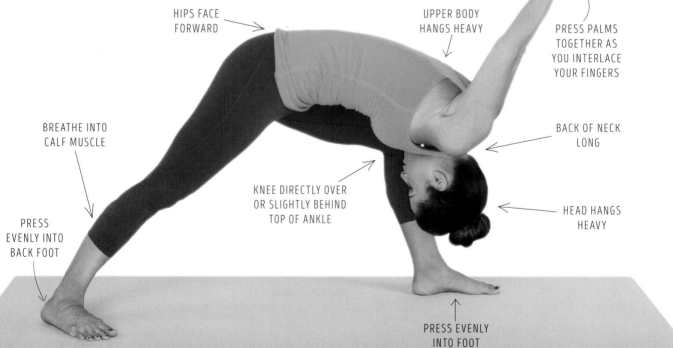

HIPS FACE FORWARD

UPPER BODY HANGS HEAVY

PRESS PALMS TOGETHER AS YOU INTERLACE YOUR FINGERS

BREATHE INTO CALF MUSCLE

BACK OF NECK LONG

KNEE DIRECTLY OVER OR SLIGHTLY BEHIND TOP OF ANKLE

HEAD HANGS HEAVY

PRESS EVENLY INTO BACK FOOT

PRESS EVENLY INTO FOOT

UTKATA KONASANA goddess pose

Goddess pose is like cow face pose in that I cannot figure out how it earned its name. I certainly do not feel like a goddess when I do it. Instead, I feel more like one of those beasts that Lindsay Lohan and friends turn into during the *Mean Girls* cafeteria scene. Anyhoo, it is what it is, and it's a great pose for building leg strength, so let's get on with it.

Begin by facing the long edge of your mat. Take a deep breath, jump your legs out wide, and turn your toes out toward the short ends of the mat. Position yourself so that your knees are directly over or slightly behind your ankles (but not in front of them, which is a quick ticket to knee problems). Then sink your hips low and lengthen through your spine as you inhale.

Cactus your arms so that they're bent about 90 degrees and spread your fingers as wide as you can. Relax your shoulders away from your ears and relax the space between your eyebrows. Breathe fully and deeply here for three to seven breaths or even longer.

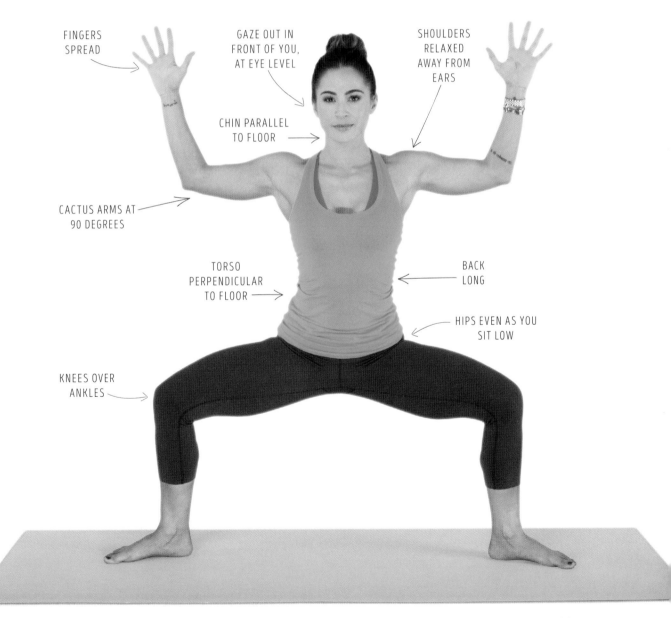

FINGERS SPREAD

GAZE OUT IN FRONT OF YOU, AT EYE LEVEL

SHOULDERS RELAXED AWAY FROM EARS

CHIN PARALLEL TO FLOOR

CACTUS ARMS AT 90 DEGREES

TORSO PERPENDICULAR TO FLOOR

BACK LONG

HIPS EVEN AS YOU SIT LOW

KNEES OVER ANKLES

MALASANA garland pose

This is a fantastic pose for athletes—runners, weightlifters, skiers. Pretty much anyone who moves is going to want to add this pose on the reg. It's particularly good for releasing tension through the backs of the calves and in the inner thighs and it's wonderful for developing ankle mobility.

Begin in mountain pose (page 106), then take your feet slightly wider than hip width apart. If you have tight ankles or calves, you'll want to stay on the balls of your feet, as shown in the modified version. If you're quite open through those areas, you can keep your feet flat on the mat.

On your next inhale, lengthen through your entire body. As you exhale, sink your hips low so that the backs of your thighs are touching your calves. Intend to keep your leg muscles engaged rather than resting in this position, which can put strain on your knees and lead to knee problems over time. Bring your hands into prayer position and position your elbows against the insides of your knees. Then, as you exhale, press out through your elbows to continue to open up your knees and inner thighs. Intend to maintain an open chest and draw your shoulder blades toward one another. Breathe for three to seven breaths before moving on.

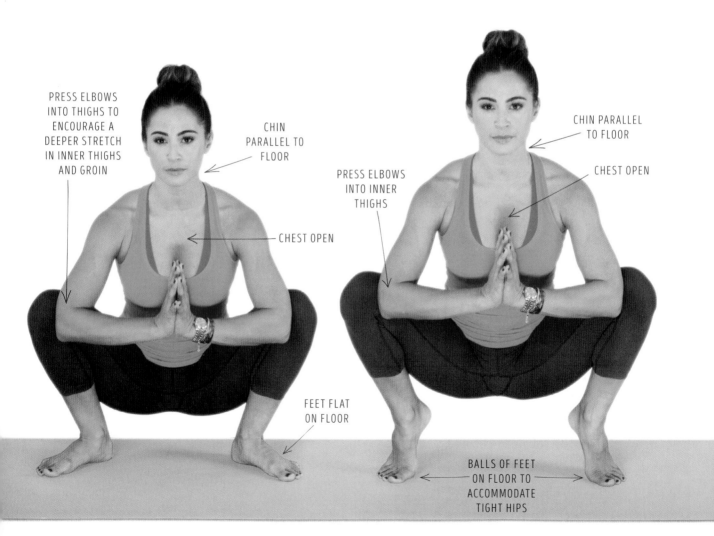

PRESS ELBOWS INTO THIGHS TO ENCOURAGE A DEEPER STRETCH IN INNER THIGHS AND GROIN

CHIN PARALLEL TO FLOOR

CHEST OPEN

FEET FLAT ON FLOOR

CHIN PARALLEL TO FLOOR

CHEST OPEN

PRESS ELBOWS INTO INNER THIGHS

BALLS OF FEET ON FLOOR TO ACCOMMODATE TIGHT HIPS

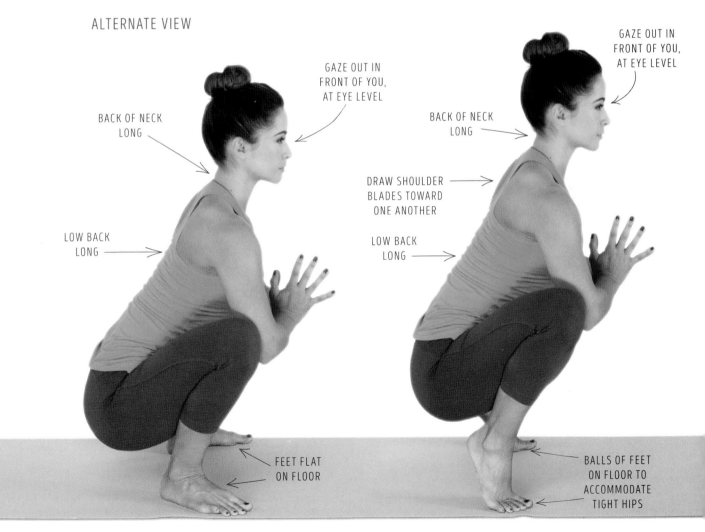

ALTERNATE VIEW

GAZE OUT IN
FRONT OF YOU,
AT EYE LEVEL

BACK OF NECK
LONG

LOW BACK
LONG

FEET FLAT
ON FLOOR

GAZE OUT IN
FRONT OF YOU,
AT EYE LEVEL

BACK OF NECK
LONG

DRAW SHOULDER
BLADES TOWARD
ONE ANOTHER

LOW BACK
LONG

BALLS OF FEET
ON FLOOR TO
ACCOMMODATE
TIGHT HIPS

BADDHA MALASANA garland pose with a bind

If you'd like to take garland pose a step further, you can add a bind. Release the prayer position of your hands and bring your right hand to the ground while using your upper arm to maintain openness in your right leg. Then lift your left arm and wrap it around your back. Wrap your right arm around your right leg until it meets your left hand. If the hands don't meet, you can use a yoga strap to connect them. If they do meet, clasp your hands and breathe, intending to keep your spine long and your chest open. Gaze out over your left shoulder with your right eye and take three to seven breaths before switching sides.

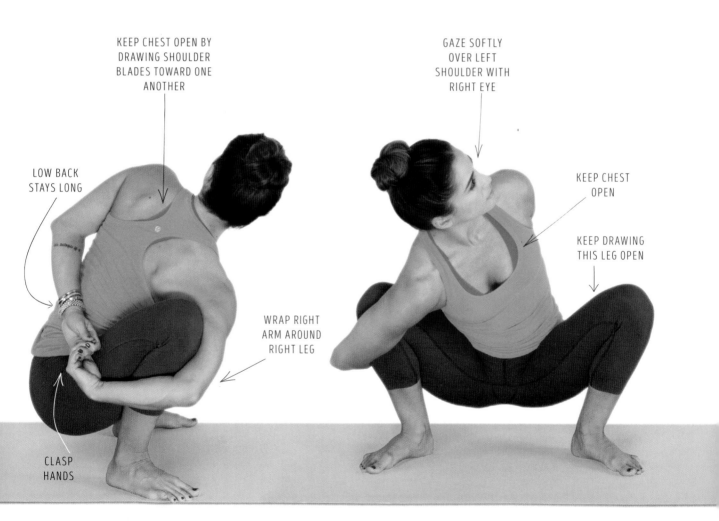

KEEP CHEST OPEN BY DRAWING SHOULDER BLADES TOWARD ONE ANOTHER

GAZE SOFTLY OVER LEFT SHOULDER WITH RIGHT EYE

LOW BACK STAYS LONG

KEEP CHEST OPEN

KEEP DRAWING THIS LEG OPEN

WRAP RIGHT ARM AROUND RIGHT LEG

CLASP HANDS

TRIKONASANA triangle pose

Triangle pose is always a class favorite—I think because it hits so many notoriously tight spots. You'll definitely feel some side-body stretching, as well as some inner-thigh and outer-hip stretching.

Start in warrior 2 (page 114) with your left leg forward. As you inhale, straighten your left leg. Make sure that your heels are in line and your right toes are facing the long edge of your mat. On your next inhale, send your torso forward toward your left toes. When you can't go any farther, exhale and rotate your arms so that your right arm is lifted to the sky and either your left fingers are on the ground or your left peace fingers are wrapped around your big toe. If you're very tight and struggling to bring your left hand to the ground, place a yoga block on whichever side works better for you. Breathe space through your entire side body and intend to keep your upper body in line with your lower body. You have the option to gaze down at the ground or up toward the sky, as shown. Breathe for at least three breaths before releasing.

FULL EXPRESSION

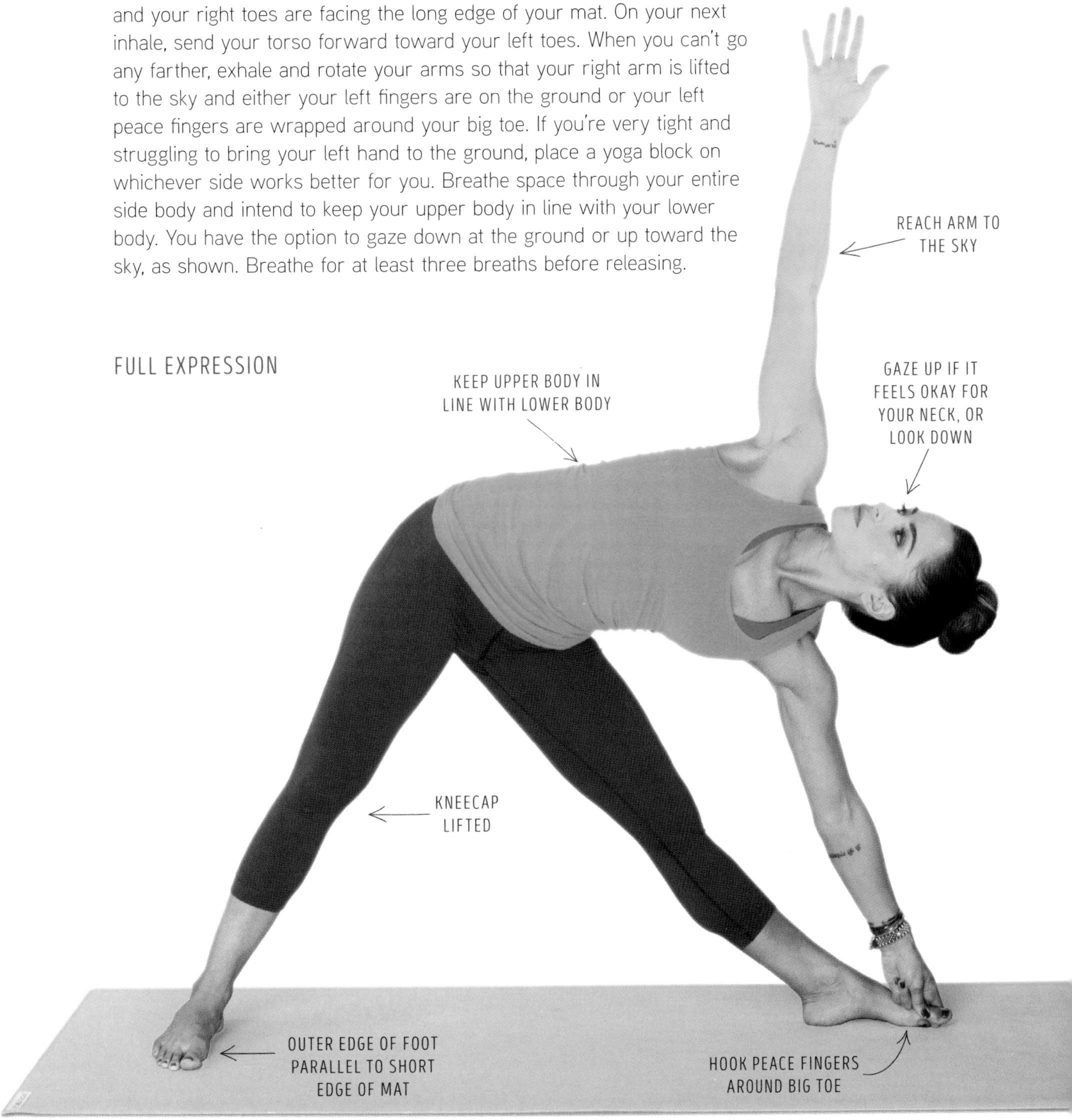

REACH ARM TO THE SKY

KEEP UPPER BODY IN LINE WITH LOWER BODY

GAZE UP IF IT FEELS OKAY FOR YOUR NECK, OR LOOK DOWN

KNEECAP LIFTED

OUTER EDGE OF FOOT PARALLEL TO SHORT EDGE OF MAT

HOOK PEACE FINGERS AROUND BIG TOE

GO DEEPER WITH A BIND

If you want to take triangle pose a step further, you can add a bind. Bend your left leg and slide your left arm behind your left knee. Then bring your right arm behind your back and reach the hands toward one another until they clasp. If the hands don't meet, you can use a yoga strap to help you. Once the hands clasp or the strap is in place, you can begin straightening your front leg. Breathe for three to seven breaths before taking it to the other side.

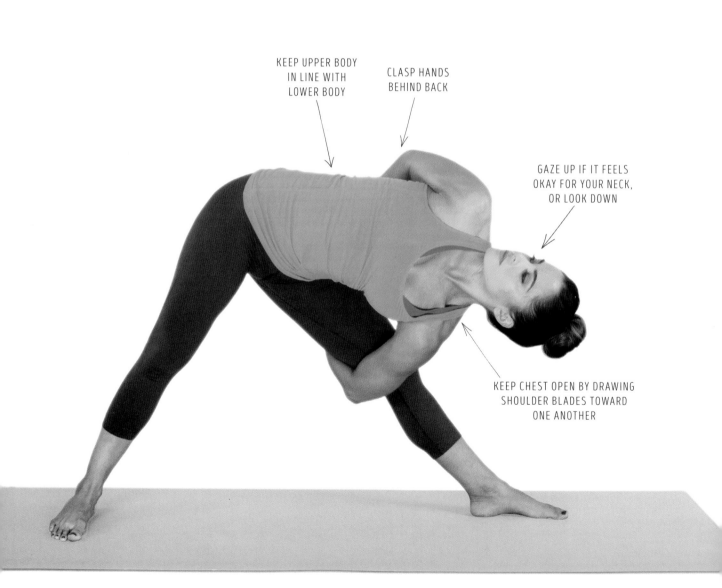

KEEP UPPER BODY
IN LINE WITH
LOWER BODY

CLASP HANDS
BEHIND BACK

GAZE UP IF IT FEELS
OKAY FOR YOUR NECK,
OR LOOK DOWN

KEEP CHEST OPEN BY DRAWING
SHOULDER BLADES TOWARD
ONE ANOTHER

UTTHITA PARSVAKONASANA extended side angle pose

This pose is particularly great for developing oblique strength, and if you add the bind, it also works to open up the chest.

Begin in warrior 2 (page 114). As you inhale, hinge from the hips and bring just your upper body as far forward as it will comfortably come. When you can't move forward any farther, exhale and rotate your arms to 12:00 and 6:00. Then, take a breath. To take it a bit further, rotate your upper arm to 2:00 as shown. Breathe for three to seven breaths before deciding whether to take it another step further by adding the bind.

To add the bind, bring your right arm down by your side and bend at the elbow as you reach behind your back and bring your left hand under your left leg and up to meet your right hand. Clasp hands (or use a yoga strap to connect them) and breathe. Intend to keep your upper body light and lifted and remember to press into your legs so that you're using your leg muscles and core strength to stay lifted. Look over your right shoulder with your left eye (as shown) if it feels okay for your neck, or look down at the ground. Breathe for three to seven breaths in this pose before taking it to the other side.

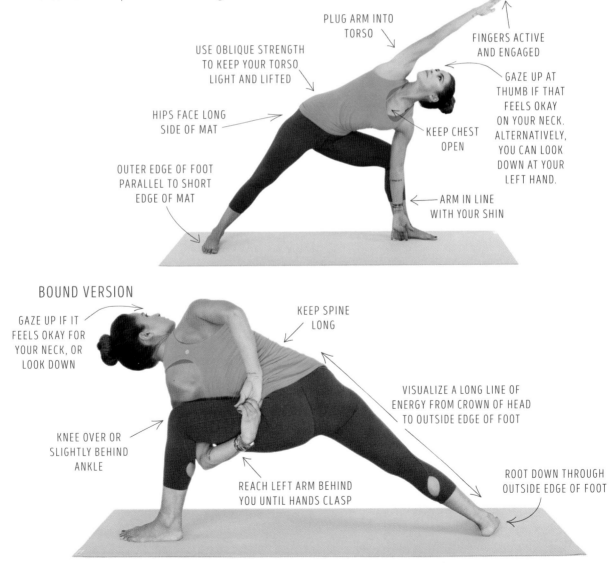

PLUG ARM INTO TORSO

FINGERS ACTIVE AND ENGAGED

USE OBLIQUE STRENGTH TO KEEP YOUR TORSO LIGHT AND LIFTED

GAZE UP AT THUMB IF THAT FEELS OKAY ON YOUR NECK. ALTERNATIVELY, YOU CAN LOOK DOWN AT YOUR LEFT HAND.

HIPS FACE LONG SIDE OF MAT

KEEP CHEST OPEN

OUTER EDGE OF FOOT PARALLEL TO SHORT EDGE OF MAT

ARM IN LINE WITH YOUR SHIN

BOUND VERSION

GAZE UP IF IT FEELS OKAY FOR YOUR NECK, OR LOOK DOWN

KEEP SPINE LONG

VISUALIZE A LONG LINE OF ENERGY FROM CROWN OF HEAD TO OUTSIDE EDGE OF FOOT

KNEE OVER OR SLIGHTLY BEHIND ANKLE

REACH LEFT ARM BEHIND YOU UNTIL HANDS CLASP

ROOT DOWN THROUGH OUTSIDE EDGE OF FOOT

UTTHITA HASTA PADANGUSTASANA A and B
standing hand-to-big-toe pose A and B

This pose feels wonderful for tight hips, but it requires a good amount of flexibility through the hamstrings. If you find yourself struggling, place a yoga strap around the middle of your foot or modify the pose by bending your lifted knee.

Begin in mountain pose (page 106). Lift your toes, spread them, and set them down for a stable foundation in this balancing pose. Look for a spot out in front of you that is at eye level and not moving and focus your gaze on this point. As you inhale, shift your weight onto your left foot as you use your core and hip flexor strength to lift your right leg. Hinge at the waist and gently wrap your right peace fingers around your right big toe as you flex the right foot. Then bring your left hand to your left hip. Avoid leaning back. Instead, use your core strength and sense of balance to remain tall. Activate your core by bringing your navel in toward your spine and up toward your heart. Broaden your collarbones and relax your shoulders away from your ears.

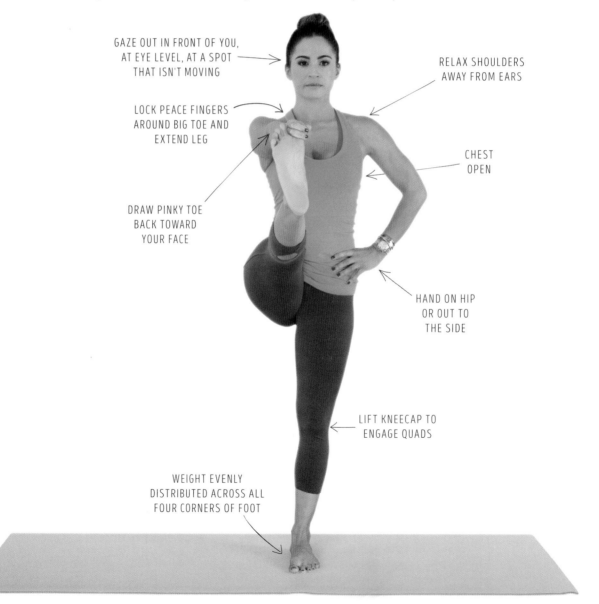

GAZE OUT IN FRONT OF YOU, AT EYE LEVEL, AT A SPOT THAT ISN'T MOVING

RELAX SHOULDERS AWAY FROM EARS

LOCK PEACE FINGERS AROUND BIG TOE AND EXTEND LEG

CHEST OPEN

DRAW PINKY TOE BACK TOWARD YOUR FACE

HAND ON HIP OR OUT TO THE SIDE

LIFT KNEECAP TO ENGAGE QUADS

WEIGHT EVENLY DISTRIBUTED ACROSS ALL FOUR CORNERS OF FOOT

Take three to seven deep breaths here in part A before opening your right leg to the right for part B. As you open the leg, slowly shift your gaze over your left shoulder. This will definitely test your balance! If you wobble or fall over, who cares? Just get back into the pose slowly and try again. Breathe for three to seven breaths in part B before inhaling and bringing your leg back out in front of you. Slowly release and then take the pose to the other side.

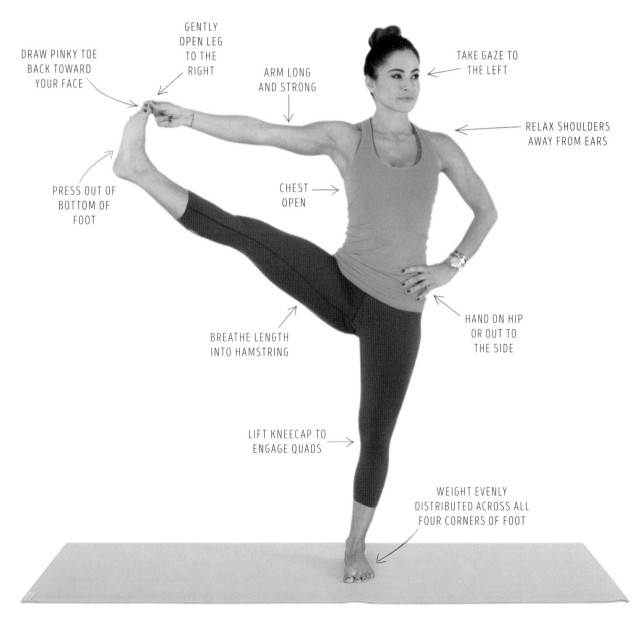

GENTLY OPEN LEG TO THE RIGHT

DRAW PINKY TOE BACK TOWARD YOUR FACE

ARM LONG AND STRONG

TAKE GAZE TO THE LEFT

RELAX SHOULDERS AWAY FROM EARS

PRESS OUT OF BOTTOM OF FOOT

CHEST OPEN

BREATHE LENGTH INTO HAMSTRING

HAND ON HIP OR OUT TO THE SIDE

LIFT KNEECAP TO ENGAGE QUADS

WEIGHT EVENLY DISTRIBUTED ACROSS ALL FOUR CORNERS OF FOOT

baby grasshopper pose

I love teaching this pose because it looks so much more complicated than it actually is. When I demonstrate it, people usually groan and sort of side-eye each other as if to say, "Is this girl crazy? We can't do that!" And I smirk and kind of giggle to myself because I know that in about ten seconds, they're all going to be surprised by the accessibility of the pose. So, if you're looking skeptically at this pose and already feeling your heart start to race with anxiety, please don't worry, because I'm about to break it down for you.

The key to baby grasshopper pose is not to overthink it. Overthinking, as a general rule, is a death sentence. Think nothing, do everything. New life mantra.

With that out of the way, begin seated on your mat with both legs straight out in front of you. Bend your right leg and place the right foot just outside your left thigh, with the toes pointing outward at about a 45-degree angle. Then twist to the left, initiating the twist from your navel, so that you're facing the long edge of your mat. Reach down with your right hand and grab hold of the bottom of your left foot or shin, depending on your flexibility. Then place your left hand next to your left hip, turning the fingers outward. Slide your left hand to the left, just outside your shoulder. From there, rock forward and backward as you press into your left hand and right foot and lift your entire body. Once you're up off the ground, bend your left elbow and stay lifted through your hips and chest. Take three to seven deep breaths here before switching sides.

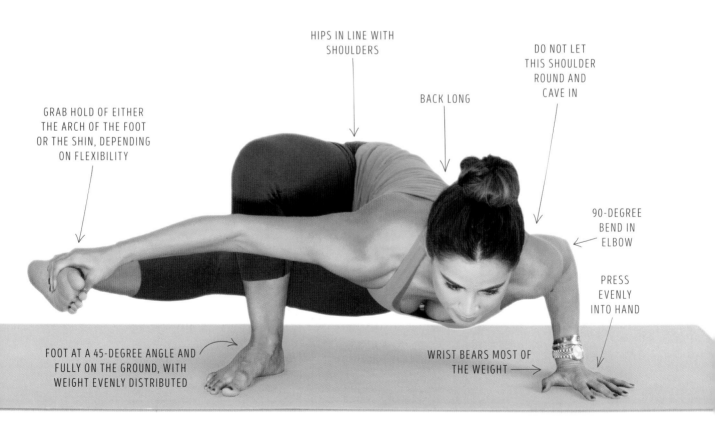

HIPS IN LINE WITH SHOULDERS

DO NOT LET THIS SHOULDER ROUND AND CAVE IN

BACK LONG

GRAB HOLD OF EITHER THE ARCH OF THE FOOT OR THE SHIN, DEPENDING ON FLEXIBILITY

90-DEGREE BEND IN ELBOW

PRESS EVENLY INTO HAND

FOOT AT A 45-DEGREE ANGLE AND FULLY ON THE GROUND, WITH WEIGHT EVENLY DISTRIBUTED

WRIST BEARS MOST OF THE WEIGHT

UTTHAN PRISTHASANA lizard pose

This pose tends to bring out a lot of emotion when I teach it in class. People either love it or loathe it. I mean, I've heard people swearing at me under their breath when I've walked by them while teaching this pose, and I get it—it's not a feel-good pose for many, especially those with tight hips. But you know what they say: the poses you hate are the ones you should do more often, so roll out your mat and let's get started.

Begin in a runner's lunge with your left leg behind you and your right foot planted on the ground. Then heel-toe your right foot an inch or two to the right to open up your hips a bit. Bring your hands onto the ground in front of you and slowly begin to make your way down to your forearms. If this is excruciating for you, grab a yoga block and place it on its side, then rest your forearms on the block.

Once your forearms are down, check your alignment. You want your shoulders to be even and your chest to stay open. To keep your chest as open as possible, avoid letting your upper back round too much. Another trick is to keep your gaze on the ground about three feet out in front of you. This focal point will help keep your spine long and your chest open. Breathe through the hips, imagining that your breath is combing through any tangles you feel in your legs. If you feel like it, you can walk your arms out even farther. Some people like to walk the arms all the way out and rest the head on the mat. Whatever works for you is cool; just try to keep the integrity of the alignment. Breathe for three to seven breaths before switching sides.

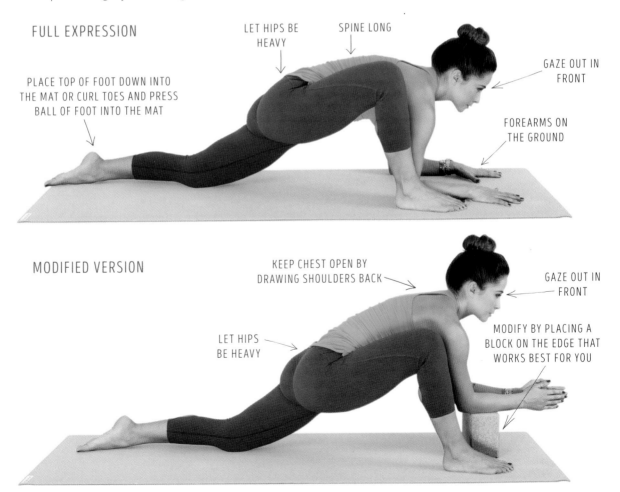

FULL EXPRESSION

LET HIPS BE HEAVY

SPINE LONG

GAZE OUT IN FRONT

PLACE TOP OF FOOT DOWN INTO THE MAT OR CURL TOES AND PRESS BALL OF FOOT INTO THE MAT

FOREARMS ON THE GROUND

MODIFIED VERSION

KEEP CHEST OPEN BY DRAWING SHOULDERS BACK

GAZE OUT IN FRONT

LET HIPS BE HEAVY

MODIFY BY PLACING A BLOCK ON THE EDGE THAT WORKS BEST FOR YOU

VASISTHASANA side plank

Side plank is a fabulous pose for strengthening your core. Solid core strength may help alleviate back pain and improve posture, so let's plank it out!

Begin in regular plank pose (page 109). As you inhale, place your left hand in the center of your mat and roll onto the knife-edge of your left foot. Stack your feet and find a spot on the ground about three feet in front of you that isn't moving. Focus your gaze here to help you maintain your balance. Then lift your hips and press into the mat with your left hand. Position your body so that your left hand is not directly underneath your left shoulder, which can irritate the shoulder girdle. Instead, aim to have the left hand slightly in front of the left shoulder. As you breathe, imagine that air is entering your body through the center of your left palm and follow the breath up through your chest and into your right fingertips. This visualization is helpful in maintaining the sensation of a lift through the body rather than letting your weight rest in your wrist and letting the hips sink—a common mistake.

Intend to keep your body light and lifted and try to keep your chest in line with your hips. Breathe fully and deeply for three to seven breaths before switching sides.

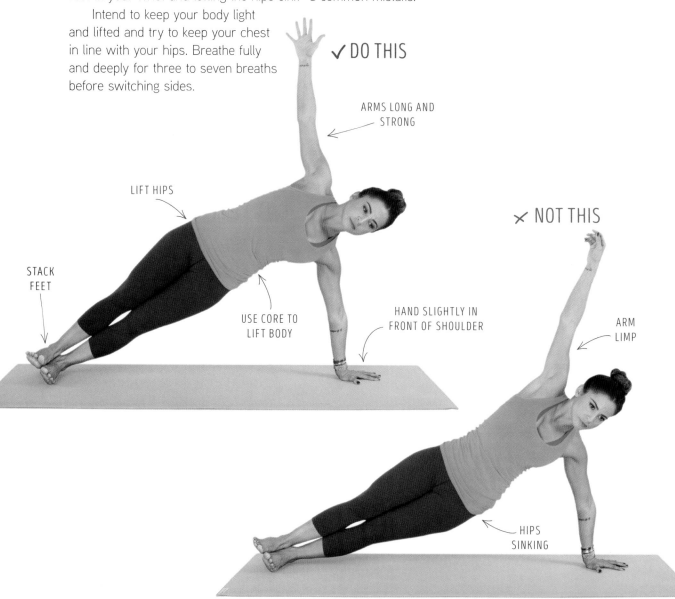

✓ DO THIS

ARMS LONG AND STRONG

LIFT HIPS

STACK FEET

USE CORE TO LIFT BODY

HAND SLIGHTLY IN FRONT OF SHOULDER

✗ NOT THIS

ARM LIMP

HIPS SINKING

MODIFIED VERSION

If you find that you're not quite ready for side plank, you can modify the pose by bringing your left knee to the ground and aligning your left shin with your knee, as shown. Press your right foot into the ground for added stability, lift your hips, and breathe.

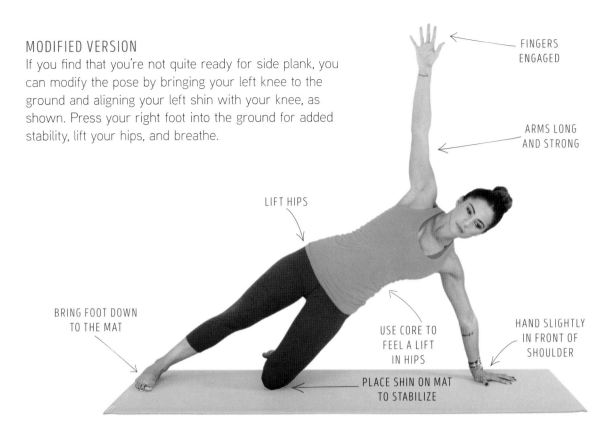

FINGERS ENGAGED

ARMS LONG AND STRONG

LIFT HIPS

BRING FOOT DOWN TO THE MAT

USE CORE TO FEEL A LIFT IN HIPS

HAND SLIGHTLY IN FRONT OF SHOULDER

PLACE SHIN ON MAT TO STABILIZE

TAKE IT DEEPER

If you find that you're ready to try an advanced variation of the pose, come into side plank and simply lift your right leg, keeping your right toes active and your right foot gently flexed, which will encourage the leg muscles to stay engaged.

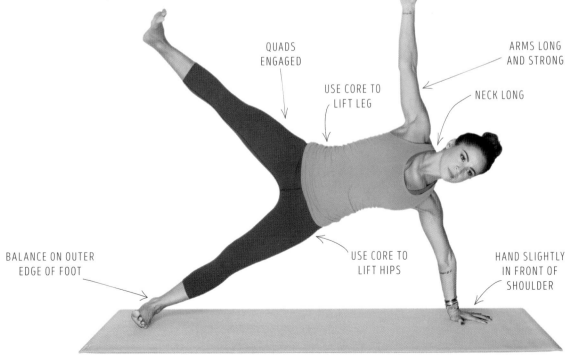

QUADS ENGAGED

USE CORE TO LIFT LEG

ARMS LONG AND STRONG

NECK LONG

BALANCE ON OUTER EDGE OF FOOT

USE CORE TO LIFT HIPS

HAND SLIGHTLY IN FRONT OF SHOULDER

VIRABHADRASANA 3 warrior 3

This pose may not look like much, but ohhh, baby! It works the entire body like no other! It's a good pose to add if you're looking to strengthen your legs and posterior chain.

Begin in mountain pose (page 106) at the back of your mat. Take a big step forward with your right foot. Keep your hands at your sides and, on your next inhale, lift your left leg and bring your torso forward until your body is making the shape of a capital T. You may want to reach back and touch your hips to make sure that they're even, as the left hip tends to lift. A trick to ensure that your left hip stays in proper alignment is to spin the left inner thigh up toward the sky and point the left toes down toward the mat. To prevent hyperextension, either micro-bend your right leg or lift your right kneecap to engage your leg muscles. To maintain your balance, gaze softly on the ground about three feet in front of you.

Once you're in the pose, you have a few options:

• Stay where you are.

• Bring your hands into reverse prayer position by bringing them behind your back and pressing the palms together with your fingers pointed toward your hips. Then, keeping the hands together, rotate them so that your fingers point toward your low back. Then rotate them one last time so that your fingers point up toward your head.

• Interlace your fingers behind your back and press your palms together, imagining that someone has a string tied around your hands and is gently pulling you backward. This is a great stretch for the chest.

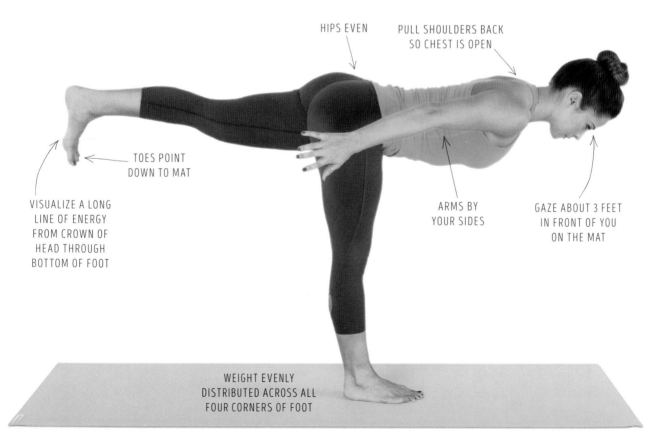

HIPS EVEN

PULL SHOULDERS BACK
SO CHEST IS OPEN

TOES POINT
DOWN TO MAT

VISUALIZE A LONG
LINE OF ENERGY
FROM CROWN OF
HEAD THROUGH
BOTTOM OF FOOT

ARMS BY
YOUR SIDES

GAZE ABOUT 3 FEET
IN FRONT OF YOU
ON THE MAT

WEIGHT EVENLY
DISTRIBUTED ACROSS ALL
FOUR CORNERS OF FOOT

VARIATION 1

HANDS IN REVERSE
PRAYER POSITION

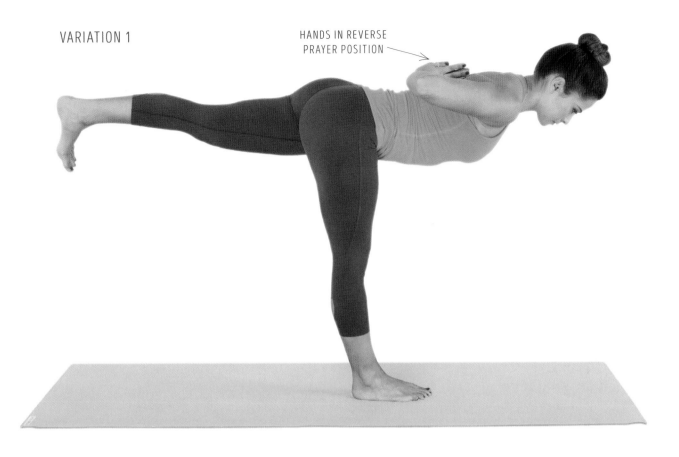

VARIATION 2

FINGERS INTERLACED AND
PALMS PRESSED TOGETHER

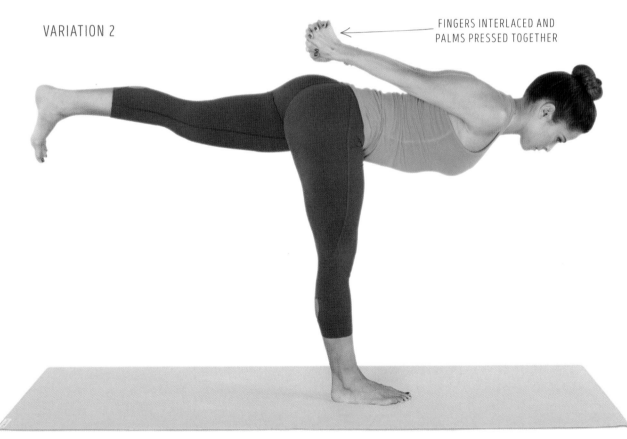

URDHVA PRASARITA EKA PADASANA (standing split) variation

All my people with tight hammies are going to want to cozy up to this pose. Now, if you're very tight, it won't be a delightful cozy-up sesh, but stick with it, as developing flexibility takes time and patience more than anything else.

Start in high lunge (page 112) with your right leg forward. As you inhale, send your torso forward and bring your hands to the ground. Use your back-body strength to lift your left leg. Be careful here. The tendency is for the left hip to open, so point your left toes toward the ground and spin your left inner thigh up toward the sky. You can also bring your left hand to the back of your hips to check that the hips are even.

Next, check your alignment. Be sure that your right hip is stacked over your right ankle. If you're prone to hyperextension, micro-bend your knee to protect your hamstring. If not, engage your quadriceps muscles. Then wrap your forearms around your right calf and pull up with your hands for a stable foundation as you lift through your back leg until you feel a good stretch in your right hamstring. Intend to keep your back long and your chest open. Take three to seven breaths before switching sides.

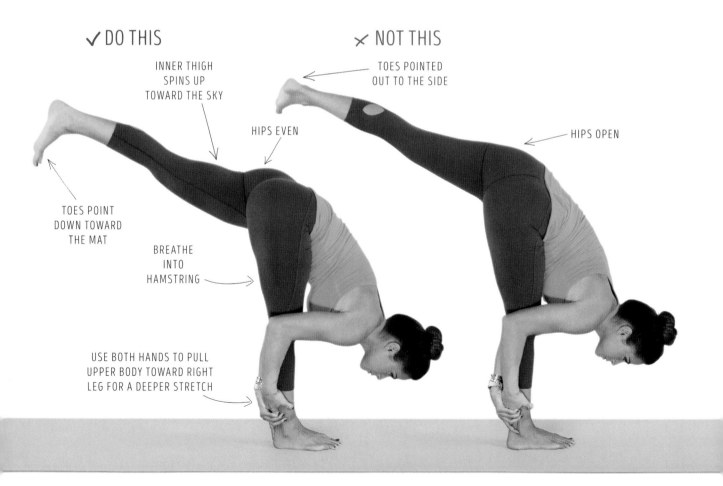

✓ DO THIS

INNER THIGH
SPINS UP
TOWARD THE SKY

HIPS EVEN

TOES POINT
DOWN TOWARD
THE MAT

BREATHE
INTO
HAMSTRING

USE BOTH HANDS TO PULL
UPPER BODY TOWARD RIGHT
LEG FOR A DEEPER STRETCH

✗ NOT THIS

TOES POINTED
OUT TO THE SIDE

HIPS OPEN

SALABHASANA dolphin pose

Dolphin pose is one of those poses that used to make me groan because I found it to be so challenging, but over time, as I've built up more strength, it's a pose that I have come to welcome with open arms and shoulders (see what I did there?). It is a pose that you'll definitely want to add if you're working on building upper-body strength. In addition to helping you build strength, this pose serves as a good way to increase range of movement through the shoulders and chest area.

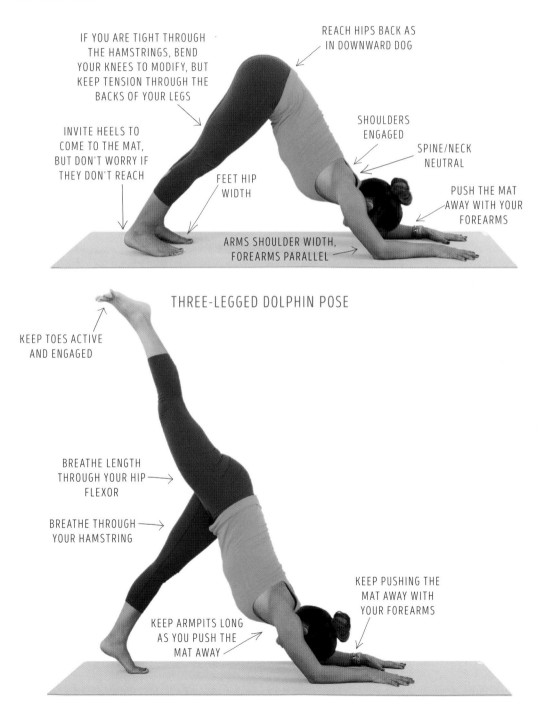

IF YOU ARE TIGHT THROUGH THE HAMSTRINGS, BEND YOUR KNEES TO MODIFY, BUT KEEP TENSION THROUGH THE BACKS OF YOUR LEGS

REACH HIPS BACK AS IN DOWNWARD DOG

INVITE HEELS TO COME TO THE MAT, BUT DON'T WORRY IF THEY DON'T REACH

SHOULDERS ENGAGED

SPINE/NECK NEUTRAL

FEET HIP WIDTH

PUSH THE MAT AWAY WITH YOUR FOREARMS

ARMS SHOULDER WIDTH, FOREARMS PARALLEL

THREE-LEGGED DOLPHIN POSE

KEEP TOES ACTIVE AND ENGAGED

BREATHE LENGTH THROUGH YOUR HIP FLEXOR

BREATHE THROUGH YOUR HAMSTRING

KEEP PUSHING THE MAT AWAY WITH YOUR FOREARMS

KEEP ARMPITS LONG AS YOU PUSH THE MAT AWAY

URDHVA MUKHA SVANASANA upward-facing dog

This pose is near and dear to my heart because it reminds me of how far I've come both on and off the mat. When I was in yoga teacher training in Thailand and still dealing with major joint issues, my wrists were too creaky to do this pose comfortably. Because I was studying Ashtanga yoga, a rigorous, athletic style, you can imagine how frustrating this was for me. Now that my joint issues and all the Lyme mess are behind me, I feel so grateful to be able to practice this pose in its entirety.

Upward dog is a tough pose that requires a good amount of strength to perform. Begin lying facedown on your mat. Bring your hands underneath your shoulders with your elbows pointing straight back behind you. From here, slide your hands down about 4 or 5 inches so that the tips of your middle fingers are in line with your armpits. Then press into your hands and the tops of your feet to lift your body. The only parts of your body that should be touching the mat are your hands and the tops of your feet.

From here, check your alignment. Your weight should be evenly distributed between your hands, and your shoulders should be gently pulled back and relaxed away from your ears. Avoid hyperextending your elbows by micro-bending your arms. Your chest should be nice and broad; if you looked at yourself in a mirror, your body would be making the shape of a sideways letter J, not a sideways letter L. Breathe length into your spine and breathe through the entire front body before releasing the pose.

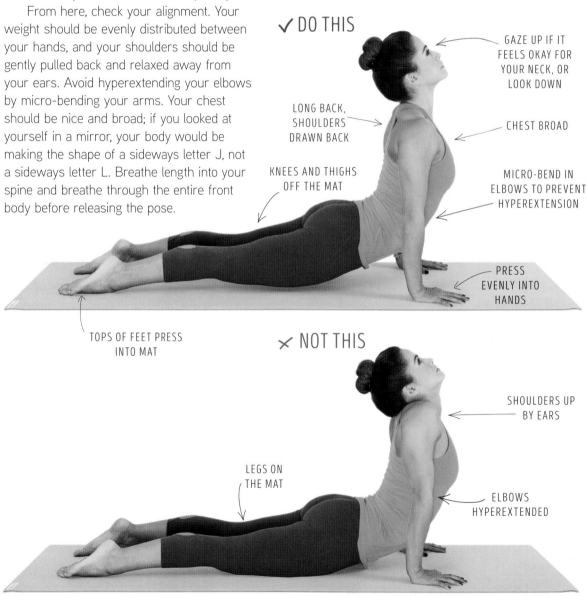

✔ DO THIS

GAZE UP IF IT FEELS OKAY FOR YOUR NECK, OR LOOK DOWN

CHEST BROAD

MICRO-BEND IN ELBOWS TO PREVENT HYPEREXTENSION

LONG BACK, SHOULDERS DRAWN BACK

KNEES AND THIGHS OFF THE MAT

PRESS EVENLY INTO HANDS

TOPS OF FEET PRESS INTO MAT

✗ NOT THIS

SHOULDERS UP BY EARS

LEGS ON THE MAT

ELBOWS HYPEREXTENDED

ARDHA PADMASANA VRKSASANA half-bound lotus tree pose

Half-bound lotus tree pose is a nice variation of one of yoga's most fundamental balancing postures, tree pose. It adds a little hip-opening action and is the stepping-stone to the half-bound lotus standing forward fold (page 200).

Begin by standing on your left leg in tree pose (page 105). Slowly reach down and take hold of your right foot. Activate your foot so that the toes are spread, which will help prevent your ankle from sickling. Nestle your right foot into your left hip crease (where your leg meets your torso). Bring your right hand to your heart center. You can keep your left hand gently on your right foot to keep it in place or, if you want more of a challenge, bring both hands into prayer position and see if you can keep your right foot in your left hip crease on its own.

Encourage your hip to open by gently guiding your knee into line with your left leg. You'll notice that this is the same leg position as seated half lotus (page 57). Take full, deep breaths for however long you like. When you're ready, gently bring your left hand to your right foot if you've moved it to prayer position and guide your foot away from your hip crease as you return to standing. Remember to take the pose to the other side as well.

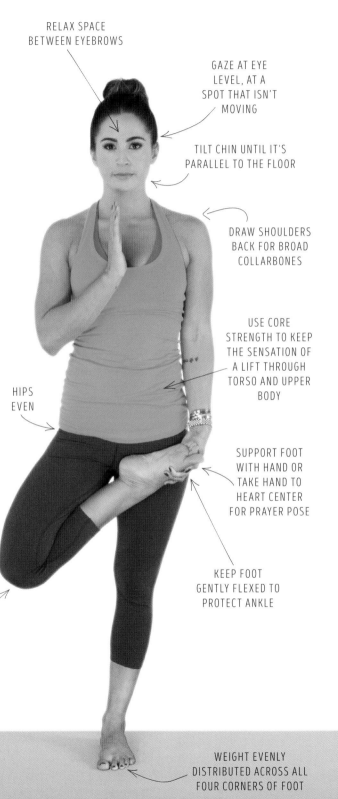

RELAX SPACE
BETWEEN EYEBROWS

GAZE AT EYE
LEVEL, AT A
SPOT THAT ISN'T
MOVING

TILT CHIN UNTIL IT'S
PARALLEL TO THE FLOOR

DRAW SHOULDERS
BACK FOR BROAD
COLLARBONES

USE CORE
STRENGTH TO KEEP
THE SENSATION OF
A LIFT THROUGH
TORSO AND UPPER
BODY

HIPS
EVEN

SUPPORT FOOT
WITH HAND OR
TAKE HAND TO
HEART CENTER
FOR PRAYER POSE

KEEP FOOT
GENTLY FLEXED TO
PROTECT ANKLE

DRAW KNEE AS CLOSE
IN LINE WITH STANDING
LEG AS YOU CAN

WEIGHT EVENLY
DISTRIBUTED ACROSS ALL
FOUR CORNERS OF FOOT

ARDHA BADDHA PADMOTTANASANA
half-bound lotus standing forward fold

This is a delicious pose for the hips and back. It requires a good bit of flexibility, so if you're not quite there yet, stay the course—eventually the pose will become accessible to you.

Begin in mountain pose (page 106). Lift your toes, spread them, and then set them down for a stable foundation. Gaze out in front of you at a spot that is at eye level and not moving. Focus your energy on that spot as you shift your weight to your left leg and begin to lift your right foot. Place your right foot in your left hip crease (where your leg meets your torso) and gently flex the foot to prevent ankle injury. On your next inhale, micro-bend your left leg and hinge at your hips as you begin to come forward in a forward fold. As you come down, you can slowly shift your gaze to the floor about three feet out in front of you. When you're in forward fold, reach your right hand around your back until it connects with your right big toe. If you're unable to connect just yet, use a yoga strap to help you. Then bring your left hand down to the ground, with the tips of your fingers in line with your toes. Invite your right knee to come in line with your left knee. Try to keep your low back long as you take your gaze to the ground, just next to your left ankle, and reach your head toward your left leg. Breathe for three to seven breaths before switching sides.

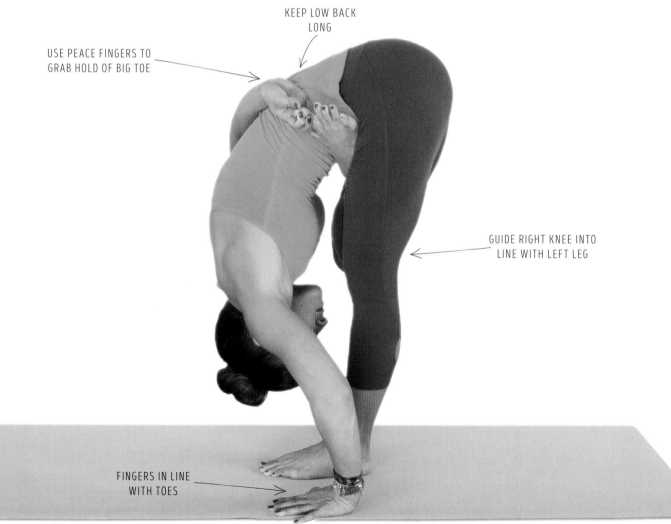

KEEP LOW BACK LONG

USE PEACE FINGERS TO GRAB HOLD OF BIG TOE

GUIDE RIGHT KNEE INTO LINE WITH LEFT LEG

FINGERS IN LINE WITH TOES

UTKATASANA (chair pose) variation standing pigeon pose

One of the things I love about yoga is the idea that poses are body shapes, and we can switch the foundations around and take these shapes to great new (literal) heights. Take standing pigeon pose, for example. Here you're looking to balance on one foot, but if you take the same position while lying on your back, it becomes an awesome supine hip opener. In the same light, you can do this exact same pose on your hands and be in a funky hip-opening arm balance. There is always somewhere to go when you're practicing, so as you move through asana, keep in mind how you can practice these poses in other ways.

Begin in mountain pose (page 106). Find a spot in front of you that's at eye level and not moving. Focus on that drishti as you lift your toes, spread them, and set them down for a stable foundation. Then shift your weight onto your right foot and lift your left leg, crossing your left ankle over your right thigh as you sink low with your hips. Bring your hands into prayer position, then check your spine, making sure that your tailbone is tucked to avoid arching your back. Keep your collarbones broad by pressing your hands together and drawing your shoulder blades toward one another. Distribute your weight evenly across all four corners of your right foot. Breathe fully and deeply for three to seven breaths before switching sides.

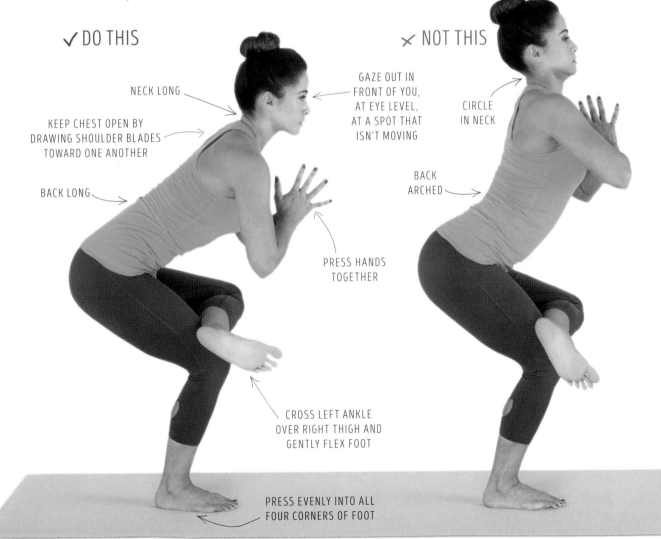

✓ DO THIS

NECK LONG

KEEP CHEST OPEN BY
DRAWING SHOULDER BLADES
TOWARD ONE ANOTHER

BACK LONG

CROSS LEFT ANKLE
OVER RIGHT THIGH AND
GENTLY FLEX FOOT

PRESS EVENLY INTO ALL
FOUR CORNERS OF FOOT

✗ NOT THIS

GAZE OUT IN
FRONT OF YOU,
AT EYE LEVEL,
AT A SPOT THAT
ISN'T MOVING

CIRCLE
IN NECK

BACK
ARCHED

PRESS HANDS
TOGETHER

EKA PADA MALASANA balancing bound wide squat

This pose will put your balance to the test, and it's a good indicator of how open your hips are. Remember that if the bind isn't accessible to you right now, you can always use a yoga strap to help your hands connect.

Begin in mountain pose (page 106). Find a spot in front of you that's at eye level and not moving. Focus on that drishti as you lift your toes, spread them, and set them down for a stable foundation. Shift your weight onto your left foot and slowly begin to lift your right leg by using your core and hip flexor strength. Bring your right knee in toward your right armpit, being mindful to either micro-bend your left leg or lift your left kneecap to engage your leg muscles and protect your hamstring. Bring your right arm out in front of you and make a thumbs-down sign with your hand. Then lean forward slightly and, keeping the thumb down, wrap your arm around your right leg. Keep your right leg lifted with your core and hip flexor strength rather than supporting the leg too much with your right arm. From here, wrap your left arm around your back and reach until both hands meet. Use a yoga strap to connect your hands if they don't meet on their own. From here, stand tall, keeping the space between your eyebrows relaxed. Breathe fully and deeply, utilizing your lungs to their fullest capacity, for three to seven breaths before switching sides.

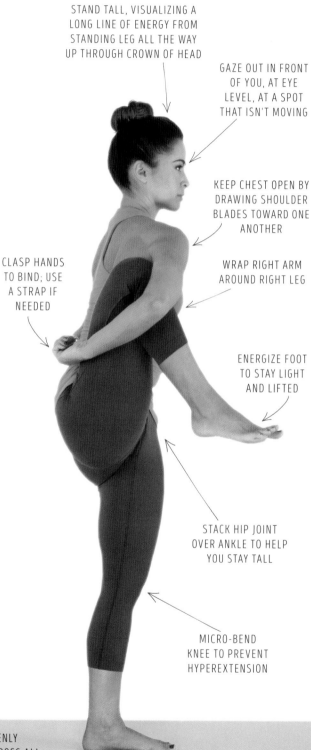

STAND TALL, VISUALIZING A LONG LINE OF ENERGY FROM STANDING LEG ALL THE WAY UP THROUGH CROWN OF HEAD

GAZE OUT IN FRONT OF YOU, AT EYE LEVEL, AT A SPOT THAT ISN'T MOVING

KEEP CHEST OPEN BY DRAWING SHOULDER BLADES TOWARD ONE ANOTHER

CLASP HANDS TO BIND; USE A STRAP IF NEEDED

WRAP RIGHT ARM AROUND RIGHT LEG

ENERGIZE FOOT TO STAY LIGHT AND LIFTED

STACK HIP JOINT OVER ANKLE TO HELP YOU STAY TALL

MICRO-BEND KNEE TO PREVENT HYPEREXTENSION

WEIGHT EVENLY DISTRIBUTED ACROSS ALL FOUR CORNERS OF FOOT

PARIVRTTA PARSVAKONASANA revolved angle pose

This pose may not look like much, but it's a beast. You might look at my face in this picture and think, "Wow, she looks so peaceful and calm." Let me just tell you that I'm a good actress—well, at least when it comes to yoga. I have a terrible poker face in 100 percent of activities off the mat, but when it comes to asana, I usually breathe through whatever nonsense I'm feeling because I use the mantra "I can do anything for ten seconds." Okay, now that we've established that this pose is tough for me, let's break it down.

Come into warrior 1 (page 113) with your hands in prayer position. From here, inhale, bring your torso forward, and twist from your navel to the right. Then set your left hand to the outside of your right foot with the fingers in line with the toes. You can use your knee for leverage. Then bring your right arm in line with your right ear, palm facing down. If your neck feels okay here, you can look up at your right thumb. Now, this is probably going to feel like madness for your left calf, and if you start to wonder what kind of tomfoolery is going on, just try to stay mindful. If it's just feeling like an intense stretch, breathe through it. If it feels like you might actually rip your calf muscle in half, you can modify the pose by lifting your back heel. Take three to seven breaths before switching sides.

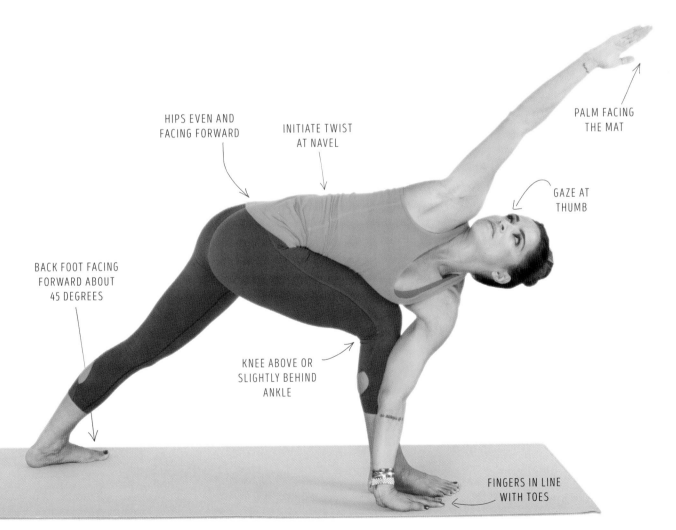

HIPS EVEN AND FACING FORWARD

INITIATE TWIST AT NAVEL

PALM FACING THE MAT

GAZE AT THUMB

BACK FOOT FACING FORWARD ABOUT 45 DEGREES

KNEE ABOVE OR SLIGHTLY BEHIND ANKLE

FINGERS IN LINE WITH TOES

GARUNDASANA eagle pose

If balancing is your jam, you'll want to acquaint yourself with eagle pose. I also recommend it for runners and weightlifters because it helps strengthen the ankle joints and improve ankle mobility, which is ideal for both marathoners and sprinters and for people who are working on their squats.

Begin in mountain pose (page 106). Pick your toes up, spread them, and set them down for a stable foundation in this balancing pose. Find a spot in front of you that is at eye level and not moving, and focus your energy on that spot as you shift your weight onto your left foot. Pick up your right leg and cross your right thigh over your left. Bend your knees deeply as if you're about to sit down in a chair behind you, and if you can, hook the top of your right foot around the back of your left calf. Open your arms wide as if you're going in for a big hug, then swoop your arms in, sliding your right arm over your left and hooking your right hand around your left. If you have a large chest or are very tight in your upper body, this position may not be accessible to you yet. In that case, press your forearms together with your arms bent 90 degrees.

Regardless of what you're doing with your arms, sit low and breathe. Tuck your tailbone slightly for a long, neutral spine and press through your heels. Keep your body upright and pull your arms down while maintaining a long, flat back. Draw your shoulder blades down and relax your shoulders away from your ears. Take three to seven full, deep breaths before switching sides.

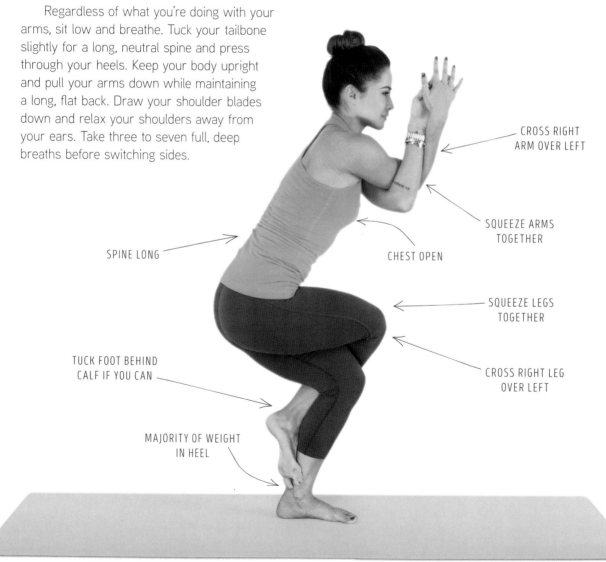

CROSS RIGHT
ARM OVER LEFT

SQUEEZE ARMS
TOGETHER

SPINE LONG

CHEST OPEN

SQUEEZE LEGS
TOGETHER

TUCK FOOT BEHIND
CALF IF YOU CAN

CROSS RIGHT LEG
OVER LEFT

MAJORITY OF WEIGHT
IN HEEL

PARIVRTTA TRIKONASANA revolved triangle pose

This pose feels incredible for tight hips and hamstrings, and the twist adds a detoxifying benefit.

Begin by standing at the back of your mat with your feet together. Take a big step forward with your left leg and turn your right foot out about 45 degrees. Straighten both legs and, as you inhale, follow your breath up through the bottoms of your feet as you simultaneously lift your kneecaps, engage your leg muscles, and get as tall as you can through the torso. As you exhale, lift your right arm out in front of you so that it is parallel to the ground and bring the back of your hand to your low back. Take another deep breath in to get as tall as you can, and as you exhale, send your upper body forward and rotate to the left, initiating the twist from your navel. Bring your right hand down to the ground with the fingers in line with your left toes. If your hand doesn't reach, use a yoga block to help you. Slowly begin to roll your left shoulder up toward the sky. If this is feeling really intense for you, you can stop here. If you're feeling great, you can lift your left arm up toward the sky. Breathe fully and deeply, working through any tension you feel. If your legs are particularly tight and you need to modify the pose to accommodate them, you can bend your front leg a little bit, but try to keep the sensation of tension in your hamstring, as if you're trying to continually straighten your leg. Take three to seven breaths before switching sides.

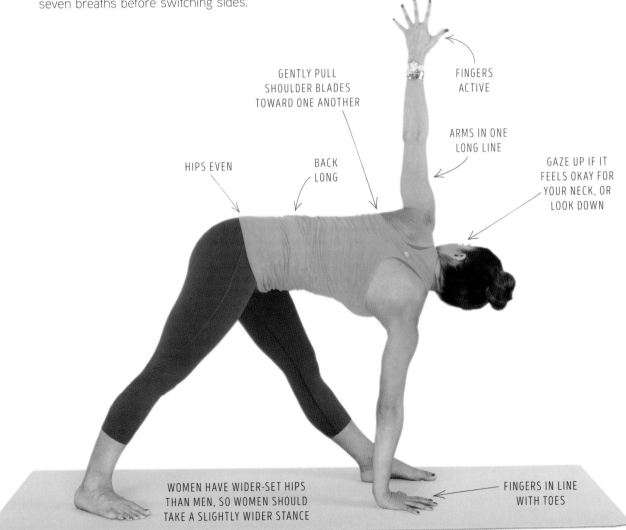

GENTLY PULL
SHOULDER BLADES
TOWARD ONE ANOTHER

FINGERS
ACTIVE

ARMS IN ONE
LONG LINE

HIPS EVEN

BACK
LONG

GAZE UP IF IT
FEELS OKAY FOR
YOUR NECK, OR
LOOK DOWN

WOMEN HAVE WIDER-SET HIPS
THAN MEN, SO WOMEN SHOULD
TAKE A SLIGHTLY WIDER STANCE

FINGERS IN LINE
WITH TOES

PARSVOTTANASANA intense stretch

They don't call this "intense stretch" for nothing. This pose, in the words of Rachel Zoe, is ba-na-nas for the hamstrings. My advice? Breathe deeply and tune in to how you feel. If you need to, back off and use the modifications offered below.

Begin by standing at the back of your mat. As you inhale, take a big step forward with your right foot. Your hips should be facing forward, and your left foot should be fully on the ground with the toes turned out about 45 degrees. Heel-toe your right foot about two inches to the right for a stable foundation. As you inhale, lengthen through your spine and lift your arms overhead, bringing your hands into prayer position. As you exhale, hinge at the hips and come forward with your torso as you reach your belly toward your right thigh. This helps prevent your low back from rounding. Reach your head toward your right leg and place the knife-edges of your hands on the ground if they reach.

Once you're in the pose, check your alignment. Make sure that your right kneecap is lifted to prevent your hamstring from hyperextending. If you are unable to straighten your leg due to tight hamstrings, just bend the leg a little. Then check in with your hips, which should be even. You can reach back with your left hand to see if your left hip has lifted a bit. If it has, pull your right hip back. This stretch will feel quite intense for your left hamstring, so be mindful. If it's too intense, just bend your right leg more deeply, which should reduce the intensity. Breathe fully and deeply for three to seven breaths before raising your torso, bending your front leg, stepping to the back of the mat, and taking it to the other side.

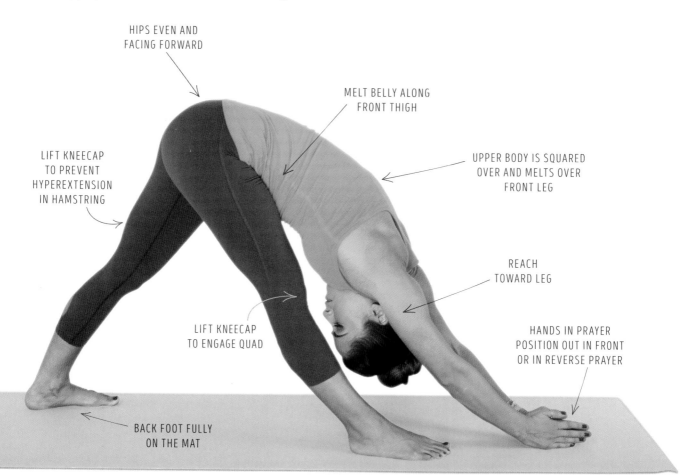

HIPS EVEN AND
FACING FORWARD

MELT BELLY ALONG
FRONT THIGH

LIFT KNEECAP
TO PREVENT
HYPEREXTENSION
IN HAMSTRING

UPPER BODY IS SQUARED
OVER AND MELTS OVER
FRONT LEG

REACH
TOWARD LEG

LIFT KNEECAP
TO ENGAGE QUAD

HANDS IN PRAYER
POSITION OUT IN FRONT
OR IN REVERSE PRAYER

BACK FOOT FULLY
ON THE MAT

PARIVRTTA ARDHA CHANDRASANA revolved half moon pose

This pose is one of those good ones that seem to have it all. Strength building? Check. Total body stretch? Check. Balance? Check.

Start in high lunge (page 112) with your left foot forward, your right leg behind you, and your arms overhead. As you inhale, send your right arm out in front of you and your left arm behind you, palms facing down and arms parallel to the ground. Initiate a twist from your navel as you look to the left. Intend to keep your chest open by drawing your shoulder blades toward one another. On the next inhale, reach forward with your torso, and when you can't come any farther forward, rotate your arms so that your right fingers are on the ground and your left arm is lifted to the sky. As you slowly walk your fingers out in front of you even more, use your back-body strength to lift your right leg. Aim to have your arms in one long line and imagine that with each breath you're sucking up air through the center of your right palm.

Gently flex your right foot and spin your right inner thigh up to the sky so that your right toes are pointed down toward the mat and your hips are even. The common mistake here is to allow the right hip to lift, so be mindful. Press out of the bottom of your right foot to keep your leg muscles engaged, then check in with your left leg, being sure to either micro-bend the knee or engage the quad muscles to protect your hamstring. Take three to seven breaths here before moving to the other side.

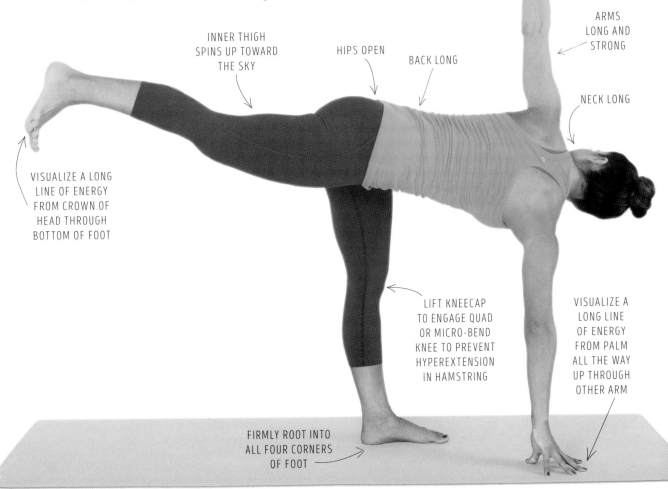

FINGERS ACTIVE

ARMS LONG AND STRONG

NECK LONG

INNER THIGH SPINS UP TOWARD THE SKY

HIPS OPEN

BACK LONG

VISUALIZE A LONG LINE OF ENERGY FROM CROWN OF HEAD THROUGH BOTTOM OF FOOT

LIFT KNEECAP TO ENGAGE QUAD OR MICRO-BEND KNEE TO PREVENT HYPEREXTENSION IN HAMSTRING

VISUALIZE A LONG LINE OF ENERGY FROM PALM ALL THE WAY UP THROUGH OTHER ARM

FIRMLY ROOT INTO ALL FOUR CORNERS OF FOOT

CAMATKARASANA wild thing

Wild thing feels as good as it looks. It opens the entire front body, challenges balance, and helps build strength in the shoulder area. It's really a full-body pose.

Begin in three-legged dog (page 175) with your left leg lifted. Continue to push the mat away as you bend your left leg and activate your toes. As you reach your left toes to the mat, slowly begin to turn on the ball of your right foot so that your right toes are pointed to the left. Lift your left arm overhead as your left toes touch down and get as long as you can from your fingertips to your toes. Let your head go if it feels okay for your neck. Continue to push the mat away with your right hand and make sure that your right shoulder is behind your right hand. Stacking your right shoulder on top of your wrist compromises the integrity of the shoulder girdle. Breathe length through your entire front body. When you're ready to release the pose, spin your right foot to face the front again as you come back into three-legged dog.

1. THREE-LEGGED DOG

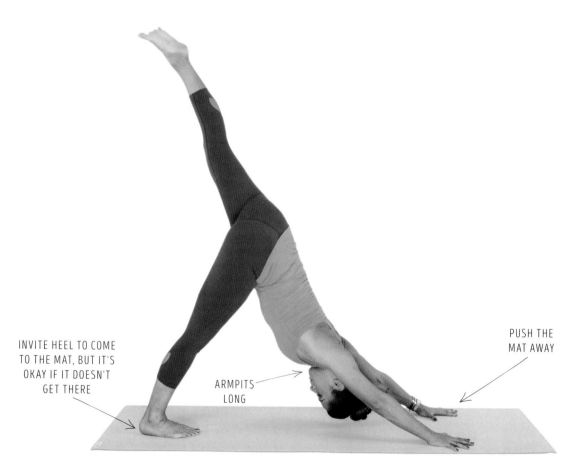

INVITE HEEL TO COME TO THE MAT, BUT IT'S OKAY IF IT DOESN'T GET THERE

ARMPITS LONG

PUSH THE MAT AWAY

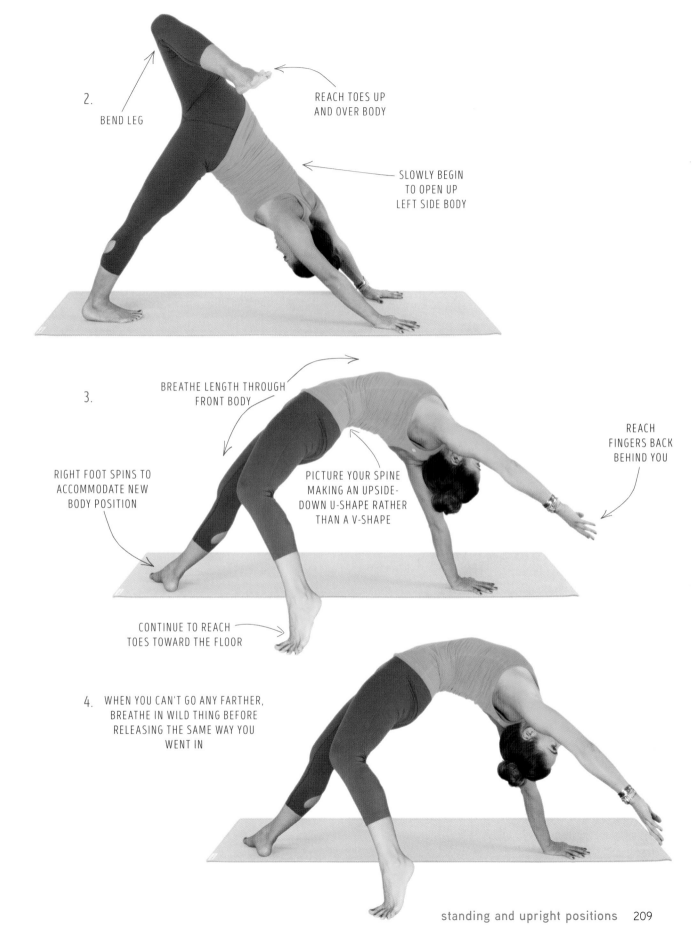

2. BEND LEG

REACH TOES UP AND OVER BODY

SLOWLY BEGIN TO OPEN UP LEFT SIDE BODY

3. BREATHE LENGTH THROUGH FRONT BODY

RIGHT FOOT SPINS TO ACCOMMODATE NEW BODY POSITION

PICTURE YOUR SPINE MAKING AN UPSIDE-DOWN U-SHAPE RATHER THAN A V-SHAPE

REACH FINGERS BACK BEHIND YOU

CONTINUE TO REACH TOES TOWARD THE FLOOR

4. WHEN YOU CAN'T GO ANY FARTHER, BREATHE IN WILD THING BEFORE RELEASING THE SAME WAY YOU WENT IN

standing and upright positions   209

URDHVA PRASARITA EKA PADASANA standing split

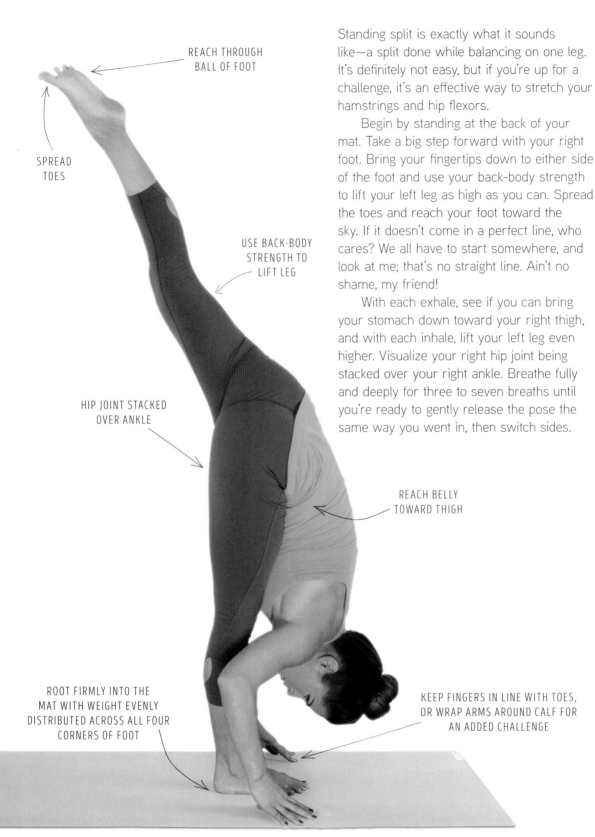

REACH THROUGH
BALL OF FOOT

SPREAD
TOES

USE BACK-BODY
STRENGTH TO
LIFT LEG

HIP JOINT STACKED
OVER ANKLE

REACH BELLY
TOWARD THIGH

ROOT FIRMLY INTO THE
MAT WITH WEIGHT EVENLY
DISTRIBUTED ACROSS ALL FOUR
CORNERS OF FOOT

KEEP FINGERS IN LINE WITH TOES,
OR WRAP ARMS AROUND CALF FOR
AN ADDED CHALLENGE

Standing split is exactly what it sounds like—a split done while balancing on one leg. It's definitely not easy, but if you're up for a challenge, it's an effective way to stretch your hamstrings and hip flexors.

Begin by standing at the back of your mat. Take a big step forward with your right foot. Bring your fingertips down to either side of the foot and use your back-body strength to lift your left leg as high as you can. Spread the toes and reach your foot toward the sky. If it doesn't come in a perfect line, who cares? We all have to start somewhere, and look at me; that's no straight line. Ain't no shame, my friend!

With each exhale, see if you can bring your stomach down toward your right thigh, and with each inhale, lift your left leg even higher. Visualize your right hip joint being stacked over your right ankle. Breathe fully and deeply for three to seven breaths until you're ready to gently release the pose the same way you went in, then switch sides.

DANDAYAMANA JANUSHIRASANA
standing head-to-knee pose

This pose is a wobbly one! The combination of major hamstring- and hip-opening components makes it tricky. The keys are to maintain focus on a solid drishti and to be mindful that your standing leg is totally engaged.

Begin in mountain pose (page 106). Lift your toes, spread them, and set them down for a stable foundation in this balancing pose. Find a spot in front of you that is at eye level and not moving. Focus your gaze on that spot as you shift your weight to your left foot. Feel your weight evenly distributed across all four corners of the foot as you lift your right leg. Interlace your fingers under the middle of your right foot. Flex the right foot gently and press out of the bottom of the foot to extend your right leg. If you're prone to hyperextension, micro-bend both knees. If not, lift both kneecaps to engage your quadriceps muscles. As you exhale, reach your belly toward your right thigh so that your low back stays long, and intend to keep your chest open. Breathe fully and deeply, and when you're ready to release the pose, go out the same way you went in before taking it to the other side.

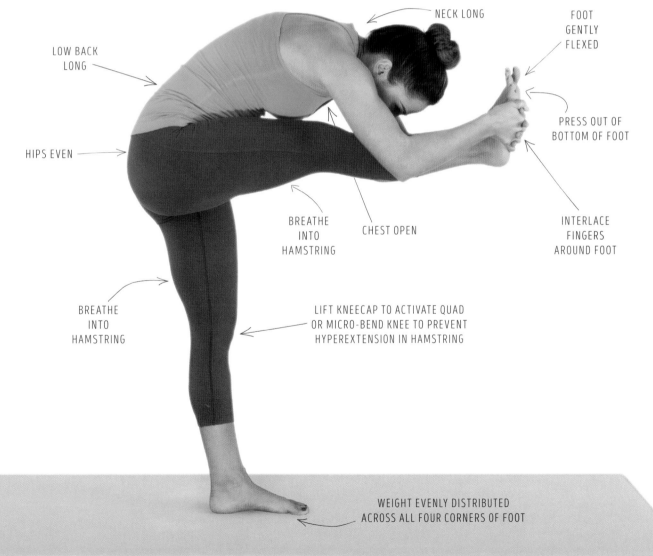

NECK LONG

FOOT GENTLY FLEXED

LOW BACK LONG

PRESS OUT OF BOTTOM OF FOOT

HIPS EVEN

BREATHE INTO HAMSTRING

CHEST OPEN

INTERLACE FINGERS AROUND FOOT

BREATHE INTO HAMSTRING

LIFT KNEECAP TO ACTIVATE QUAD OR MICRO-BEND KNEE TO PREVENT HYPEREXTENSION IN HAMSTRING

WEIGHT EVENLY DISTRIBUTED ACROSS ALL FOUR CORNERS OF FOOT

MANDUKASANA frog pose

There are a number of variations of frog pose, but this is the one that I put into my classes most often. Like lizard pose (page 191), I find that people have strong feelings about this one: they either love it or are in agony! My best advice is to breathe through whatever it is you're experiencing and ask yourself if you're feeling actual pain or just tightness—there is a difference. If it's tightness, continue to breathe through it. If it's pain, come out of the pose.

To enter, sit on your shins with your knees and ankles together. Come onto all fours and slowly widen your knees, keeping your ankles in line with your knees. If you're on a regular yoga mat, this position can be tough on the knees. If you need more padding, place a folded blanket underneath each knee. Then bring your forearms down onto the ground with your palms together. Breathe fully and deeply and see if you can feel gravity pull your hips toward the ground with each exhale. Stay here for up to a minute. When you're ready to release the pose, bring your big toes together, followed by your knees, and then sit back on your shins.

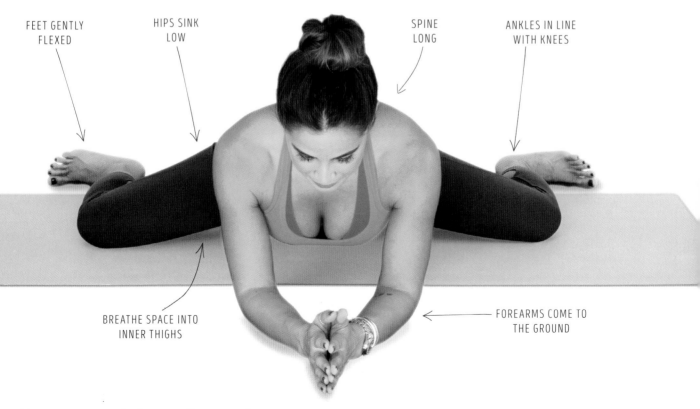

FEET GENTLY FLEXED

HIPS SINK LOW

SPINE LONG

ANKLES IN LINE WITH KNEES

BREATHE SPACE INTO INNER THIGHS

FOREARMS COME TO THE GROUND

SUPTA MATSYENDRASANA supine spinal twist

Supine spinal twist is one of my favorite poses. It's relaxing because it requires very little effort, and it always leaves me feeling incredible. The twisting component makes it detoxing and gently rejuvenating.

Begin by lying on your back with your left leg bent. With your palms facing up, open your arms so that they are perpendicular to your body. From here, twist to the right, initiating the twist from your navel, and bring your left leg up and over your body. Bring your right hand to the outside of your left thigh and gently press it down. Look over your left shoulder with your right eye. For a deeper stretch in your chest, you can bend your left arm 90 degrees; otherwise, keep it perpendicular to your body. With each exhale, feel gravity pulling your left shoulder and left leg farther toward the ground and visualize a "wringing out" of your center. Take three to ten breaths here before rolling back to center and taking it to the other side.

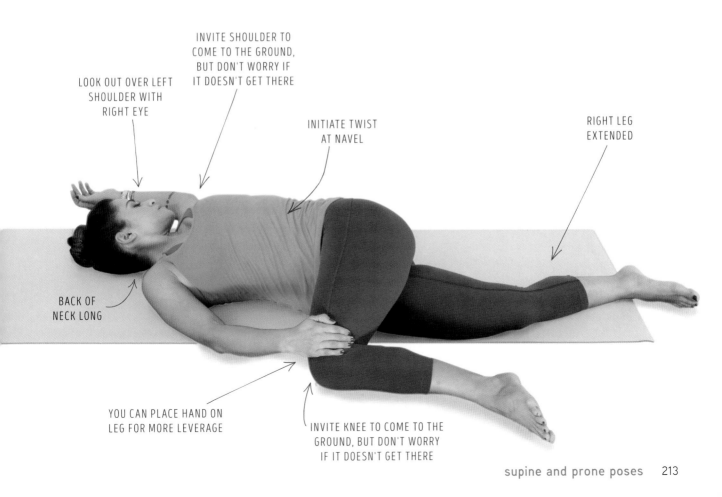

LOOK OUT OVER LEFT SHOULDER WITH RIGHT EYE

INVITE SHOULDER TO COME TO THE GROUND, BUT DON'T WORRY IF IT DOESN'T GET THERE

INITIATE TWIST AT NAVEL

RIGHT LEG EXTENDED

BACK OF NECK LONG

YOU CAN PLACE HAND ON LEG FOR MORE LEVERAGE

INVITE KNEE TO COME TO THE GROUND, BUT DON'T WORRY IF IT DOESN'T GET THERE

PURVOTTANASANA upward plank pose

True story: In yoga teacher training, we had to memorize a number of poses by their Sanskrit names. I was studying one day in preparation for our final test and trying to figure out which poses I would remember. When I stumbled upon purvottanasana, I burst out laughing. Purvottanasana, to me, sounded like "pervert," and given that you throw your head back and stick your pelvis in the air, a lightbulb went off! That's the story of how I know the name purvottanasana, and I'm pretty sure that from now on, you'll remember it, too. You're welcome.

Begin by sitting on your mat in staff pose (page 98) with your feet hip width apart.

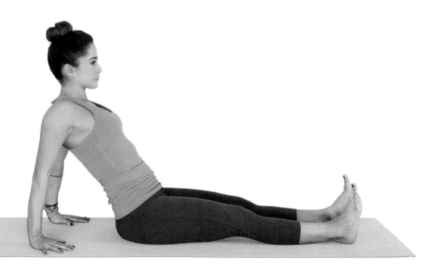

1.

On your next exhale, lean back, bringing your hands about eight inches behind you, with your fingers spread and facing your body. As you inhale, press into your hands and heels to lift your hips off the mat.

2.

Reach the bottoms of your feet toward the mat and lift your hips higher. If it feels okay for your neck, let your head go. Continue to press evenly through your hands and breathe through the fronts of your shoulders. Take three to seven breaths here before coming down the same way you went in.

LET HEAD GO BACK IF IT FEELS OKAY FOR YOUR NECK

BREATHE INTO FRONTS OF SHOULDERS AND THROUGH CHEST

LIFT HIPS

PRESS BOTTOMS OF FEET INTO THE MAT

WEIGHT EVENLY DISTRIBUTED THROUGH HANDS

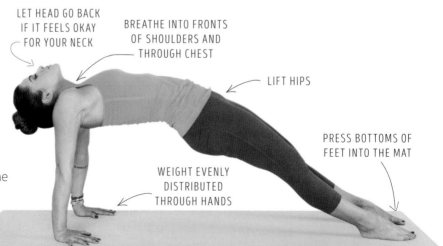

3.

SALABHASANA A locust pose A

The posterior chain (the muscles along the back of the body) often gets ignored. Why do we want to work the posterior chain? Because strong hamstrings, glutes, and backs help support our bodies in our daily lives and may help prevent injuries when we're doing everyday things. Locust pose helps build strength in the back body, and for that reason I'm psyched to introduce it to you.

Begin by lying on your stomach with your arms at your sides and your feet hip width apart. Take a deep breath in and, as you exhale, peel your chest, arms, and legs off the mat. Gaze at a spot on the ground in front of you and try to get as long as you can while you lift as high as you can. Visualizing length through your spine will help you avoid compressing your low back. Take as many breaths as you can here before relaxing onto the mat.

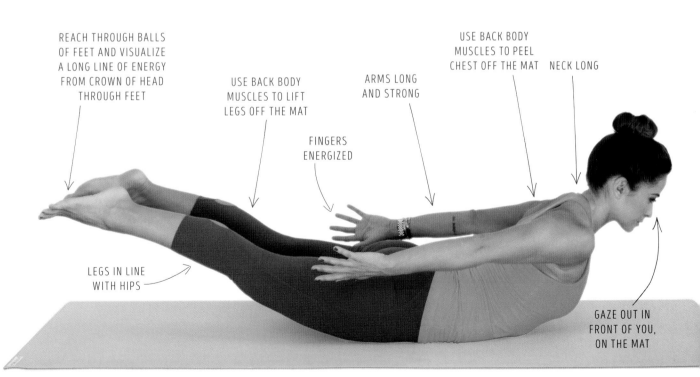

REACH THROUGH BALLS OF FEET AND VISUALIZE A LONG LINE OF ENERGY FROM CROWN OF HEAD THROUGH FEET

USE BACK BODY MUSCLES TO LIFT LEGS OFF THE MAT

FINGERS ENERGIZED

ARMS LONG AND STRONG

USE BACK BODY MUSCLES TO PEEL CHEST OFF THE MAT

NECK LONG

LEGS IN LINE WITH HIPS

GAZE OUT IN FRONT OF YOU, ON THE MAT

MATSYASANA fish pose

Fish pose is a nice opener for the chest, and it's a pose that I always add to my heart-opening and back-bending classes. The trick is to visualize a string tied around your chest and imagine that you are being pulled up by that string. That visualization should give you the sense of a gentle lift that creates a small yet significant bend in your upper back. The variation that you see here has my legs at about a 45-degree angle. This is how I learned it in teacher training, but a simpler version has the legs fully on the ground, so keep that in mind as an option if you find you're struggling to keep the legs up.

Begin by lying on your back. If you're wearing your hair up, take out your ponytail or bun because you'll be placing that part of your head on the mat. Using that image of a string tied around your chest, imagine that you're being lifted up by that string. Use your core strength to keep yourself light and lifted. Bring the back of your head (the place where you'd wear a high ponytail) to the mat, placing minimal weight on the head to avoid compressing your neck. As you inhale, bring your arms up so that they're parallel to your legs. Interlace the fingers and release your index fingers as you exhale. Breathe here for three to seven breaths before releasing.

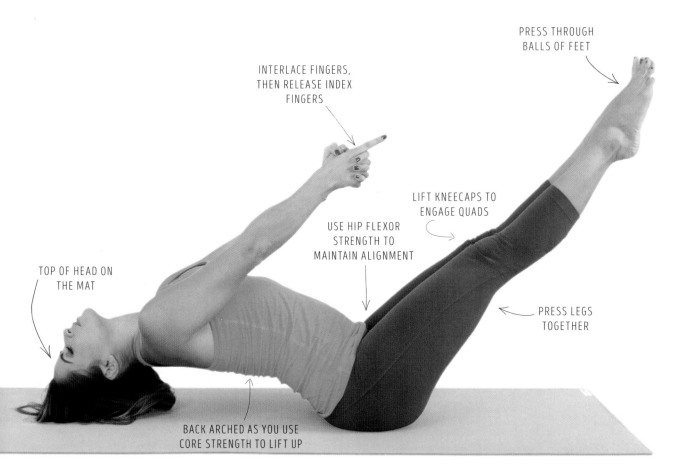

PRESS THROUGH
BALLS OF FEET

INTERLACE FINGERS,
THEN RELEASE INDEX
FINGERS

LIFT KNEECAPS TO
ENGAGE QUADS

USE HIP FLEXOR
STRENGTH TO
MAINTAIN ALIGNMENT

TOP OF HEAD ON
THE MAT

PRESS LEGS
TOGETHER

BACK ARCHED AS YOU USE
CORE STRENGTH TO LIFT UP

SUPTA VIRASANA reclined hero pose

All you runners out there are going to want to get down with this pose because it opens up the quads like no other. If you have knee problems, though, you will likely want to avoid it. Everyone should move slowly and mindfully in every pose, but particularly in this one, which puts the knees in a somewhat delicate position.

Begin in hero pose (page 94). Bring your hands behind you on the mat and slowly begin to ease your upper body down toward the ground. Move slowly and carefully and keep your heart lifted to bring length through your entire back and front body. Place your upper back on the mat and bring your arms overhead. The back of your neck should be flush against the mat. Breathe through your quads and torso, aiming to work through any tension you are feeling. Take three to seven breaths and, when you're ready to release, bring your arms to your sides, press into your forearms to lift your back off the mat, and return to hero pose.

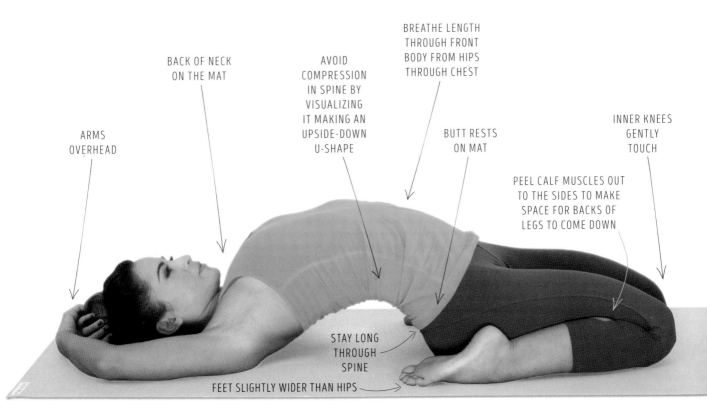

BREATHE LENGTH THROUGH FRONT BODY FROM HIPS THROUGH CHEST

BACK OF NECK ON THE MAT

AVOID COMPRESSION IN SPINE BY VISUALIZING IT MAKING AN UPSIDE-DOWN U-SHAPE

INNER KNEES GENTLY TOUCH

ARMS OVERHEAD

BUTT RESTS ON MAT

PEEL CALF MUSCLES OUT TO THE SIDES TO MAKE SPACE FOR BACKS OF LEGS TO COME DOWN

STAY LONG THROUGH SPINE

FEET SLIGHTLY WIDER THAN HIPS

SALAMBA SARVANGASANA supported shoulder stand

This nice little inversion is supposed to be particularly energizing and rejuvenating for both the mind and the body, so if you find yourself in a midday slump, I recommend taking a little break and popping up into this pose for a few minutes—especially if you work in an office among a bunch of people. Extra gold stars for that!

Now, sometimes people's necks feel a little, um, funky, in this position. "Funky" is never a way we want to describe how our neck feels, so if you have issues, place a folded blanket underneath your back, with the edge of the blanket in line with the tops of your shoulders. If your neck is fine, you don't need to use a blanket.

Begin by lying on your back with your knees bent. Bend your arms and bring your hands to your low back as you lift your legs, then shimmy your elbows in so that they support you. Magnetize your elbows so that they don't slip out to the sides. "Magnetizing" is just what it sounds like—it should feel like your elbows are pulling toward one another, but you're not actually moving them. Keeping this imaginary tension between your elbows will help make your foundation more stable. Gaze toward your belly button as you lift through your legs, press your big toe mounds together, and spread your toes. Zip your legs up and reach through the balls of your feet as you breathe. To avoid compromising your neck, do not turn your head when you're in this position. Stay here for up to five minutes, breathing fully and deeply.

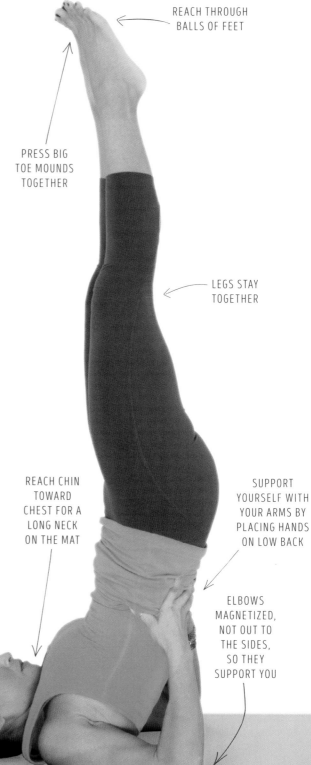

REACH THROUGH BALLS OF FEET

PRESS BIG TOE MOUNDS TOGETHER

LEGS STAY TOGETHER

REACH CHIN TOWARD CHEST FOR A LONG NECK ON THE MAT

SUPPORT YOURSELF WITH YOUR ARMS BY PLACING HANDS ON LOW BACK

ELBOWS MAGNETIZED, NOT OUT TO THE SIDES, SO THEY SUPPORT YOU

GAZE TOWARD NAVEL

TO AVOID COMPROMISING NECK, DO NOT TURN HEAD WHILE IN THIS POSITION

ROOT INTO UPPER ARMS FOR STABILITY

PADMA SARVANGASANA lotus shoulder stand

If shoulder stand is becoming a snooze-fest and you're ready to spice it up, you can add lotus with your legs.

Begin in supported shoulder stand (opposite). Slowly bend your legs and bring your right foot in toward your left hip crease and then your left foot in toward your right hip crease. Breathe length through your spine. From here, you can either stay in stillness or play around with bringing your knees toward and away from your face. Breathe in the pose for up to two minutes before reversing the positions of your legs.

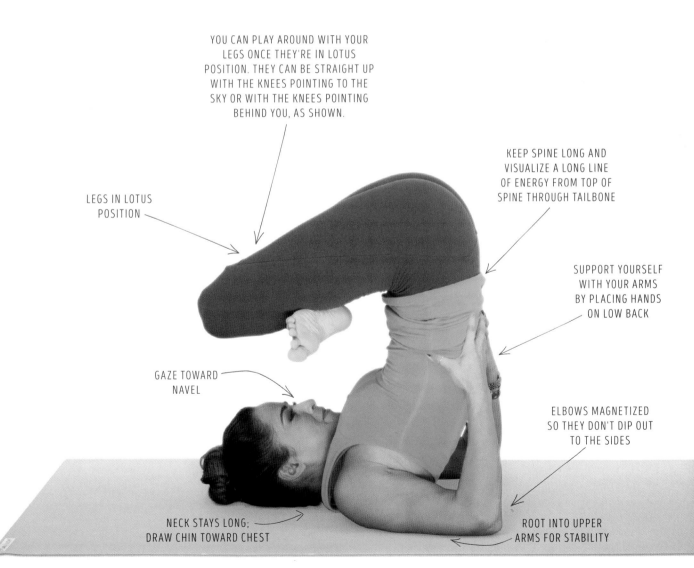

YOU CAN PLAY AROUND WITH YOUR LEGS ONCE THEY'RE IN LOTUS POSITION. THEY CAN BE STRAIGHT UP WITH THE KNEES POINTING TO THE SKY OR WITH THE KNEES POINTING BEHIND YOU, AS SHOWN.

KEEP SPINE LONG AND VISUALIZE A LONG LINE OF ENERGY FROM TOP OF SPINE THROUGH TAILBONE

LEGS IN LOTUS POSITION

SUPPORT YOURSELF WITH YOUR ARMS BY PLACING HANDS ON LOW BACK

GAZE TOWARD NAVEL

ELBOWS MAGNETIZED SO THEY DON'T DIP OUT TO THE SIDES

NECK STAYS LONG; DRAW CHIN TOWARD CHEST

ROOT INTO UPPER ARMS FOR STABILITY

SUPTA PADANGUSTHASANA A AND B
reclining hand-to-big-toe pose A and B

This supine position feels wonderful for tight legs and can easily be modified for people who are super tight.

Begin by lying on your back with your legs extended. As you inhale, tilt your pelvis back slightly to glue your low back to the mat. On your next inhale, lift your right leg. If you're very tight and would like to do the modified version, wrap a yoga strap around the arch of your right foot and grab hold of it as close to the foot as you can. If you aren't using a strap, wrap your peace fingers around your right big toe. Bring your left hand to the top of your left hip and press in to prevent it from lifting. On your next inhale, peel your head and upper back off the mat, drawing your head toward your leg. As you breathe, use your biceps strength to gently pull your leg toward your head. Take three to seven breaths here in part A before opening up your leg to the right for part B.

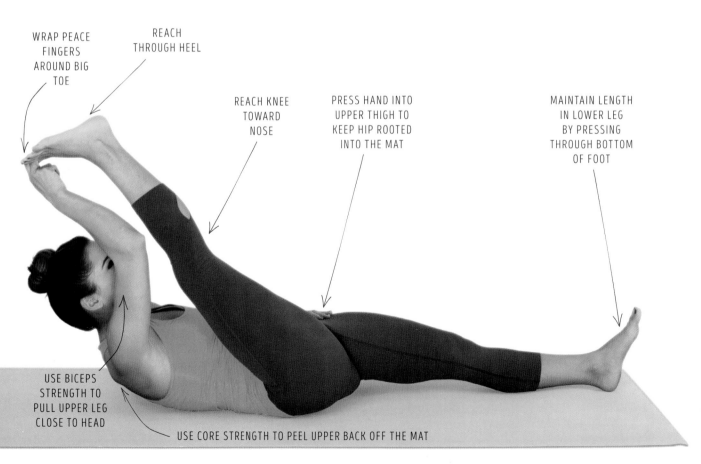

WRAP PEACE FINGERS AROUND BIG TOE

REACH THROUGH HEEL

REACH KNEE TOWARD NOSE

PRESS HAND INTO UPPER THIGH TO KEEP HIP ROOTED INTO THE MAT

MAINTAIN LENGTH IN LOWER LEG BY PRESSING THROUGH BOTTOM OF FOOT

USE BICEPS STRENGTH TO PULL UPPER LEG CLOSE TO HEAD

USE CORE STRENGTH TO PEEL UPPER BACK OFF THE MAT

This is where your left hand comes into play. Often, this shift to the right makes the left hip rise. Encourage your left hip to stay glued to the mat by pressing into the hip with your left hand. Gently flex your right foot to activate the leg muscles as you gently take your gaze over your left shoulder. Breathe fully and deeply for three to seven breaths before bringing your right leg back to center, releasing the pose, and taking it to the other side.

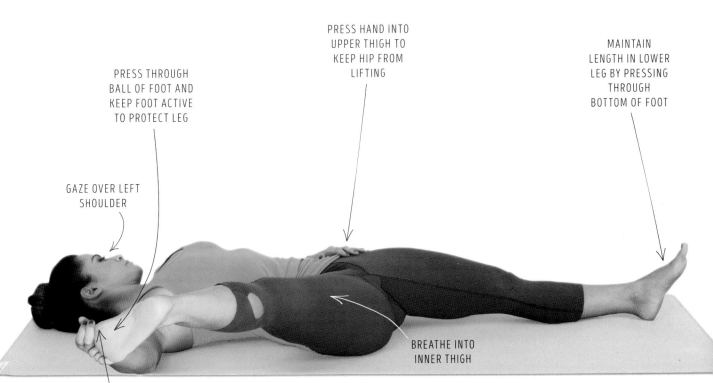

PRESS HAND INTO
UPPER THIGH TO
KEEP HIP FROM
LIFTING

MAINTAIN
LENGTH IN LOWER
LEG BY PRESSING
THROUGH
BOTTOM OF FOOT

PRESS THROUGH
BALL OF FOOT AND
KEEP FOOT ACTIVE
TO PROTECT LEG

GAZE OVER LEFT
SHOULDER

BREATHE INTO
INNER THIGH

WRAP PEACE FINGERS AROUND BIG TOE

BAKASANA crow pose

If you've ever dreamed of flying, crow pose is essentially your ticket to making your dreams come true. It's one of the first arm balances that I teach to intermediate students because it is quite accessible and is what I consider to be the stepping-stone to all major arm balances.

To begin, squat low and place your hands on the mat about shoulder width apart. One of the most common mistakes I see is placing the hands too close together, so double-check that your hands are truly shoulder width. Then lift your hips and walk your feet as close to your arms as you can. Gently perch your knees as high up on your arms as you can. If your knees won't come higher than your elbows, it just means that you are quite tight through the hips and should work on more hip opening before going further.

Once you've perched your knees high up on your arms, it's time to set your gaze. This is really important because you're liable to fall over if you look straight down. True story: My yoga teacher broke her nose that way, so please heed my caution! Instead of looking straight down, look about three feet out in front of you.

With your gaze out in front, magnetize your elbows. Imagine that your elbows have a tension between them—so much so that if someone tried to push your elbows out to the sides, they wouldn't budge. This imaginary magnetization helps protect your wrists. If you allow your elbows to splay, a common mistake, you are dumping the weight into the outsides of your wrists, which is super painful and can cause injury.

✓ DO THIS

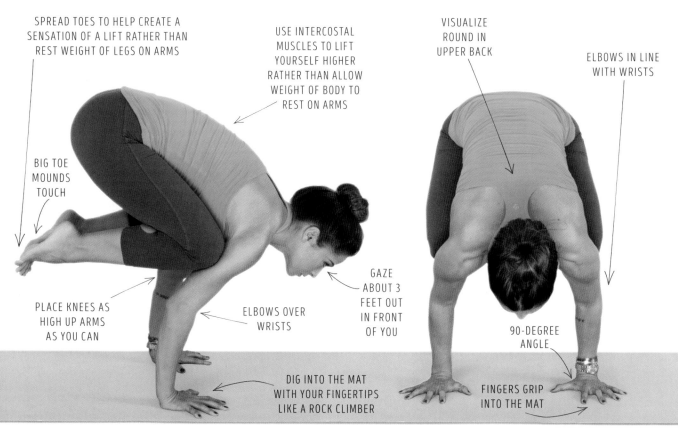

SPREAD TOES TO HELP CREATE A SENSATION OF A LIFT RATHER THAN REST WEIGHT OF LEGS ON ARMS

USE INTERCOSTAL MUSCLES TO LIFT YOURSELF HIGHER RATHER THAN ALLOW WEIGHT OF BODY TO REST ON ARMS

VISUALIZE ROUND IN UPPER BACK

ELBOWS IN LINE WITH WRISTS

BIG TOE MOUNDS TOUCH

PLACE KNEES AS HIGH UP ARMS AS YOU CAN

ELBOWS OVER WRISTS

GAZE ABOUT 3 FEET OUT IN FRONT OF YOU

DIG INTO THE MAT WITH YOUR FINGERTIPS LIKE A ROCK CLIMBER

90-DEGREE ANGLE

FINGERS GRIP INTO THE MAT

The next step is lift off. First things first: do not jump! I repeat, do not jump! Instead, lift just one foot. You may wobble with one foot lifted, and that's cool. It's just your hands calibrating what's going on. Stick with it and don't panic.

Then test what happens when you slowly, gently, and carefully lift the other foot. When it comes up, press your hands into the mat even more and visualize a round beginning to form in your upper back. This round indicates that you are utilizing your intercostal muscles and that you are using upper-body and core strength to lift up rather than resting the weight of your body on your arms.

Spread your toes, which helps create the sensation that you're lifting up. Grip into the mat like you're a rock climber for better stability. Keep your gaze softly out in front of you and imagine that someone has a string wrapped around your torso and is pulling you up. Breathe fully and deeply for however long feels good before slowly releasing.

✕ NOT THIS

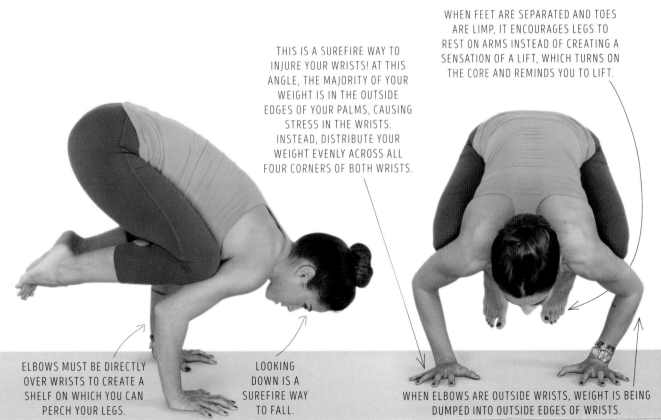

THIS IS A SUREFIRE WAY TO INJURE YOUR WRISTS! AT THIS ANGLE, THE MAJORITY OF YOUR WEIGHT IS IN THE OUTSIDE EDGES OF YOUR PALMS, CAUSING STRESS IN THE WRISTS. INSTEAD, DISTRIBUTE YOUR WEIGHT EVENLY ACROSS ALL FOUR CORNERS OF BOTH WRISTS.

WHEN FEET ARE SEPARATED AND TOES ARE LIMP, IT ENCOURAGES LEGS TO REST ON ARMS INSTEAD OF CREATING A SENSATION OF A LIFT, WHICH TURNS ON THE CORE AND REMINDS YOU TO LIFT.

ELBOWS MUST BE DIRECTLY OVER WRISTS TO CREATE A SHELF ON WHICH YOU CAN PERCH YOUR LEGS.

LOOKING DOWN IS A SUREFIRE WAY TO FALL.

WHEN ELBOWS ARE OUTSIDE WRISTS, WEIGHT IS BEING DUMPED INTO OUTSIDE EDGES OF WRISTS.

arm balances and inversions   223

PARSVA BAKASANA side crow pose

Side crow is a really fun pose and another one I consider to be a stepping-stone to interesting transitions and other playful arm balances. It requires a solid amount of openness and flexibility through the torso and hips, so be aware of that. If you give it a go and it's just not happening for you, you likely need to work on your flexibility in those areas.

I usually teach two variations of side crow. One is considered the modified version, but it's only a modified version if you have pretty open hips—otherwise it's a beast. The other variation is the full expression, which requires a good amount of upper-body strength but not as much hip openness. What I'm trying to say is that some people are going to find the so-called modified version harder than the traditional, full expression, so I suggest that you give both variations a try to see which works better for you.

"Modified" Version

Begin by squatting low with your feet and knees together and your heels raised. Keeping your feet where they are, swing your knees to the right. Then place your hands on the mat, shoulder width apart. Make sure that they are truly shoulder width; one of the common mistakes I see is placing the hands too close together. Spread your fingers, grip into the mat as if you're a rock climber, and use your fingertips to help find your balance. On your next inhale, lift your hips and perch your stacked knees as high up on your right arm as you can. Then perch your stacked hips as high up on your left arm as you can. Keep your arms in "wax on, wax off" position. While you definitely want upper-body and core strength to be what holds you up, the fact is that this position sets you up so that you can rest your body weight on your arms, so keeping your arms pulled in will help create a more stable foundation. Slowly come forward until one foot lifts, followed closely by the other foot. Keep your gaze on the ground about three feet out in front of you and continue using your fingertips to maintain your balance. Take three to seven deep breaths here before switching sides.

MODIFIED VERSION   ALTERNATE VIEW

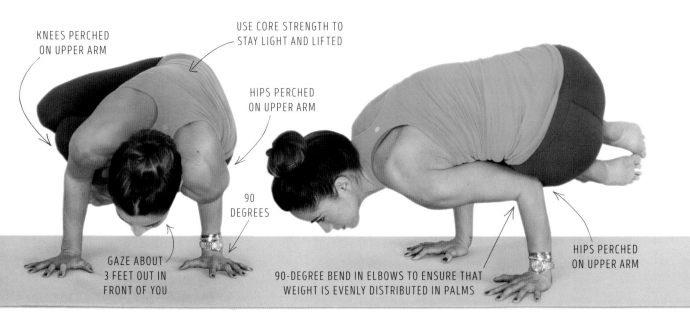

KNEES PERCHED
ON UPPER ARM

USE CORE STRENGTH TO
STAY LIGHT AND LIFTED

HIPS PERCHED
ON UPPER ARM

90
DEGREES

GAZE ABOUT
3 FEET OUT IN
FRONT OF YOU

90-DEGREE BEND IN ELBOWS TO ENSURE THAT
WEIGHT IS EVENLY DISTRIBUTED IN PALMS

HIPS PERCHED
ON UPPER ARM

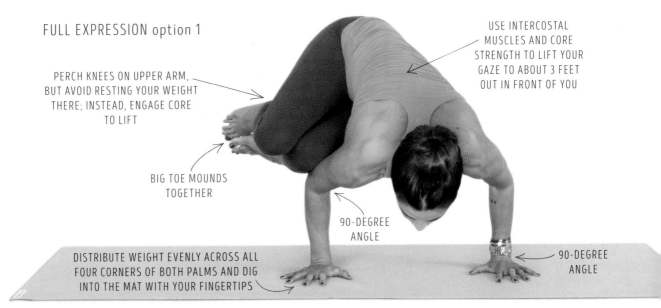

FULL EXPRESSION option 1

PERCH KNEES ON UPPER ARM, BUT AVOID RESTING YOUR WEIGHT THERE; INSTEAD, ENGAGE CORE TO LIFT

USE INTERCOSTAL MUSCLES AND CORE STRENGTH TO LIFT YOUR GAZE TO ABOUT 3 FEET OUT IN FRONT OF YOU

BIG TOE MOUNDS TOGETHER

90-DEGREE ANGLE

90-DEGREE ANGLE

DISTRIBUTE WEIGHT EVENLY ACROSS ALL FOUR CORNERS OF BOTH PALMS AND DIG INTO THE MAT WITH YOUR FINGERTIPS

Full Version

Begin by squatting low with your feet and knees together and your heels raised. Keeping your feet where they are, swing your knees to the right. Then place your hands on the mat, shoulder width apart. Make sure that they are truly shoulder width; one of the common mistakes I see is placing the hands too close together. Spread your fingers, grip into the mat as if you're a rock climber, and use your fingertips to find your balance. On your next inhale, lift your hips and perch your stacked knees as high up on your right arm as you can. Then look about three feet out in front of you on the ground and slowly begin to come forward, lifting one foot and then the other. Keep your elbows magnetized, as if there's an invisible tension between them. This helps prevent the elbows from splaying out to the sides, which indicates that your weight is being dumped into the outer edges of your palms and can be dangerous for your wrists.

If you feel great here, you can extend your legs for an added challenge. Keep your hips light and lifted and visualize a round in your upper back, imagining the space between your shoulder blades inflating. Take three to seven deep breaths here before switching sides.

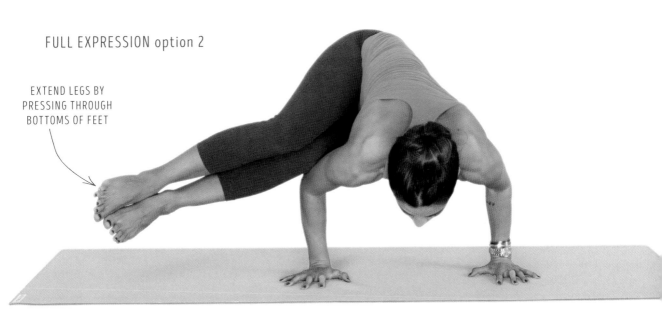

FULL EXPRESSION option 2

EXTEND LEGS BY PRESSING THROUGH BOTTOMS OF FEET

ASTAVAKRASANA eight-angle pose

This is one of my favorite poses to teach because it always throws people off—but in the best way. When I demonstrate it, I usually get eye-rolls and "I can't do that" mumbles, but then something incredible happens. People try it and realize that it's a lot easier than it looks! Eight-angle pose does require a good amount of hip flexibility, so if you're struggling with it, work on hip openness. It also requires a bit of upper-body strength, so if you're having trouble holding yourself up, keep working on building upper-body strength with poses like downward-facing dog (page 100).

Begin seated with your left leg bent with the knee on the ground and your right leg bent with the bottom of the foot on the ground. Lift your right leg and place the back of the knee as high up on your right arm as you can. Clamp your right leg around your right arm and squeeze it tightly so that it stays put. Open your arms about six inches wider than shoulder width and cross your left foot over the top of your right foot. Place your hands flat on the ground with the fingers spread as wide as possible. "Plug in" to the mat to ensure that your weight is evenly distributed, particularly between your thumbs and index fingers. Squeeze your elbows in toward your body and lean forward until your hips lift up. Continue bringing your chest down and your hips up. Squeeze your legs together and press out of the bottoms of your feet to extend the legs. Visualize your shoulders being even and avoid allowing your left shoulder to round. Take three to seven deep breaths in this position before switching sides.

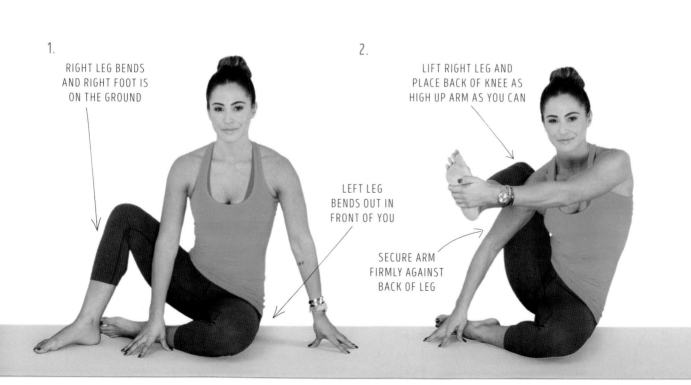

1.

RIGHT LEG BENDS AND RIGHT FOOT IS ON THE GROUND

LEFT LEG BENDS OUT IN FRONT OF YOU

2.

LIFT RIGHT LEG AND PLACE BACK OF KNEE AS HIGH UP ARM AS YOU CAN

SECURE ARM FIRMLY AGAINST BACK OF LEG

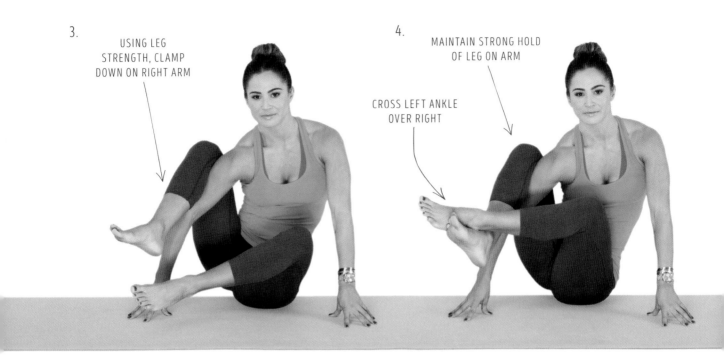

3. USING LEG STRENGTH, CLAMP DOWN ON RIGHT ARM

4. MAINTAIN STRONG HOLD OF LEG ON ARM

CROSS LEFT ANKLE OVER RIGHT

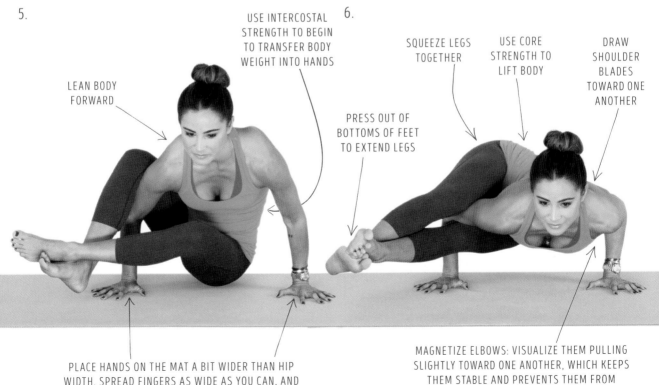

5. LEAN BODY FORWARD

USE INTERCOSTAL STRENGTH TO BEGIN TO TRANSFER BODY WEIGHT INTO HANDS

PLACE HANDS ON THE MAT A BIT WIDER THAN HIP WIDTH, SPREAD FINGERS AS WIDE AS YOU CAN, AND BEGIN TO PUSH INTO HANDS TO LIFT UP

6. SQUEEZE LEGS TOGETHER

USE CORE STRENGTH TO LIFT BODY

DRAW SHOULDER BLADES TOWARD ONE ANOTHER

PRESS OUT OF BOTTOMS OF FEET TO EXTEND LEGS

MAGNETIZE ELBOWS: VISUALIZE THEM PULLING SLIGHTLY TOWARD ONE ANOTHER, WHICH KEEPS THEM STABLE AND PREVENTS THEM FROM SPLAYING OUT TO THE SIDES

EKA PADA GALAVASANA (flying pigeon pose) variation
baby flying pigeon pose

This is one of my favorite poses because it's a vehicle to so many amazing places on the yoga journey. I know, that was borderline cheesy. I cheese it up sometimes—I'll own that. Bear with me.

This pose requires upper-body strength, core strength, and some hip flexibility, so keep that in mind if you find yourself struggling.

Start in standing pigeon pose (page 201) with your left ankle crossed over your right thigh, and hinge at the hips as you bring your hands shoulder width apart. Check to be sure that the hands are shoulder width; the hands being too close together is one of the common mistakes I see. Spread your fingers as wide as you can. Take your gaze to the ground about three feet out in front of you as you rise up off your right heel. Tip forward until your left shin perches on your arms. Aim to perch your shin as high up on the arms as you can and spread your toes. Spreading the toes helps encourage the lower body to stay active and engaged. Using your right toes, send your body forward until your shoulders are past your wrists and your elbows are in line with your wrists. Round your upper back and imagine that someone has a string wrapped around your torso and is lifting you up. This visualization will encourage you to use your core strength to lift your body rather than allow the weight of your body to rest on your arms. Use your fingertips to help find your sense of balance and breathe fully and deeply for three to seven breaths before switching sides.

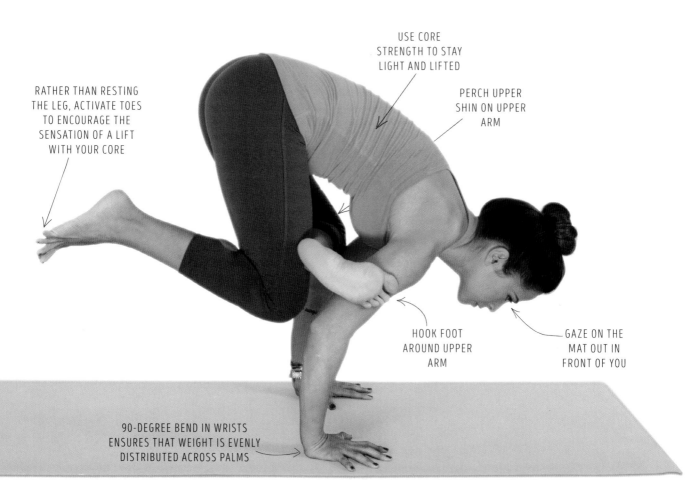

USE CORE STRENGTH TO STAY LIGHT AND LIFTED

PERCH UPPER SHIN ON UPPER ARM

RATHER THAN RESTING THE LEG, ACTIVATE TOES TO ENCOURAGE THE SENSATION OF A LIFT WITH YOUR CORE

HOOK FOOT AROUND UPPER ARM

GAZE ON THE MAT OUT IN FRONT OF YOU

90-DEGREE BEND IN WRISTS ENSURES THAT WEIGHT IS EVENLY DISTRIBUTED ACROSS PALMS

SALAMBA SIRSASANA supported headstand

Headstand is up there with crow pose (page 222) in that it's one of the first arm balances I teach. I love them both because they can take you so many places in the yoga practice.

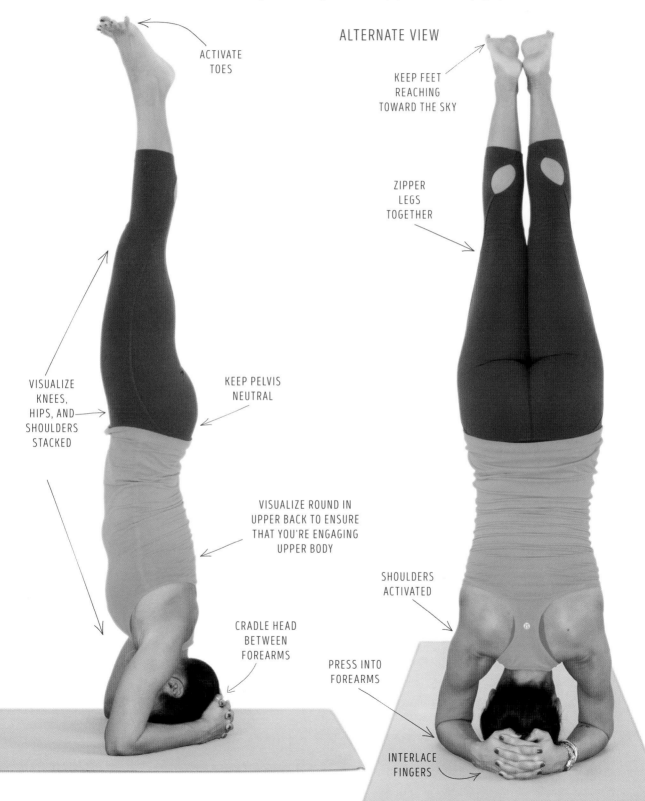

ACTIVATE
TOES

ALTERNATE VIEW

KEEP FEET
REACHING
TOWARD THE SKY

ZIPPER
LEGS
TOGETHER

VISUALIZE
KNEES,
HIPS, AND
SHOULDERS
STACKED

KEEP PELVIS
NEUTRAL

VISUALIZE ROUND IN
UPPER BACK TO ENSURE
THAT YOU'RE ENGAGING
UPPER BODY

SHOULDERS
ACTIVATED

CRADLE HEAD
BETWEEN
FOREARMS

PRESS INTO
FOREARMS

INTERLACE
FINGERS

Before you start, you need to find the proper place on your head that will be placed on the mat. To find it, place the heel of your hand on your face where your eyebrows begin. Then lay your palm flat on your forehead. Your middle finger should end at the crown of your head. Tap that spot a few times with your middle finger so you know to place that part of your head on the mat.

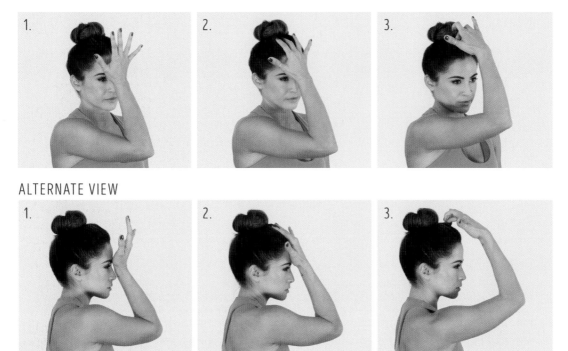

ALTERNATE VIEW

Begin by sitting on your shins, then bring your forearms to the mat and grab opposite biceps. Really grab the biceps, not the elbows; one of the most common mistakes I see is the arms being too far apart. Grabbing the biceps ensures that your arms are in great alignment. Keeping your elbows there, let go of your biceps, bring your hands out in front of you, and interlace the fingers, pressing the knife-edges of your hands into the mat. As you press your forearms into the mat, notice that your upper back rounds. This helps engage the shoulder girdle and upper body, which supports your weight rather than allowing all that weight to be dumped into your head (which you want to avoid!). Bring the crown of your head (where your middle finger tapped) down so that your hands are cradling the back of your head.

Then straighten your legs and walk your feet as close to your body as you can. This requires major hamstring flexibility, so if it's tough for you, keep working on opening up your hammies. When you feel that your pelvis is directly over your head, lift one leg. Keep pressing into your forearms as you spread your toes and use your hamstring strength to lift your other leg off the mat. Do not jump! Instead, move super slowly and use your core strength to come into the pose. I always tell people who are new to headstand to make a V with the legs—that is, to split the legs so that when viewed from the side, the body is making the shape of the letter Y. In this position, the legs act like a seesaw, and you can use them to find balance. Spread your toes and move slowly. When you find your balance, you can work on bringing your legs together and squeezing the inner thighs together.

The majority of your weight should be in your forearms, so keep pushing the mat away from you. Breathe fully and deeply for as long as it feels good. When you're ready, gently release and come into child's pose (page 93). Avoid coming up too quickly, as the blood can quickly go to your head and cause you to feel a bit faint.

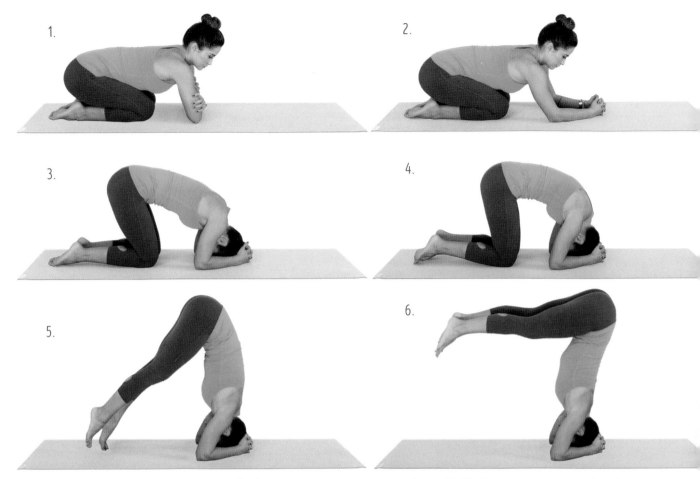

1. Grab opposite biceps, not opposite elbows (a common mistake) so that you can position your elbows underneath you in a way that fully supports your body.

2. Once you grab opposite biceps, keep your elbows where they are and take your hands out in front of you as you interlace your fingers.

3. Place the top of your head on the mat as described on page 230 and press into your forearms to engage your shoulders and create a small round in your upper back.

4. Round more and begin to lift your hips.

5. Straighten your legs and walk your feet forward until your hips come over your head.

6. Slowly and gently begin to transfer the weight to your arms as you use core and back strength to lift your legs. Avoid jumping or kicking. If you'd like to come up with one leg lifted, hop off the bottom foot rather than using momentum and kicking with your lifted leg. Kicking with the lifted leg doesn't use control and can be dangerous, as you'll flip over if you kick too hard. Find control and move with intention.

7. Bring the legs all the way up and squeeze your inner thighs together as you visualize your head, pelvis, and ankles in one line.

MUKTA HASTA SIRSASANA A tripod headstand

Do you want to know a secret? Tripod headstand was impossible for me for years! In fact, I really only started doing it about a year ago. For some reason, supported headstand (page 229) was so much more accessible to me than tripod, but oddly, many of my friends feel the opposite! So keep that in the back of your mind. If supported headstand eludes you, maybe tripod will be your jam.

Setup for Tripod Headstand

It's important to set up correctly for every pose, but it's especially important for tripod. I like to visualize a large triangle drawn on my mat. In fact, when I teach this pose, I have my students draw one with their finger. Do "wax on, wax off" with your arms, then place your hands on the mat. Your hands go on each corner at the base of the triangle, and your head (that same place where your middle finger taps, as described in supported headstand) goes at the top.

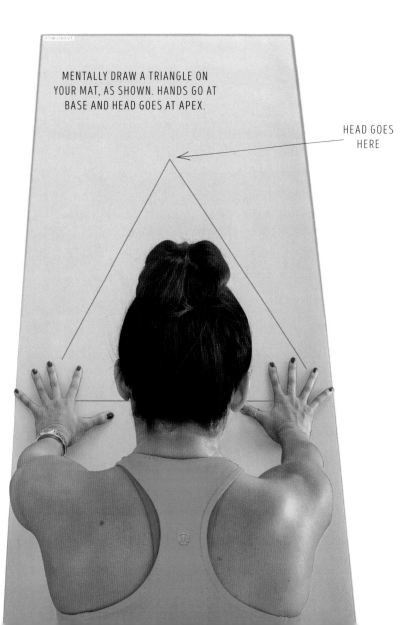

MENTALLY DRAW A TRIANGLE ON YOUR MAT, AS SHOWN. HANDS GO AT BASE AND HEAD GOES AT APEX.

HEAD GOES HERE

Once your head is down, check that your arms are still in "wax on, wax off" position. Do not let your elbows splay out to the sides. Spread your fingers and grip into the mat. From here, you have a few options for entering the pose. Here are my top three:

• Lift your hips and extend your legs, then walk your feet as close to your head as you can. When you feel like your pelvis is over your head, lift one leg and spread the toes. Use your back-body strength to lift the other leg and slowly zipper the legs together.

• Perch one knee on each arm and press into your arms until you feel that your pelvis is over your head. From here, slowly use your intercostal and upper-body strength to lift your feet.

• Lift your hips and extend your legs, then walk your feet as close to your head as you can. Press into your toes until you feel like your pelvis is over your head. From here, use your hamstring strength to float your legs together up to the sky.

Whichever way you choose to come up, always move slowly and keep the majority of your weight in your arms. Maintain the sensation of "wax on, wax off" in your arms, and breathe fully and deeply. When you're ready to release the pose, slowly bring your legs to the ground and come into child's pose (page 93). Avoid lifting your head all the way up too quickly after a headstand, as it may cause you to feel faint.

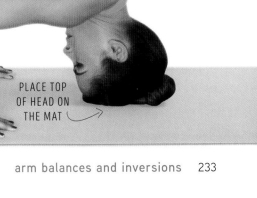

ACTIVATE TOES TO KEEP THE SENSATION OF A LIFT THROUGH ENTIRE BODY

ZIPPER LEGS TOGETHER

MAKE ARMS SO STRONG THAT THEY WOULDN'T MOVE IF SOMEONE TRIED TO PUSH THEM

ACTIVATE INTERCOSTAL MUSCLES AND CORE TO KEEP TORSO LIGHT AND LIFTED

MAGNETIZE ELBOWS TO MAINTAIN A SOLID, STABLE FOUNDATION

SPREAD FINGERS AND GRIP INTO THE MAT WITH FINGERTIPS

PLACE TOP OF HEAD ON THE MAT

DEVADUUTA PANNA ASANA fallen angel pose

I'm not going to lie to you; this pose always terrified me. It looks so dangerous for your neck, right?! I thought for sure that this is how it would all end for me. I was convinced that my neck would snap in half. But, as with nearly everything we worry about, none of those fears came true. Life lesson, my friend. My point is, if you're scared, I get it. But do it anyway (after you've built up some upper-body strength and have a solid arm-balance practice). You'll likely be pleasantly surprised by what you can do when you get out of your own way.

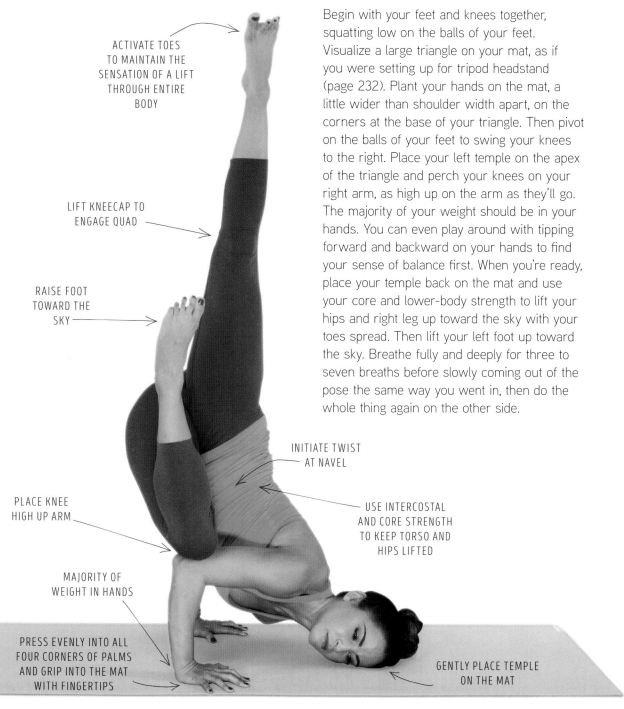

ACTIVATE TOES
TO MAINTAIN THE
SENSATION OF A LIFT
THROUGH ENTIRE
BODY

LIFT KNEECAP TO
ENGAGE QUAD

RAISE FOOT
TOWARD THE
SKY

PLACE KNEE
HIGH UP ARM

MAJORITY OF
WEIGHT IN HANDS

PRESS EVENLY INTO ALL
FOUR CORNERS OF PALMS
AND GRIP INTO THE MAT
WITH FINGERTIPS

INITIATE TWIST
AT NAVEL

USE INTERCOSTAL
AND CORE STRENGTH
TO KEEP TORSO AND
HIPS LIFTED

GENTLY PLACE TEMPLE
ON THE MAT

Begin with your feet and knees together, squatting low on the balls of your feet. Visualize a large triangle on your mat, as if you were setting up for tripod headstand (page 232). Plant your hands on the mat, a little wider than shoulder width apart, on the corners at the base of your triangle. Then pivot on the balls of your feet to swing your knees to the right. Place your left temple on the apex of the triangle and perch your knees on your right arm, as high up on the arm as they'll go. The majority of your weight should be in your hands. You can even play around with tipping forward and backward on your hands to find your sense of balance first. When you're ready, place your temple back on the mat and use your core and lower-body strength to lift your hips and right leg up toward the sky with your toes spread. Then lift your left foot up toward the sky. Breathe fully and deeply for three to seven breaths before slowly coming out of the pose the same way you went in, then do the whole thing again on the other side.

HALASANA plow pose

This pose feels incredible on my back. It is an inversion that I love to do at the end of a long day.

Begin in supported shoulder stand (page 218). Extend your arms (or interlace your fingers and press your forearms into the ground) and bring your legs overhead, pressing the balls of your feet into the mat behind you. Keep your legs active, seeing if you can feel a good strength through the backs of your hips and hamstrings. As you breathe, visualize space being created in the back of your rib cage. Breathe here for three to seven breaths. When you're ready to release the pose, gently push through the balls of your feet to lower your spine vertebra by vertebra. Use your arms as brakes as you lower down and challenge yourself to go slower than you want to go.

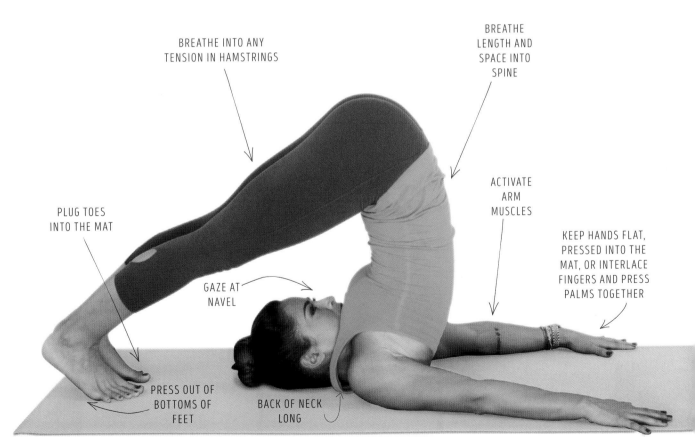

BREATHE INTO ANY
TENSION IN HAMSTRINGS

BREATHE
LENGTH AND
SPACE INTO
SPINE

ACTIVATE
ARM
MUSCLES

PLUG TOES
INTO THE MAT

KEEP HANDS FLAT,
PRESSED INTO THE
MAT, OR INTERLACE
FINGERS AND PRESS
PALMS TOGETHER

GAZE AT
NAVEL

PRESS OUT OF
BOTTOMS OF
FEET

BACK OF NECK
LONG

URDHVA DHANURASANA wheel pose

Wheel pose is a longtime favorite of mine because it's a nod to my childhood gymnastics days. The key is to have lots of openness through the front body, especially in the hip flexors, armpits, and chest. If you're struggling with this pose, continue to work on those areas. Once the flexibility is there, the full expression will appear.

Begin by lying on your back. As you inhale, bend your legs, bringing your feet as close to your pelvis as you can. Your feet should be hip width apart and your toes pointed straight out in front of you. Do not allow them to splay out to the sides, which can create unnecessary pressure through the knees and trigger an injury. If you struggle with this, place a block between your lower thighs and squeeze it as you move through the pose. The need to squeeze your legs will help prevent your toes from splaying and ultimately will help protect your knees.

From here, bend your arms so that your elbows are pointed straight up to the sky, your palms are flat on the ground on either side of your ears, and your fingers are pointed toward your traps. If you have trouble pointing your elbows straight up to the sky, your triceps are tight, so work on opening up through the shoulders, chest, armpits, and triceps.

When you're ready, take a deep breath in and press into your feet and hands to lift your entire body off the ground. If it feels okay for your neck, gaze between your thumbs toward the mat. Feel that your knees are pointing straight out in front of you and not splaying to the sides. Breathe length through your entire front body, from your knees through your armpits. Imagine that if you were looking into a mirror placed to your side, your body would be making an upside-down U-shape rather than a V-shape. That is, avoid compression in your low back by breathing length between the vertebrae in your spine. Take three to seven breaths in this pose. When you're ready to release, slowly lower your body to the ground.

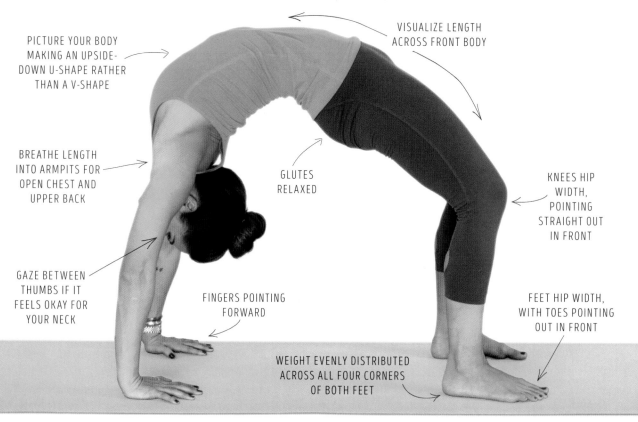

PICTURE YOUR BODY MAKING AN UPSIDE-DOWN U-SHAPE RATHER THAN A V-SHAPE

VISUALIZE LENGTH ACROSS FRONT BODY

BREATHE LENGTH INTO ARMPITS FOR OPEN CHEST AND UPPER BACK

GLUTES RELAXED

KNEES HIP WIDTH, POINTING STRAIGHT OUT IN FRONT

GAZE BETWEEN THUMBS IF IT FEELS OKAY FOR YOUR NECK

FINGERS POINTING FORWARD

FEET HIP WIDTH, WITH TOES POINTING OUT IN FRONT

WEIGHT EVENLY DISTRIBUTED ACROSS ALL FOUR CORNERS OF BOTH FEET

KARNAPIDASANA knee-to-ear pose

This pose requires major flexibility through the spine but is really fun to do between plow pose (page 235) and supported shoulder stand (page 218).

    Begin in supported shoulder stand. Slowly bend your knees, lowering them toward your ears. Keep your gaze toward your navel to protect your neck, and keep your feet light and lifted to encourage your body to stay engaged and lifted. Press your arms into the ground with the hands flat, as shown, or interlace the fingers and press the knife-edges of your palms into the mat. As you breathe, imagine that you're creating space between the vertebrae in your spine. Take three to seven breaths in this pose before moving on.

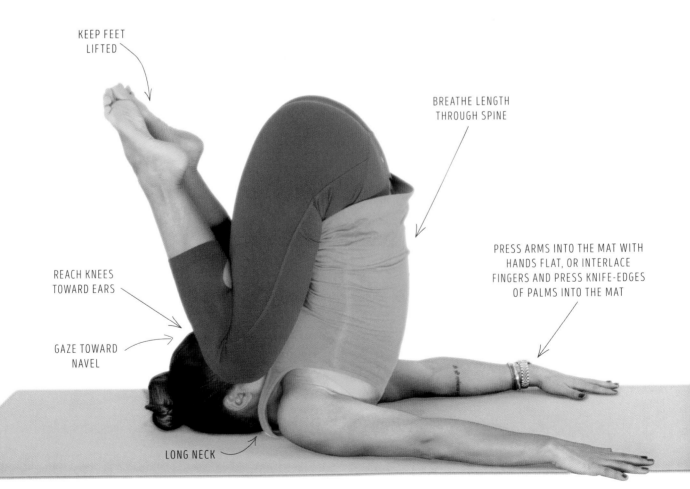

KEEP FEET LIFTED

BREATHE LENGTH THROUGH SPINE

PRESS ARMS INTO THE MAT WITH HANDS FLAT, OR INTERLACE FINGERS AND PRESS KNIFE-EDGES OF PALMS INTO THE MAT

REACH KNEES TOWARD EARS

GAZE TOWARD NAVEL

LONG NECK

sequence 1

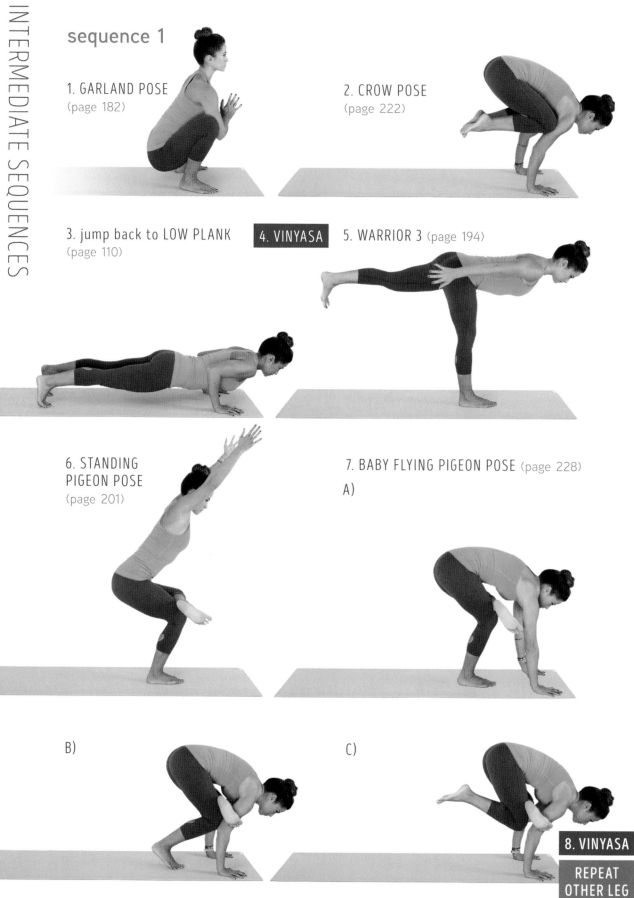

1. GARLAND POSE
(page 182)

2. CROW POSE
(page 222)

3. jump back to LOW PLANK
(page 110)

4. VINYASA

5. WARRIOR 3 (page 194)

6. STANDING PIGEON POSE
(page 201)

7. BABY FLYING PIGEON POSE (page 228)

A)

B)

C)

8. VINYASA

REPEAT OTHER LEG

sequence 2

1. SIDE CROW POSE (page 224)

A)

B)

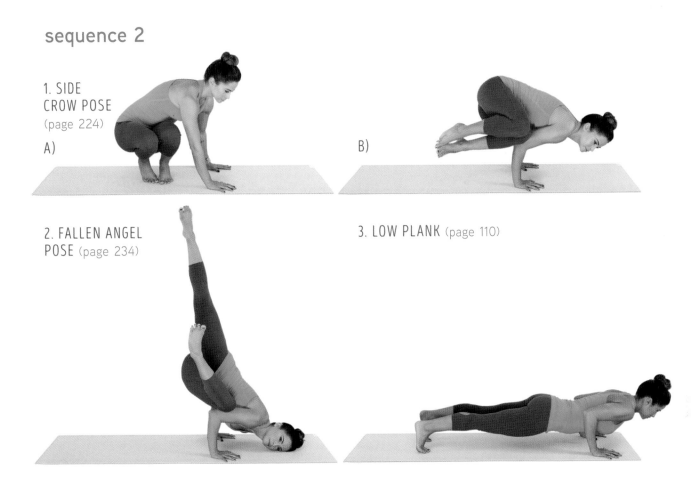

2. FALLEN ANGEL POSE (page 234)

3. LOW PLANK (page 110)

4. SIDE PLANK with lifted leg (page 193)

5. VINYASA

REPEAT OTHER LEG

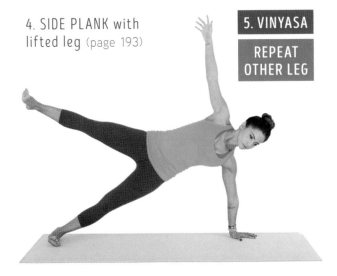

sequence 3

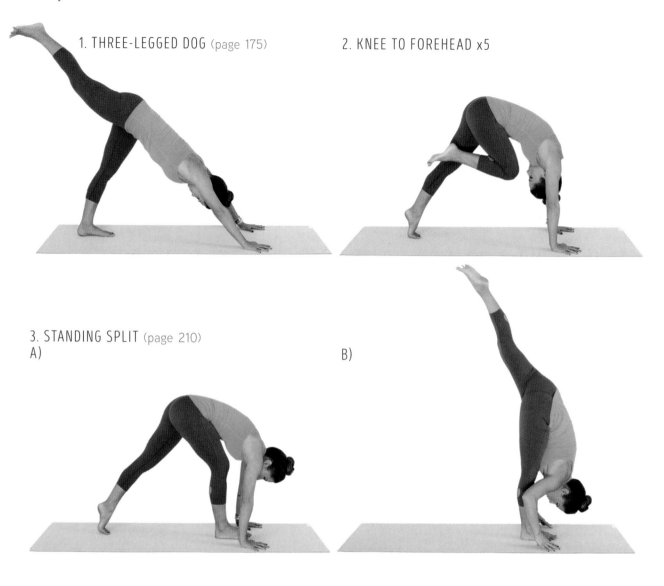

1. THREE-LEGGED DOG (page 175)

2. KNEE TO FOREHEAD x5

3. STANDING SPLIT (page 210)
A)

B)

4. HALF SPINAL TWIST (page 172)
A)

B)

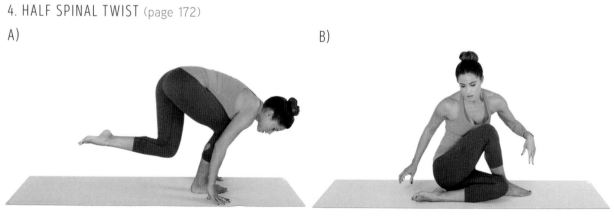

C)

5. WIDE-LEG FORWARD FOLD A (page 120)

A)

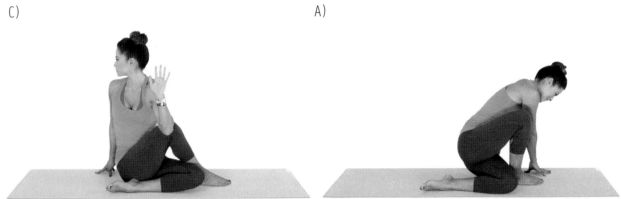

B)

6. VINYASA

REPEAT OTHER SIDE

sequence 4

1. TRIPOD HEADSTAND
(page 232)

A)

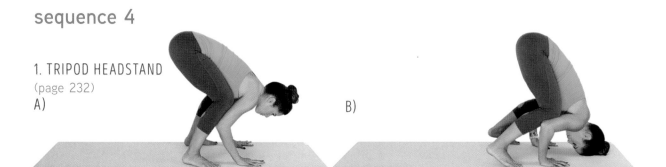

B)

C)

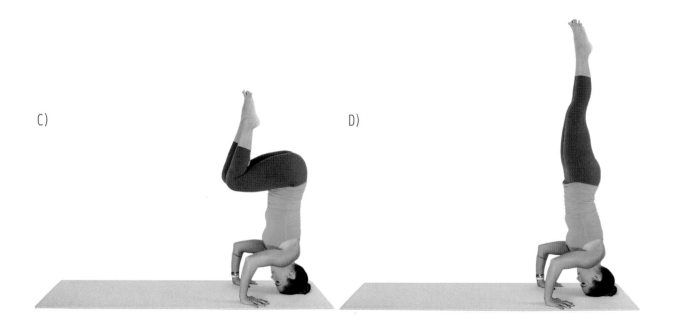

D)

2. CROW POSE (page 222)

A)

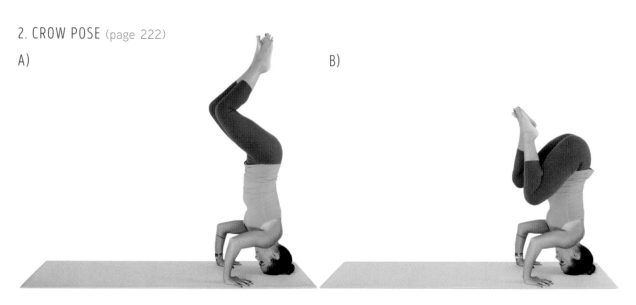

B)

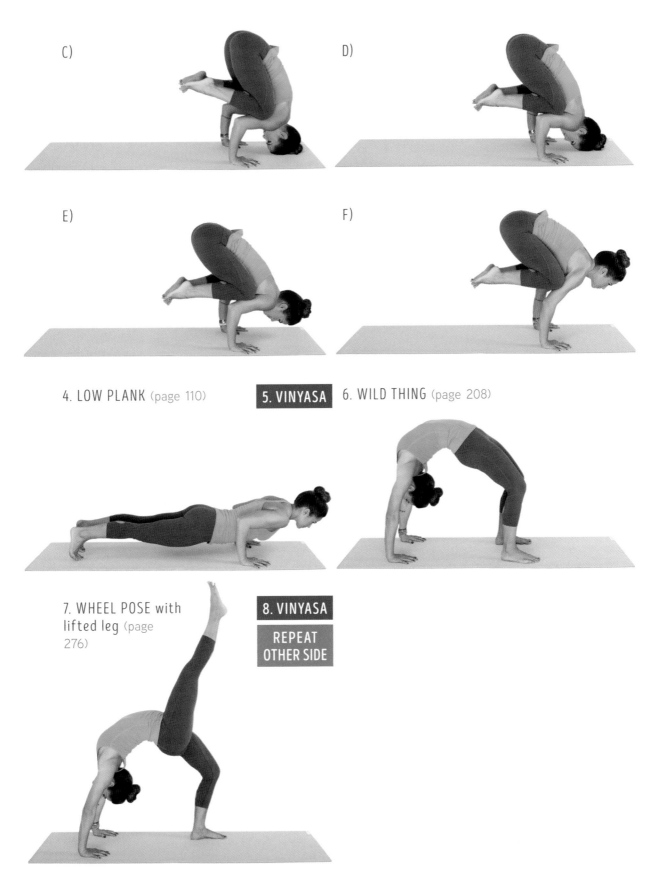

C)

D)

E)

F)

4. LOW PLANK (page 110)

5. VINYASA

6. WILD THING (page 208)

7. WHEEL POSE with lifted leg (page 276)

8. VINYASA

REPEAT OTHER SIDE

sequence 5

1. EAGLE POSE
(page 204)

2. WARRIOR 1
(page 113)

3. VINYASA

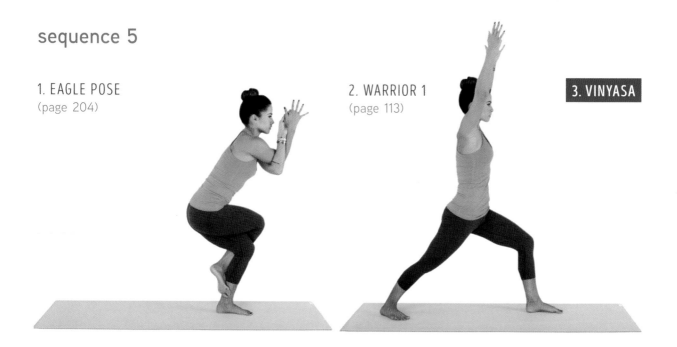

4. PIGEON POSE
(page 97)

5. MERMAID POSE
(page 164)

6. VINYASA

REPEAT OTHER SIDE

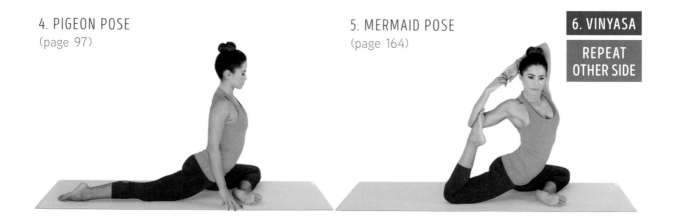

moving on
March 2012

The hotel room I'm in is one that I will remember forever. It is an oversized suite with a bathtub made of tiny tiles. The windows overlook lush Thai grounds that are bursting with Skittles-colored flowers, and just beyond is the bright blue sea. I have completed my yoga teacher training and am taking a few days to myself in Phuket before heading back to Germany to meet Greg and pack up our stuff for our nineteenth move in six years together. It is the off-season, and we are excited to go home.

I will remember this room for the views. For the incredible tub. For the glorious air-conditioning. For the remarkable handmade teak furniture. And for the amount of pain I experience. It's 6 a.m., and I am writhing in excruciating pain. My entire body feels like it is seizing up. I moan audibly, trying to breathe through it, and momentarily wonder if I could pass out from the pain. I am sweating profusely and my sheets are soaked, yet I feel chilled to the bone. My arms lock up and I sob loudly, giving into it all.

In twenty minutes, it's over. This exact episode has repeated itself every morning and night for the last three weeks. I get out of bed, shuffle to my luggage, and pop three Aleve pills to deal with my joint pain. These are the first of nine Aleve pills that I take each day, and it doesn't occur to me that this might be bad for me. In addition to the Aleve, I am still taking a heavy dose of antibiotics along with an anti-yeast pill, and with all the pills I'm popping it's really no wonder that I feel like the walking dead.

****

Back in Germany, I am trying to help Greg pack. All his teammates and their wives and girlfriends left a few weeks ago, and the off-season is well underway. We're both eager to get our summer started before we have to deal with contract negotiations for the next hockey season.

I am trying to pack my clothing, but I can barely lift my arms because they feel like anchors. Once they come parallel to the ground, they freeze up, and I can't lift them any higher. My whole body feels stiff and painful. I ask Greg to rub my shoulders.

"Candace," he says incredulously, "your shoulders are as hard as rocks!" His hands cup my traps and he digs his thumbs into the space between my shoulder blades, but my back feels frozen. No matter how hard he presses, his thumbs can't make any headway in loosening up my muscles. Tears run down my face and I collapse into him, apologizing for not being able to help him pack.

"I can tell you're really hurting," he says quietly, wiping away my tears.

"Can you get me some Aleve from the medicine cabinet?" I ask.

A few days later, our apartment is packed up, but I can't sit up to eat. Every time I sit up, pain runs up through my chest, and I have this weird gurgly burping that won't stop. As soon as I lie down, I feel relief. As a result, I eat lying down.

The ride to the airport is stressful because Buckles is panicking. He's next to me in the backseat doing his half-cry, half-bark thing for the entire drive down the Autobahn to Munich International Airport. Trying not to pass out from the pain in my stomach, I resort to laying myself over the dog to find slight relief.

We get to the airport and are dropped off with our life's possessions in six hockey bags. We stand at the oversized baggage area to check in. I tell Greg that I need to lie down and go lie in the waiting area, sprawled over three chairs.

Minutes later, I decide to ask the lady at the desk if there's a doctor at the airport. *Maybe if I could get something to make this stomach pain go away*, I think, *I'd feel a whole lot better.*

The blond in the booth looks at me and says, "You really can't fly if you're sick—but I'll call the doctor."

I walk away and lie down on the chairs again, in too much pain to argue with her.

The next thing I know, four paramedics with a stretcher come racing into the waiting area and rush to my side. The people around me form a circle. The paramedics take my vitals and talk back and forth in stern German before one looks me in the eye and says, "Appendicitis."

They start to wheel me away, and I can see the concern in Greg's eyes. "Don't worry," he says. "I'll have them get the dog back from the plane and then I'll come find you." The paramedics hurry me outside into an ambulance and whisk me to a hospital.

At the hospital they do all sorts of tests, and it is determined that I do not have appendicitis, but I need to stay put for observation.

"What? But I need to go home. I had a flight today, and I really just need to get home," I plead with the doctor.

I feel like I'm in a scene from *Grey's Anatomy*. The doctor is an older man with a very German face— defined jawbone, piercing blue eyes, and blond hair. He is surrounded by four very young-looking medical students. One of the students picks up my folder and reads a little report about me to the group. I pick out German words here and there.

"*Nein,*" the doctor snaps at me. "You are not allowed to eat. You must stay here for obserwation. When you, uh, pass shtool, you can go. You must pass shtool."

Pass shtool, pass shtool, I repeat to myself, furrowing my brow and trying to figure out what in the world that means.

"Pass shtool?" I ask.

"Yah. Pass shtool—in zee toilet."

Oh God. Now I have eighty-five questions, none of which I will ask because I am chicken shit, but, like, how are they supposed to *know* when I pass shtool? Am I supposed to show them like a small child who is being potty-trained? If I don't drag someone into the bathroom with me, are they going to think I'm lying? Can I just lie and tell them that I've already *passed shtool*? I just want to go home!

In Germany, medical stuff is done differently. You can pay for private healthcare, or a public healthcare policy will be given to you. Private care comes with a lot of perks, like private hospital rooms. Greg and I have public healthcare, which means that right now I'm being wheeled into a room with three other people.

The old woman in the bed across from me is about eighty years old, with dementia. The woman next to her is a drunk sleeping off her latest bender. I only know this because the sixty-year-old woman in the bed next to me tells me so with animated eyes. She speaks enough English to give me the rundown of the room and tells me that she has lung cancer. She has purple hair and a kind smile, and she thinks it's bullshit that I am not allowed to eat.

"How are you supposed to pass shtool if you are not allowed to eat?" she clucks to herself. Then she says, "Psst!" and gives me a tissue wrapped around three shortbread cookies.

The old woman who has dementia wakes up and shouts "*ALO!*" in a singsong voice.

"*Scheisse,*" swears my new friend. "Ziss voman vill drive us crazy," she warns.

"*ALO!*" shouts the old woman.

I stare up at the ceiling, on which there is a brightly painted mural showing people of all colors holding hands and encircling the globe.

"*ALO!*" shouts the old woman.

My new friend yells at the poor old lady to be quiet, and the old lady responds by trying to rip out her IV. She is panicking and screaming in German, and my friend is urging her to stop it. My friend looks at me and says, "Call zee nurse! Press zee button!" Wide-eyed, I repeatedly press the red button on the side of my bed.

"*ALO!*" shouts the old woman as she rips her IV out. The IV tube flies out of her arm and waves around the room like a flag in the wind. IV fluid spurts out, and I can see her arm starting to bleed.

Two nurses rush in and scold her as they each grab hold of an arm. A third nurse rushes in with a needle, and they sedate her and secure her arms with Velcro straps. In a minute, all is quiet.

Twenty minutes later, Greg rushes through the door.

"Oh my God," he says, out of breath. "Are you okay?! I can't believe I found you!"

"What do you mean?" I ask, holding my gurgling stomach as he grabs a wooden chair from the center of the room and sets it by my bedside. I quickly introduce him to my purple-haired friend, and they nod to each other.

"Well, after you left the airport, I explained the situation to the lady at the desk, and she had to put a call through to get the dog back from the plane and recall our baggage. Then she said she would watch our bags while I went to the hospital, but when I tried to get a cab, no one would take me with the dog. The lady at the desk said she couldn't watch him, so I pleaded with this random lady who was running a coat check. I still have no idea who she is or why there's a coat check at the airport, but she has Buckles."

"You left our dog with a complete stranger?!" I ask, half amused and half annoyed.

"I didn't have a choice! I thought your appendix was exploding!" he laughs. "I don't even have this lady's phone number, so I need to get back in about an hour before her shift is over."

"You've *got* to be kidding me," I say, shaking my head but smiling in gratitude. Sometimes things just come together in the most beautiful way.

"So what's the deal?" he asks. "Obviously you don't have appendicitis."

"They have no idea. They told me I look fine and can leave when I poop, but they won't feed me anything, so I'm just sort of ho-humming it until I go to the bathroom."

"They can't find anything wrong with you? Did you tell them about the Lyme and all the medication?"

"No," I sigh, "the doctor doesn't seem very patient, and I don't think anyone speaks English well enough to understand it all. It's such a long history and such a new disease, I feel like if I tell them it will just make them want to keep me here longer. I just want to go home."

"Yeah," he says, picking a piece of dog hair off his jacket.

"I haven't taken my medicine, either," I say, looking at him carefully. "I think my body has just had enough. Like maybe it's all just too much to handle. These antibiotics are such a heavy dose, and I've been on them for over a year now. Maybe that's why my body is seizing up and freaking out."

"So maybe you should just stay off them until we can get you in with the Lyme doctor and see what she says. Maybe it's time for all this to be over."

"One can only hope," I smile.

"*ALO!*" shouts the 80-year-old woman with dementia, who has just woken up.

Greg catches my eye and we both burst out laughing at the absurdity of our situation.

****

A week later I'm back at my Lyme doctor's office in Pawling, New York. This appointment will cost nearly six hundred dollars out of pocket, since our health insurance doesn't cover the controversial, long-term antibiotic Lyme treatment.

In the time that I've been on antibiotics, I have eliminated twenty-one of my twenty-two symptoms. The lingering twenty-second symptom is joint pain. It isn't debilitating like it was in Thailand. Rather, it's like a persistent, minor rash—mostly annoying and sometimes embarrassing. I can't do simple things, like

open a jar of pasta sauce. The inflammation in my fingers makes it hurt to grip a steering wheel. I cringe when I have to shake hands with people. All my life I've admired a firm handshake, but a firm handshake sends a zap of pain through my hand and up my arm that makes me pull my hand back in agony. At times, it's painful to walk the dog because my knees feel creaky and unstable, and each step feels like a hammer to my kneecaps.

The only new symptom I have is the weird seizing-up-in-the-night thing coupled with the gurgly stomach burp thing that comes and goes and is alleviated by lying down.

"So what are your thoughts?" I look into my doctor's bright brown eyes after explaining the ordeal I've been through over the past few weeks, hoping for answers I can count on.

"Well," she says, removing her glasses and rubbing the bridge of her nose, "Lyme is persistent. It can come back. The seizing-up thing, the night sweats, those are consistent with Lyme co-infections." She names a particular co-infection.

"But I tested negative for that," I point out.

"Yes, but sometimes these co-infections can hide and come out at different times. I would suggest going back on antibiotics."

My brow furrows and I am irritated.

"But there were twenty-two symptoms. And now there is just one remaining, and one weird one that only started after treatment. Don't you think these could be caused by something else?" I can hear my voice getting testy.

"No," she shakes her head, sure of herself. "Lyme is tricky. It affects different things. This could be the Lyme coming back."

My heart is starting to race, but not from anxiety or panic. This heartbeat is like a marching drum. I want to stand up and shout at her to *work with me!* Humor me for five seconds! Consider other possible causes! Quit with your tunnel vision! Treat me like a person and not a case study!

But it's like Girlfriend is wearing Lyme goggles. It's all she can see. And it becomes very clear to me that she wants to treat the symptom and not explore and find the root cause of my one lingering symptom and one new symptom. In my heart of hearts, I know that it's time to move on and continue my journey to health without her.

"I'm not going to start back up on antibiotics," I

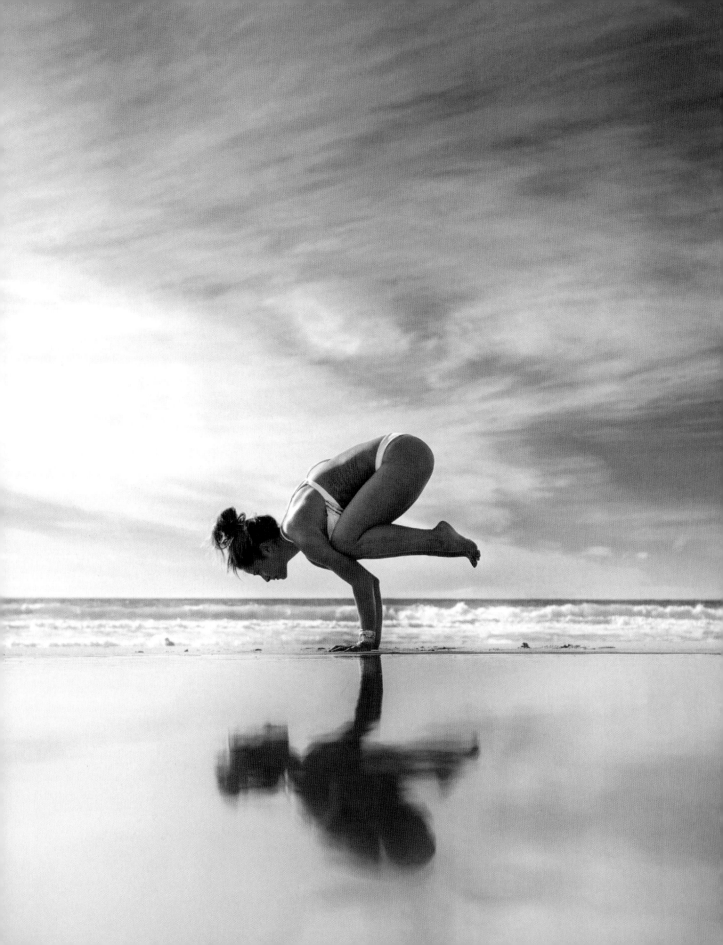

say evenly. "I really, truly feel that my body has had enough of the medication. It's heavy-duty stuff. I feel drained from it. I feel like it's done its job. There's more to be done, yes, but I don't think antibiotics are the answer."

I stand up and gather my things. This part of my journey, I know, is over.

She raises her eyebrows and shrugs. "Listen, it's your body, so you certainly can do what you choose to do. But in my clinical experience, Lyme comes back."

My eyes narrow because it feels like she's threatening me.

Not if I have anything to say about it, I think.

NAMASLAY COMMANDMENT #1:
BELIEVE IN YOURSELF.

I pivot and walk out the door. Two days later, Greg and I are packed and driving to Florida for the rest of the off-season.

****

I'm a firm believer that the three best cures for anything are a good night's sleep, sunshine, and "vitamin sea." My time in Florida provides all of them, and within three weeks my joint pain is gone, and so are the night sweats and the episodes of seizing muscles, which, in looking back, I have a feeling were caused from the obscene amount of Aleve I was taking daily in Thailand. I am teaching yoga on the beach to a small group of people every Sunday.

I obsess over what I will teach and jot down notes on index cards. I don't charge anything because I'm still a newbie. I do my best and have fun gaining experience. I blog every day, and I learn how to insert Google ads into my YouTube videos, so now I am making like .00000001 cent per view, but I don't really care because it's all fun to me.

I'm just thrilled to be enjoying life. Sure, sometimes things are off. My stomach isn't gurgling anymore and I don't feel any pain, but it gets bloated now and then. I mean *really* bloated, to the point where I take a picture and text it to my cousin Emily and say, "I'm not even pushing it out!"

I turn to the side and look in the mirror. I look like I'm pregnant. I quarter-turn to the left and it's amusing for approximately three seconds until I realize that it actually really hurts. My stomach is painfully distended, protruding so far that I look like one of those children you see on TV suffering from dysentery and malnutrition.

Could I have just one day where nothing is wrong? I silently plead. *No joint pain, no Lyme issues, no stomach issues, just one day where I can go through the entire day without thinking about my health?!*

Two months later

It's a sunny Sunday morning in August and I wake with a start. My eyes flick open, and for a second I'm confused. I'm in that weird space where you're awake but not fully present, and I need a second to figure out my whereabouts.

My eyes blink away the sleepiness and I look around the room. Greg is turned away from me, fast asleep, breathing fully and deeply, not a care in the world. A huge armoire across from our bed spans the width of the room, with cheap IKEA mirrors pasted on the doors. I stare at my distorted reflection and finally remember that I am back in Germany.

I need to get ready to teach my Sunday morning yoga class. Teaching yoga in German is simultaneously the most hysterical and most humiliating thing ever to happen to me because, well, I don't actually *speak* German. Sure, I can ask "How are you?" and "How much does this cost?" I can order tea and say, perfectly, "I'm sorry, but my German is bad; do you speak English?" My charades game is on point, but my German for yoga class? Pretty much nonexistent.

The incredible thing is that my students don't seem to care. They think it is *süß* that I butcher their language. After Googling, I learn that *süß* means "sweet."

Each week I use Google Translate to teach myself a new phrase and write it down in my notebook:

Inhale

Exhale

Look forward

Bring your right foot forward

Spread your toes

"Spread your toes" gets a good laugh out of the class because I mispronounce the German word for "spread" and accidentally say, "Splash your toes." They correct me, and I laugh unabashedly because it's just yoga, and, even though I am mildly embarrassed, they make me feel like a hero for even trying.

Germany is behind the times when it comes to the yoga culture. There isn't a studio on every corner like there is in the U.S. There are a few studios in bigger cities, but most of them offer very gentle hatha yoga or Bikram. My vinyasa power flow is set to music and is new and exciting to the people in the class, so they don't care that their weirdo American teacher speaks German like a three-year-old.

I look forward to every Sunday morning. There is a sense of community among our little group. They begin to feel like family. Their positivity and no-bullshit German way of expressing themselves lift me up. And I need lifting up. Because I am *still* battling health issues.

This morning, I slowly push myself up, swing my legs off the bed, and set my feet down. My stomach gurgles and feels heavy and full. I stand up and look down. My stomach is so distended that I can't see my toes. I try to suck it in, but it won't move. It's as hard as a rock and hurts so, so badly. It crosses my mind that I should stick a pin to it and see if it pops like a balloon.

I waddle to the bathroom and brush my teeth.

Another thing has cropped up recently: acne. Not just a simple little pimple that shows up after a night out or around my period. This is different. I have a deep cystic pimple on my forehead. It feels like there is a giant marble under my skin. When I bend over to grab a washcloth from the cabinet under the sink, I can feel the pimple pulsating like it has a heartbeat of its own.

A few days later, another cystic pimple is forming on the other side of my forehead. When I turn to the side, it almost looks like I'm sprouting a unicorn horn. I snicker at that thought, which feels better than crying, but I can feel depression starting to pull me back under. Between my constantly bloated and painful stomach and the erupting acne, I feel miserable and defeated.

Because I'm in small-town Germany where there aren't many English speakers, I don't want to see a doctor. It seems like it would be a bigger ordeal than it's worth, and how would I even explain all the drama that I've been through in the past two years?

Instead, I turn to Google.

I am a master Internet detective. Ask any of my friends, and they'll vigorously nod their heads in agreement. Need me to stalk your ex? Find the social media accounts of that cute guy you saw at the gym last week? Change your LSAT scores? Well, no promises on that last one, but I can do just about anything else.

In a five-minute jaunt through cyberspace, I stumble upon Chinese face mapping. In Chinese medicine, the skin is believed to be the body's biggest detoxing organ, so acne signifies that something unhealthy is going on internally. Each part of the face, according to Chinese face mapping, corresponds to a different part of the body.

I roll my eyes at this and chuckle because my mom used to bring "healers" to our house when I was a kid. She'd have Reiki treatments, acupuncture, and "energy work," whatever that is. I always scoffed and said that she was wasting her money, but sitting here, staring at the Chinese face map, I feel a pang of guilt. The forehead, according to this map, corresponds to the digestive tract.

What a coincidence, a little voice in my head says. *You're having stomach problems.* Maybe there's some truth to the old saying that mother knows best.

I sit up tall and roll up my sleeves, feeling like I'm about to solve a crime. I sit there for a second, take a sip of tea, and think, *I know I have the power to help myself; I just need to be smart about it. How can I get to the bottom of this?*

I furiously bang away at my keyboard, entering key phrases as I try to uncover the mystery of my stubborn health issues:

why is my stomach bloating
Lyme disease stomach bloating
antibiotics stomach bloating
acne stomach issues
acne on forehead related to stomach
acne from antibiotics stomach issues

I continue this for hours, taking notes and evaluating sources, and finally I think I have some answers.

Greg walks in from the rink. He is no stranger to my symptoms, to how much pain I am in, to how emotionally fragile I feel. He has never once complained about our situation. He has spent tens of thousands of his personal money on my medical bills. When I bring this up, he reminds me that it's our money, but to me it always feels like his since I don't—can't—contribute to our income. He is a saint personified for dealing with me.

"Can we talk?" I ask him, prepared with my findings. He follows me into the living room and sits on the couch as I prepare my evidence.

"According to my *painstaking* research," I say with a smile, because he knows what an Internet stalker I can be, "the antibiotics and all that Aleve I took in Thailand have ruined my gut, causing what's known as leaky gut. The result is that I have poor digestion and feel stomach pain and bloating pretty much all the time. Apparently, it's also the root cause of the breakouts I've been seeing." I wave my hand over my forehead, exhibit A.

"So what can we do about this? How do you repair the gut?" he asks.

"Well, there's this diet. It's referred to as a 'healing' diet because it's short-term—two years max—and it's meant to repair the gut lining. It doesn't allow for any grains, not even quinoa, and it has an emphasis on fermented foods like sauerkraut and homemade yogurt to help populate the gut with healthy bacteria. It shouldn't be hard to do because we don't really eat bread, pasta, or processed food anyway."

"Cool. I bet my gut could use some healing, too," he says in a playful tone of voice. He gets up to go to the kitchen, finished with the conversation. "I'll do it with you," he calls over his shoulder, and I could cry because I don't know what I've done to deserve someone so kind.

The diet is called the GAPS diet, and it was created by Dr. Natasha Campbell-McBride. I order her book online, and without my even asking him to, Greg reads it from cover to cover after I've finished.

The diet becomes my life. Our lives. I follow it to a T like my life depends on it, mostly because I truly believe that my life *does* depend on it and also because, more than anything, I desperately want to feel normal. Greg does it with me when we are together, though on road trips for hockey games he eats whatever is served.

The girlfriends and wives of the other hockey players on Greg's team extend invites to their girls' nights, where they have cookie-decorating parties or brownies-and-champagne gatherings. This is our first year with this team and I don't know any of these women very well, so I feel awkward having to explain the whole saga behind my health.

I *want* to fit in and take part, but it feels like a lose-lose situation no matter what I do or say. How do I explain, without sounding like a total asshole, that yes, I will decorate the cookies at the cookie-decorating party, but no, I will not eat them? That I can't drink alcohol, so I will just bring my own ginger lemon tea instead of sharing in the champagne? I don't like having to describe my health issues over and over again, so I decline most of the invitations, isolate myself, and focus on the diet, the blog, and my yoga classes. It just seems easier for everyone involved if I leave myself out.

I lose a few friends over my own isolation, but I quickly learn that there comes a time when you have to do what's best for you. Those who understand will be there for you, and those who don't get it probably aren't a good match for you as friends anyway.

There's a saying that I keep coming across: "Every day we have two options: to step forward into growth or step back into safety." I certainly wasn't growing. Isolating myself meant that I was staying inside the comfort zone. But for what it's worth, I'll say this: the safety zone has its place. Stay in the safety zone when:

- You're dealing with an illness.
- You feel emotionally and physically unstable.
- You're in the middle of figuring your shit out.

The lesson, I realize, is that taking care of yourself is the number-one priority. Being sick, I am pretty useless. I'm not a great wife, friend, daughter, or sister. I am stressed out and distracted by my health problems. I can't be present for anyone. And then I am stressed out about not being present and not being a good wife, friend, daughter, or sister. And that triggers more stress, and it just snowballs until finally I want to scream that enough is enough! I take advantage of the freedom to say no and take care of myself.

NAMASLAY COMMANDMENT #10:
TAKE NO SHIT.

What a glorious thing.

What a freeing thing.

What a delicious thing it is to take care of yourself without guilt.

In the first six weeks of following the GAPS diet, my skin starts to clear up, the painful bloating goes away, and my body starts to feel healthier than it has in years. I drink bone broth for the first time. I feel it go down, coating my insides like a fresh coat of paint on a spackled wall. It warms me from the inside out. I close my eyes, savoring the moment. It feels like an IV has been administered, and I swear that when I open my eyes the colors are brighter, my energy level is higher, and my glass is half full again.

Without any persuasion from me, Greg researches how to ferment our own vegetables and make homemade yogurt and sour cream. He makes delicious soups with bone broth, tops them with a dollop of homemade sour cream, and sets the bowl on the table as I plug away at my blog.

My blog is still a hobby, but I am quickly realizing that it can be a vehicle to bigger things.

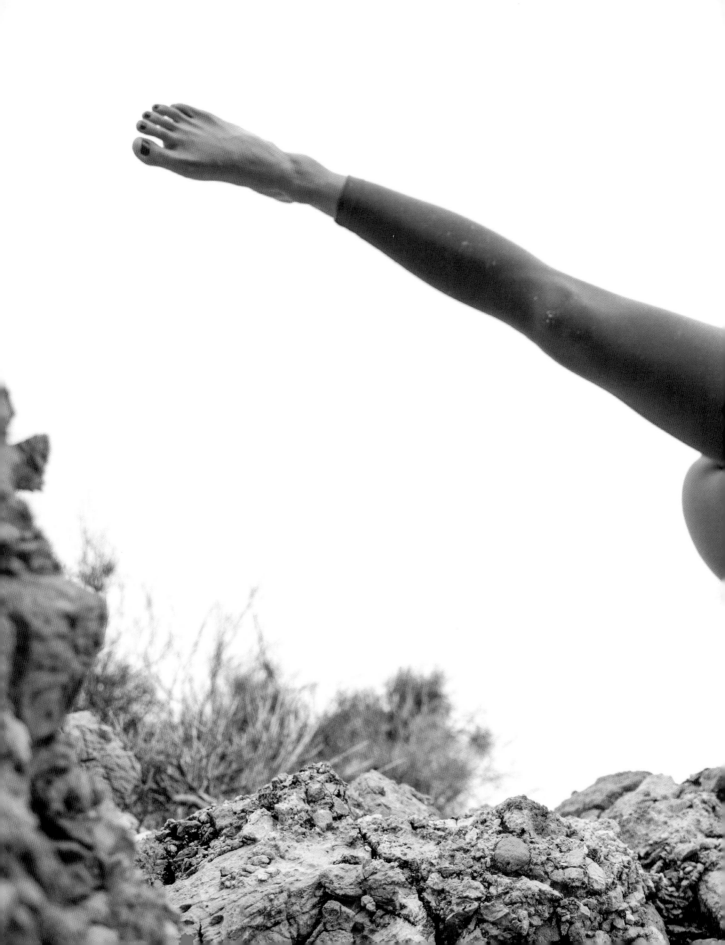

CHAPTER 5:

the advanced practice

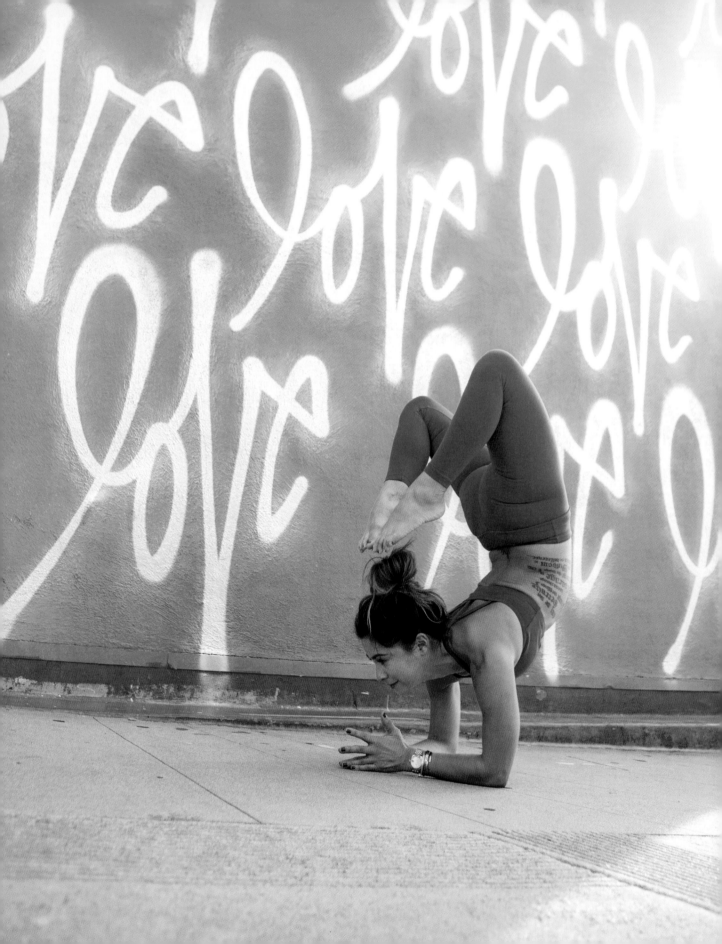

On a cold February morning, I sit down at the dining room table and open my laptop. I treat my blog like a job, and it's 7:59 a.m. I've walked the dog and am ready to tackle my emails. I log in and see a message from a woman named Sophie, a Parisian living in Greece, where Greg and I have decided to go for our winter break in a few weeks. She'd like to meet and says that it might be amazing to work together.

She offers to arrange for me to teach a workshop at Bhavana, the most prominent yoga studio in Athens. I am both terrified and thrilled, which I take to mean that I should do it. I mean, all the best things in life are both terrifying and thrilling, no?

Sometimes you have to get out of your own way and just go for it. Set fear aside and jump in.

NAMASLAY COMMANDMENT #7:
BE A HELL YEAH PERSON.

Our flight from Berlin to Athens departs at 6:00 a.m.

When I get very little sleep, I am a miserable human being. I am angry and irritable. My stomach hurts. I feel dizzy and have dry mouth. I'm certain that I'd fare better if I were suffering from the worst hangover of my life, but here I am, stuffed into my tiny seat on Ryanair, my back flush against the seat and my eyes closed as I focus on my breathing.

There is a woman in the row behind me who is either mentally unstable, drunk, or on drugs. She is at least fifty years old, and she is not wearing shoes. Her hair is matted down and she looks like she's been through the trenches, but she is singing loudly in German, happy as a clam. Somehow she's scored an entire row to herself and is lying across the seats, tapping her bare foot on the back of my seat to the beat of her song.

I sigh audibly. I want to turn around and give her one of my signature Looks. It's a Look I learned from my mom, who is the queen of giving Looks. Actually, I'm pretty sure all moms are the queens of Looks. You know the Look I'm talking about. As a kid, one Look and you knew you'd better knock it off or else.

But I don't give her a Look. I'm too worried that it will cause a confrontation. Plus, my anxiety is at an all-time high from the lack of sleep.

Greg thinks the whole situation is funny and tells me to relax, which does nothing but irritate me. Nothing makes a person less likely to relax than telling said person to relax.

When we land, we race to meet the driver Sophie has arranged for us. I've learned to say "hello" and "thank you" in Greek, which gets a good chuckle out of him. He drives us past ornate ancient statues and incredible marble buildings that make me wish I had paid more attention in history class. There's nothing quite like seeing the stuff from your textbooks in real life.

"This is incredible," Greg murmurs as we speed down the road. As we approach a stoplight, he turns to me and asks, "So after the class we're going out with Sophie?"

"Yeah," I respond. "In her email she said she had quit her high-stress job in Paris, sold everything, and moved to Greece. She wants to start organizing yoga retreats. Wouldn't it be crazy if she asked me to work with her and we did a retreat in Greece?"

"Yeah, that'd be awesome. How do you know her again? From the blog?"

"I don't know her at all, actually. She just wrote an email from the submission form on my blog."

"That's pretty incredible that she reached out and then set up this whole workshop for you," he says.

The light turns green and we're off to our AirBnB rental, a cozy little apartment with views of the Acropolis. The view is so gorgeous that for a second I'm sure this is a dream.

I quickly change into my yoga clothes and there's a knock at the door: Sophie.

Sophie is tall and lanky, with beautifully tanned skin, honey-colored hair, and bright brown eyes. She has a throaty voice and an infectious laugh. She is beautiful in the way that every French woman I know is effortlessly chic.

"*Bonjour!*" she exclaims, kissing me on each cheek. "How was your trip? Did my driver pick you up on time? Everything okay? Hi, you must be Greg!"

"Yes, the driver was perfect, thank you so much for arranging to have us picked up!" I say.

"Perfect, I'm so pleased. Shall we go to the studio?" she asks.

Together we walk to Bhavana, and the entire time I'm trying to act cool, normal, like I'm not nervous about teaching at the most prestigious yoga studio in Athens. I've never been to this studio, but I've heard of it because all the prominent yoga teachers I follow on social media have been guest instructors there. I still can't believe that they're allowing me to teach. I'm suffering from impostor syndrome.

I have tried on my own to teach at various studios in the U.S. and abroad and am often met with some variation of the following email:

Thank you for your interest in leading a workshop at our studio. However, in order to control the quality of teaching that we offer to our students, we do not allow outside teachers to come in, but we wish you the best. Namaste.

I quickly realize that the majority of the studios out there are preaching about how important it is to be inclusive but are not heeding their own advice. So being invited to teach at Bhavana is a big deal to me.

Sophie lights a cigarette and waves the smoke away, saying, "I'm sorry, I'm terrible! I know it's not very Zen of me to be smoking before yoga, but . . . pfff." She shrugs and I laugh, instantly loving her for being so unapologetically who she is.

I could learn a thing or two from this girl, I think.

We walk into Bhavana and the receptionist greets me with the biggest hug, like she's been waiting years for this encounter. She offers me tea and leads me into the studio. The room is drenched in morning light, and incense is burning. She shows me the speaker, asks if I need help hooking up my computer for my playlist, and then leaves me to get ready.

As the students gather and chat outside the empty room, I take a deep breath. Looking around, I feel an overwhelming sense of gratitude and pride. This is not just an opportunity for me to gain experience and connect with others. It's a nod to my health struggles—to my having endured such lengthy medical treatment, fulfilled the promise to myself to travel to Thailand for yoga teacher training, dealt with my subsequent health issues after getting off the medication for Lyme disease, and begun my road to recovery on a healing diet. It's a nod to the growing reach of my blog, which is how Sophie found me, and an acknowledgment of the possibility of other incredible opportunities in the future. To me, this is not just a two-hour class and a way for me to make a little money. This is a testament

to my repeatedly getting back up after being knocked down and shouting, "Yes, I *can!*"

I am so overcome with gratitude that I have to take a second to focus on my breathing so I don't start crying right before the class begins.

As the students begin to file in, I plug in my computer, roll my shoulders back, and sit down on my mat. My heart beats so loudly, I swear I can hear it. I smile at everyone.

They sit there, staring back at me expectantly. I close my eyes and take another deep breath, feeling the nerves wash over me.

Inhale. *You have nothing to prove.*

Exhale. *And everything to share.*

I open my eyes and welcome the students to the workshop. "So, let's begin," I say, and press play on my playlist.

After class, I stay and chat with some of the students. They are warm and kind and thank me profusely, which makes me melt inside.

I did it! I think. *I not only didn't screw up, but they actually enjoyed it!*

They make me promise to come back, and we exchange hugs.

Afterward, Sophie and I get coffee. Well, she gets coffee and I get tea, since I'm still on the GAPS diet. She explains that she worked in corporate PR and communications for years and gave up the crazy busy Paris life for the more laid-back Greek island life.

"I would love to deezgus zee possibility of hosting a retreat togezzah," she says, blowing the smoke from her cigarette over her shoulder and waving it away with her hand.

I look at Greg and laugh. "Babe!" I say. "What was it that I told you in the cab this morning?"

He chuckles and tells Sophie that I mentioned how cool I thought that possibility would be.

Now, years later, after organizing a number of retreats for me in Ibiza and Greece, Sophie has become one of my dearest friends. It's one of those great friendships where we can go for weeks or months without speaking and then pick up right where we left off when we finally reconnect. We have laughed together and cried together. She has taught me invaluable business lessons, and I have taught her intricacies of yoga poses. She is like a sister to me, and it all stemmed from a little email she wrote through the submission form on my yoga blog that I never thought anyone would read.

Having an advanced yoga practice is like being an adventure seeker. You've traveled to many places and done some crazy things. You've met incredible people along your journey. It hasn't been easy. There were times when you felt overwhelmed, frustrated, exhausted, and sore. You may have questioned your sanity when making the decision to go. But, looking back, you realize that you wouldn't change a thing. And the best part? There's so much more that you want to see and do.

World travelers, like advanced yoga practitioners, know a lot. They can order tea in Mandarin and ask where the bathroom is in French. They know that on Mondays admission to many museums is free and that Tuesday is the best day of the week to fly. But they also know that they don't know it all. It's impossible to know it all.

NAMASLAY COMMANDMENT #3:
CONTINUE TO LEARN.

Similarly, advanced yoga students know that one of the tricks to handstand is to engage the fingertips, and that to lift the back leg in flying pigeon it's important to utilize the posterior chain. Advanced students know a number of pranayama practices and understand that when you're tired, the most advanced form of yoga is a good, long savasana. They also know that there's still a great deal to learn and that to continue to grow, they must continue to practice.

If you've got an advanced asana practice but have hit a plateau in your growth, I urge you to sign up for a master class or an advanced workout. Keep taking classes at your local studios. Bounce around and try different instructors. Try different styles of yoga. Keep growing, but keep your beginner mindset, remembering that every time you step on the mat you have the opportunity to learn something new.

USTRASANA camel pose

Confession: This pose used to make me rage. If you're familiar with Bikram yoga, you know that it comes toward the end of class when you're feeling particularly weak and exceptionally sweaty, as if you've been dragged through a pond of your own perspiration and then forced to run a marathon. Throw in this deep backbend, and if you don't come out of it feeling lightheaded and sort of stabby, then you, my friend, are a hero in my book.

Begin seated on your shins with your knees hip width apart and your feet in line with your knees. Then lift your hips so that your body is perpendicular to the floor. Bring your hands to the backs of your hips and press your hips forward as you lean back and lift your chest. It's important to feel the sensation of a lift in the chest so that you don't compress your low back.

Continue to lean back farther. Stay here or, if you're ready for the full expression of the pose, bring your hands to your feet. Cup your heels with your palms and let your head go if it feels okay for your neck. Breathe length through your entire front body from your knees to your neck, and intend to use your lungs to their fullest capacity. Continue to lift your heart, imagining that your body is making a capital D-shape. Take three to seven breaths before exiting the pose.

I recommend coming out of camel pose quickly. If you come out too slowly, the blood tends to rush to your head, and passing out is something you're probably going to want to avoid. I also recommend going directly into child's pose rather than hanging out in a seated posture. Bringing your head right down to the mat is really calming and should help you avoid that whole OMG-I'm-gonna-pass-out feeling.

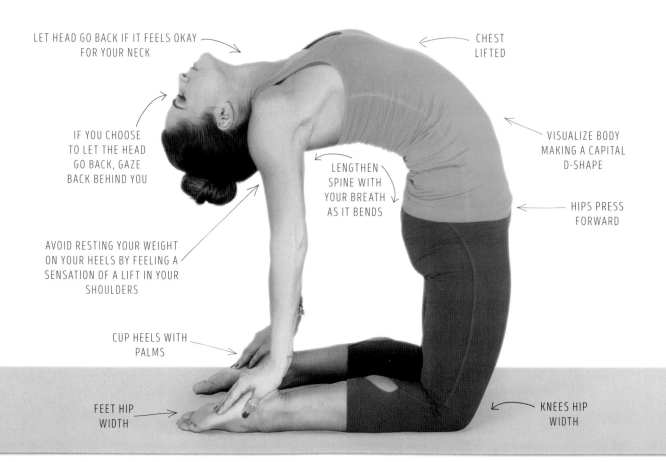

LET HEAD GO BACK IF IT FEELS OKAY FOR YOUR NECK

CHEST LIFTED

IF YOU CHOOSE TO LET THE HEAD GO BACK, GAZE BACK BEHIND YOU

VISUALIZE BODY MAKING A CAPITAL D-SHAPE

LENGTHEN SPINE WITH YOUR BREATH AS IT BENDS

HIPS PRESS FORWARD

AVOID RESTING YOUR WEIGHT ON YOUR HEELS BY FEELING A SENSATION OF A LIFT IN YOUR SHOULDERS

CUP HEELS WITH PALMS

FEET HIP WIDTH

KNEES HIP WIDTH

BANDHA PADMASANA bound lotus pose

This gorgeous seated pose feels incredible, but it requires a lot of openness through the chest and hips. If you're struggling, use a yoga strap or just do a half bind.

Begin seated on the floor with your legs out in front of you. Bend your right leg and send your right foot to the left across your torso. Position your right knee in the crook of your right elbow and your right foot in the crook of your left elbow. With the right ankle and knee joints even, slowly flex your right foot and spread the toes to help prevent ankle sickling. Then slowly bring your right foot into your left hip crease (where your leg attaches to your torso). Keep your right foot flexed as you bend your left leg and bring the left knee into the crook of your left elbow and the left foot into the crook of your right elbow. With the left ankle and knee joints even, slowly flex your left foot and guide it into your right hip crease. Sit very tall and breathe.

On your next inhale, lengthen through your spine. Then, as you exhale, wrap your left arm behind your back and reach until your left peace fingers connect with your left big toe. Take a deep breath in. As you exhale, wrap your right arm around your back and reach until your right peace fingers connect with your right big toe. Breathe fully and deeply for as long as it feels comfortable before slowly exiting the same way you went in. Then take it to the other side, with the other leg on top.

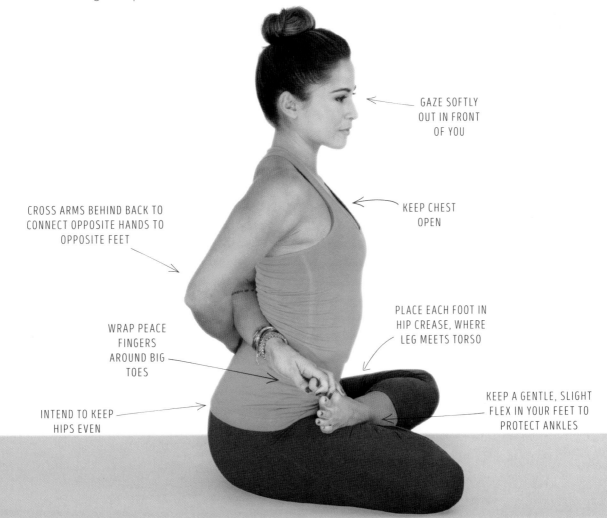

GAZE SOFTLY OUT IN FRONT OF YOU

KEEP CHEST OPEN

CROSS ARMS BEHIND BACK TO CONNECT OPPOSITE HANDS TO OPPOSITE FEET

WRAP PEACE FINGERS AROUND BIG TOES

PLACE EACH FOOT IN HIP CREASE, WHERE LEG MEETS TORSO

INTEND TO KEEP HIPS EVEN

KEEP A GENTLE, SLIGHT FLEX IN YOUR FEET TO PROTECT ANKLES

HANUMANASANA monkey pose

The splits are always on people's bucket lists. I don't know why, because they're freaking hard and make me want to cry. I kid, I kid. Splits are awesome for people who have worked hard on opening up their hamstrings and hip flexors. It's definitely a pose you've got to have patience with and work consistently at, but I promise that if you do both, it should become attainable.

If you're new to the splits or just particularly tight, I recommend starting off with blocks. I like using these ergonomic Bhoga blocks because they provide a great grip for my hands.

Start in a runner's lunge with your right leg forward and slowly bring your right leg straight, keeping the toes engaged (this encourages the rest of the leg to stay engaged, which may help prevent hyperextension). From here, slowly take your left leg behind you, keeping the toes curled. Curling the toes gives you a bit more control and may prevent hip flexor injury that can occur if you slide right down into the splits. Press into the blocks to control the speed with which you come into the pose. Breathe for as long as you can stand (ha!), then press into the block and use your core strength to lift your legs and release the pose. Give it a try with the other leg forward just to keep things even.

MODIFIED VERSION

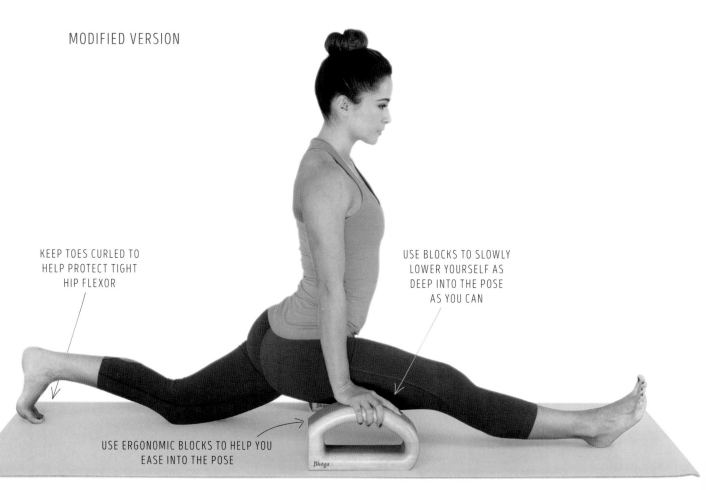

KEEP TOES CURLED TO HELP PROTECT TIGHT HIP FLEXOR

USE BLOCKS TO SLOWLY LOWER YOURSELF AS DEEP INTO THE POSE AS YOU CAN

USE ERGONOMIC BLOCKS TO HELP YOU EASE INTO THE POSE

If you're ready to give it a try without the blocks, you'll start the same way—in a runner's lunge—and then slide your right leg forward and your left leg back, keeping the toes curled. When you're fully down, you can uncurl your back toes and bring the top of the foot onto your mat.

Intend for your hips to face forward, and breathe fully and deeply for as long as it feels comfortable before switching sides. When you're ready to release the pose, press evenly into both hands, engage your core strength, and rise to standing.

FULL EXPRESSION

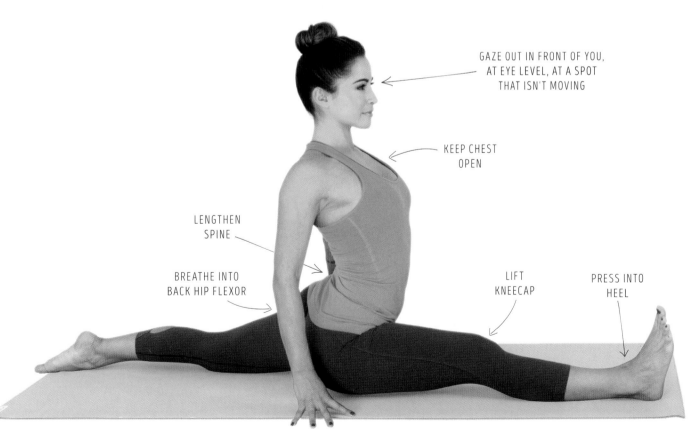

GAZE OUT IN FRONT OF YOU, AT EYE LEVEL, AT A SPOT THAT ISN'T MOVING

KEEP CHEST OPEN

LENGTHEN SPINE

BREATHE INTO BACK HIP FLEXOR

LIFT KNEECAP

PRESS INTO HEEL

HANUMANASANA variation monkey pose variation

If you're ready to take your splits a step further, you can lift your back leg by looking back and grabbing hold of your back foot with the same-side hand. Then you can decide whether you'd like to take mermaid arms (page 164) or flip the grip like in dancer's pose (page 179). It's totally up to you—make it your own beautiful pose! Breathe for as long as you comfortably can before switching sides.

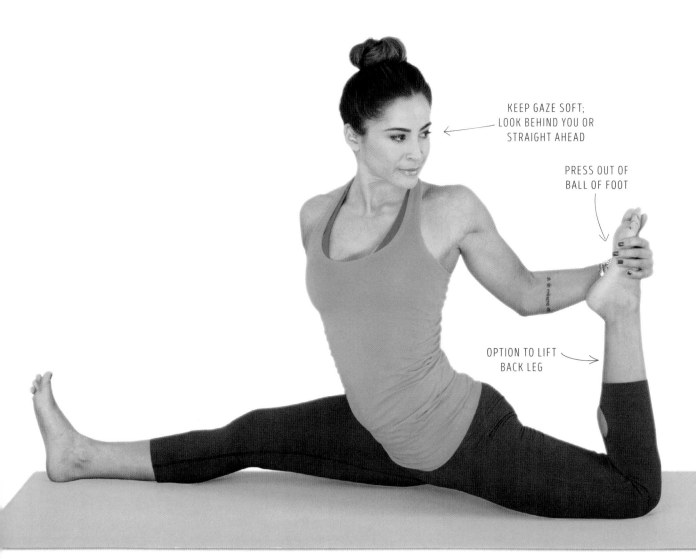

KEEP GAZE SOFT;
LOOK BEHIND YOU OR
STRAIGHT AHEAD

PRESS OUT OF
BALL OF FOOT

OPTION TO LIFT
BACK LEG

EKA PADA RAJAKAPOTASANA king pigeon pose

King pigeon pose is the next step after mermaid pose because it requires just a bit more openness in the chest.

    Begin in pigeon pose (page 97) with your left leg forward, your right leg back, and your hips facing forward. Then, as you inhale, bend your right leg and grab hold of your right foot with your right hand. Flip your grip so that your right elbow is pointed up toward the sky. On your next inhale, lift your left arm, bend at the elbow, and reach back until your hand comes in contact with your right foot. Breathe length through your front body, visualizing your spine as a backward letter C instead of a sideways V. Breathe for three to seven breaths before switching sides.

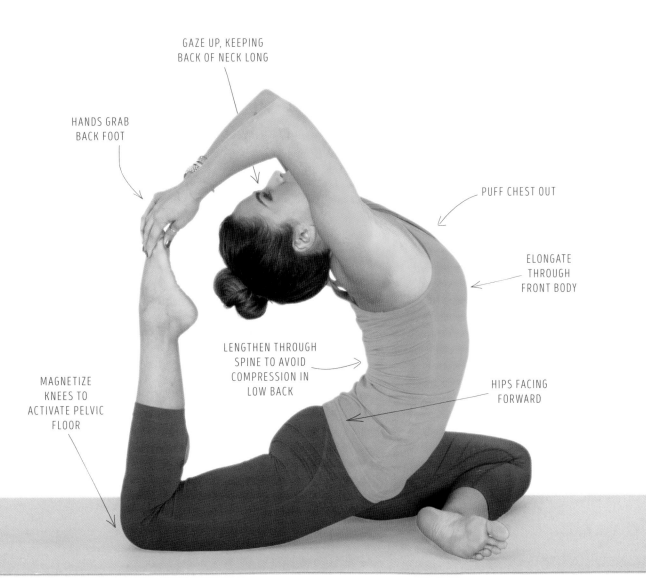

GAZE UP, KEEPING BACK OF NECK LONG

HANDS GRAB BACK FOOT

PUFF CHEST OUT

ELONGATE THROUGH FRONT BODY

LENGTHEN THROUGH SPINE TO AVOID COMPRESSION IN LOW BACK

MAGNETIZE KNEES TO ACTIVATE PELVIC FLOOR

HIPS FACING FORWARD

PARIVRTTA SURYA YANTRASANA compass/sundial pose

Compass pose is another good pose to open up the side body.

   Begin with your right leg bent and your right foot flat on the ground. Bend your left leg and place the outside of your knee on the ground in front of you, with the knee bent at about 45 degrees. If you're very open through the hips, you can keep both hips on the ground. If not, shift your weight to your left side, letting the right hip lift. Regardless of what you do with your right hip, nestle your right arm into the crook of your right knee as you press your hand into the ground. Then lift your right leg and, as you inhale, reach overhead with your left arm until it meets the outer edge of your right foot. Look out underneath your left armpit and breathe space between your left ribs. Take three to seven breaths before switching sides.

   If you're very tight, you may need to modify this pose with the use of a yoga strap. Just wrap the strap around the arch of your right foot and take hold of the strap in your left hand as you inch your way forward to find a nice stretch in your side body.

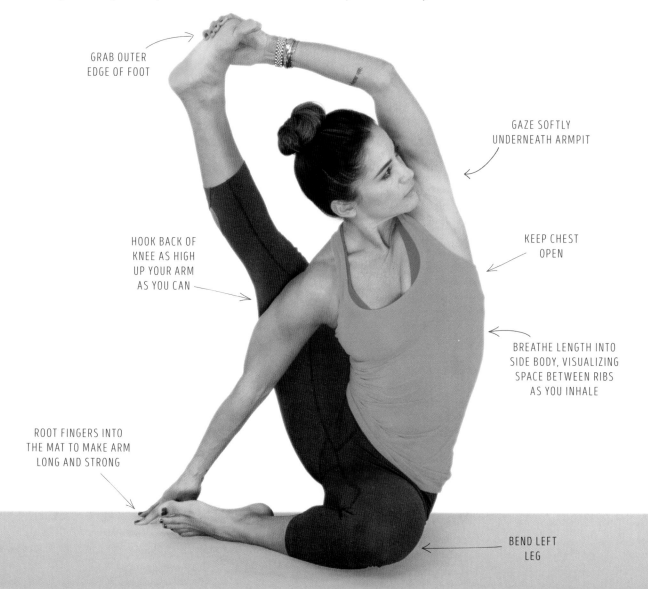

GRAB OUTER EDGE OF FOOT

GAZE SOFTLY UNDERNEATH ARMPIT

HOOK BACK OF KNEE AS HIGH UP YOUR ARM AS YOU CAN

KEEP CHEST OPEN

BREATHE LENGTH INTO SIDE BODY, VISUALIZING SPACE BETWEEN RIBS AS YOU INHALE

ROOT FINGERS INTO THE MAT TO MAKE ARM LONG AND STRONG

BEND LEFT LEG

BHARADVAJASANA sage twist

This gentle, detoxifying twist requires a bit of flexibility through the chest and solid range of motion through the torso. It's excellent for people who are parked at a desk day in and day out and really helpful for golfers, baseball players, hockey players, and other athletes whose core skills include twisting.

Begin seated on your mat. Bend your left leg behind you so that the left foot is next to your left hip. You may need to push the flesh of your calf muscle out to the left. Then bend your right leg and bring the right foot into your left hip crease. Gently flex your right foot and spread the toes to prevent your ankle from sickling.

On your next inhale, sit tall. As you exhale, twist from your belly button as you shift your gaze over your right shoulder. Slide your left hand under your right knee with the palm on the mat and the fingers pointing toward your body. Intend to keep your shoulders even and your chest open. Take another deep breath in to elongate through your spine, and as you exhale, reach your right arm around your back until your hand connects with your toes. This is the full expression of the pose. Breathe fully and deeply for three to seven breaths before switching sides.

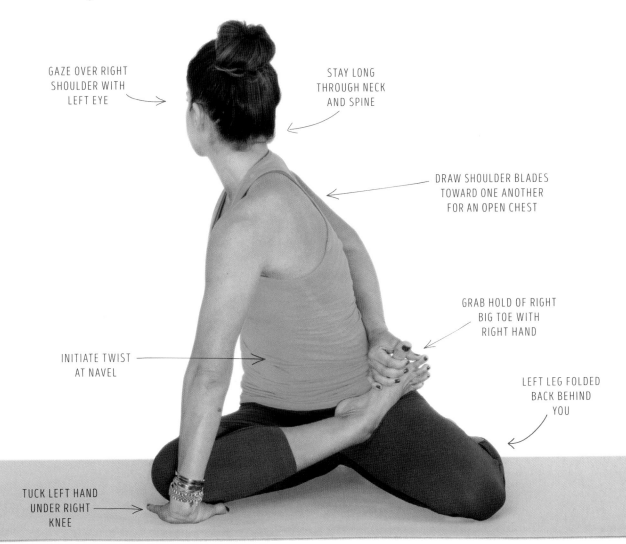

GAZE OVER RIGHT SHOULDER WITH LEFT EYE

STAY LONG THROUGH NECK AND SPINE

DRAW SHOULDER BLADES TOWARD ONE ANOTHER FOR AN OPEN CHEST

GRAB HOLD OF RIGHT BIG TOE WITH RIGHT HAND

INITIATE TWIST AT NAVEL

LEFT LEG FOLDED BACK BEHIND YOU

TUCK LEFT HAND UNDER RIGHT KNEE

UBHAYA PADANGUSTHASANA big toe pose

This hip-opening pose may have you cracking up because if you're anything like me, it'll take a couple of rocks and rolls before you get it. No worries, it's just yoga—there's no one to impress. If you fall out of it, who cares? Rock and roll, baby!

Begin in boat pose (page 158). Slowly begin to bend your knees and reach forward, wrapping your peace fingers around your big toes. Once your fingers are securely hooked around the big toes, activate your toes and press through the bottoms of your feet to straighten your legs as much as you can. Keep your low back long, your chest open, and your shoulder blades pulled in toward one another to ensure that your back is in proper alignment and that you're stretching your hips and hamstrings rather than your back. If you can't straighten your legs, it's no big deal; it just means that your hamstrings are tight. Do what you can and let that be enough.

FULL EXPRESSION

MODIFIED VERSION

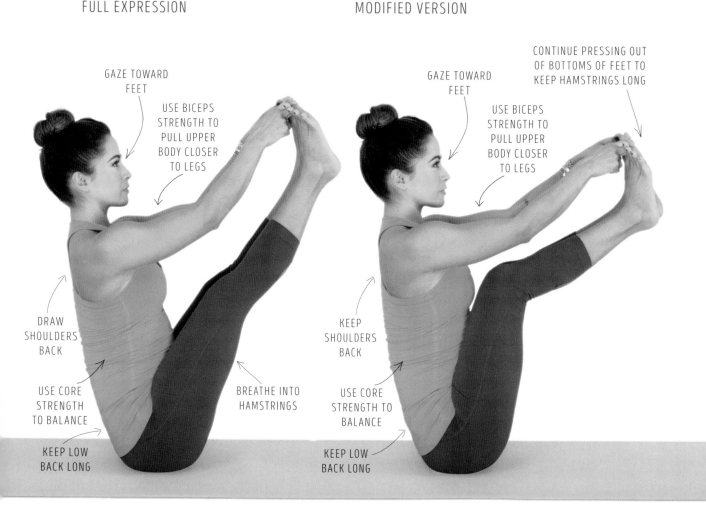

GAZE TOWARD FEET

USE BICEPS STRENGTH TO PULL UPPER BODY CLOSER TO LEGS

DRAW SHOULDERS BACK

USE CORE STRENGTH TO BALANCE

KEEP LOW BACK LONG

BREATHE INTO HAMSTRINGS

CONTINUE PRESSING OUT OF BOTTOMS OF FEET TO KEEP HAMSTRINGS LONG

GAZE TOWARD FEET

USE BICEPS STRENGTH TO PULL UPPER BODY CLOSER TO LEGS

KEEP SHOULDERS BACK

USE CORE STRENGTH TO BALANCE

KEEP LOW BACK LONG

UPAVISTHA KONASANA seated wide-leg forward fold

FULL EXPRESSION

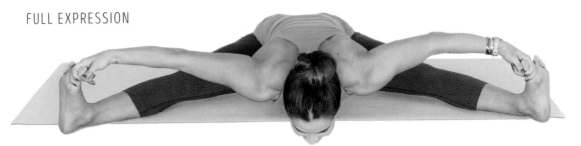

This pose is a great way to start opening up the hips and inner thighs.

To begin, sit tall and spread your legs as wide as you comfortably can. Rotate your inner thighs up toward the sky so that your toes are pointing upward (the tendency is for them to point slightly inward). Keep the toes spread and active (this will help keep your leg muscles engaged, which should help protect your hamstrings from any hypermobility).

The full expression of the pose is to grab hold of your big toes with your peace fingers and come forward with your chin on the ground and your chest as open as possible. But if this isn't your jam right now (and who cares if it's not; ain't no shame in where you are!), do a modification. There are two modifications, and the one you choose will depend on your hip opening. Here's how to check:

• Bring your hands to your hips. If your hips naturally tilt forward and your low back stays somewhat straight because you're already quite flexible, then bring your hands down to the ground in front of you.

• Bring your hands to your hips. If your hips tilt backward and your low back rounds, you're pretty tight in the hips. (So what? We all have to start somewhere.) You want your hips to tilt forward, so bring your hands to the ground behind you and press into the mat, as shown. You'll likely feel an immediate something in your inner thighs. Just breathe and work through it. The keys to developing flexibility are patience and consistency. If this is excruciating for you, place a folded blanket underneath your sitting bones. Often, a bit of height offers some relief.

MODIFIED VERSION

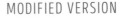

KEEP COLLARBONES BROAD

KEEP LOW BACK LONG

PRESS FINGERTIPS INTO THE MAT BEHIND YOU TO HELP TILT YOUR PELVIS FORWARD

NATARAJASANA king dancer's pose

This is the next step after regular dancer's pose. You flip the grip (which, admittedly, can be a little tricky), then do a major backbend. While standing on one leg. No big deal. You got this. Ready?

Begin in dancer's pose (page 179) with your right hand grabbing hold of the inside arch of your right foot. Then pull your right foot in toward you a bit more and slide your right hand up and over the top of the right foot so that your right elbow is pointing straight up toward the sky.

This is a major backbend, so breathe and ensure that your upper back is opening up so you aren't compromising your low back. Slowly lift your left arm and bend the elbow so it's pointed up to the sky. Then continue to reach back until your left fingers meet your right foot.

Once both hands are connected to your foot, relax your shoulders away from your ears and imagine that if you were looking at yourself in a mirror from the side, your back would be making a U-shape, not a V-shape. Doing this will help elongate your spine, which should help you avoid compression in your low back. Breathe deeply through your entire front body, and remember to either lift your left kneecap to engage your quads or micro-bend your left knee to avoid hyperextending your hamstring. Breathe fully and evenly for three to seven breaths before releasing and taking it to the other side.

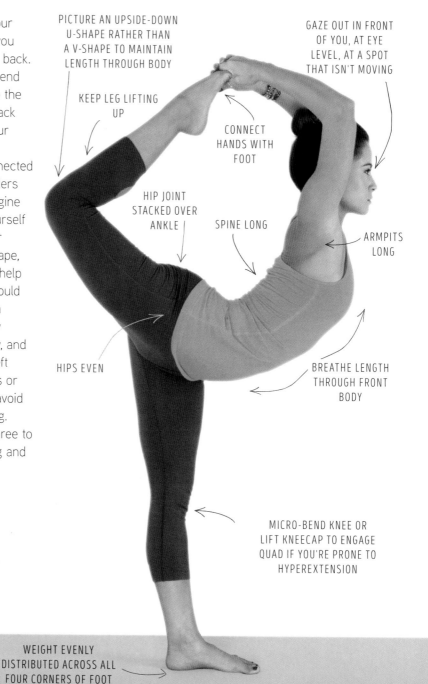

PICTURE AN UPSIDE-DOWN U-SHAPE RATHER THAN A V-SHAPE TO MAINTAIN LENGTH THROUGH BODY

KEEP LEG LIFTING UP

GAZE OUT IN FRONT OF YOU, AT EYE LEVEL, AT A SPOT THAT ISN'T MOVING

CONNECT HANDS WITH FOOT

HIP JOINT STACKED OVER ANKLE

SPINE LONG

ARMPITS LONG

HIPS EVEN

BREATHE LENGTH THROUGH FRONT BODY

MICRO-BEND KNEE OR LIFT KNEECAP TO ENGAGE QUAD IF YOU'RE PRONE TO HYPEREXTENSION

WEIGHT EVENLY DISTRIBUTED ACROSS ALL FOUR CORNERS OF FOOT

PADANGUSTASANA toe stand

This is a really fun balancing pose. Unless you're superhuman, you're likely to fall a few times, which will have you either laughing or pulling your hair out. Given the choice, I prefer the former, and you always have a choice, so just try to remember to keep your cool. It's called a yoga practice, not a yoga perfect. Sorry, that was cheesy.

Anyway, to begin, come into mountain pose (page 106). Then find a spot out in front of you at about eye level that isn't moving and gaze there. Lift your left toes, spread them as wide as you can, and set them down. Then shift all your weight onto your left foot and use your core and hip flexor strength to lift your right leg, bringing your right foot into your left hip crease. Slightly flex the right foot and spread the toes to protect your ankle and avoid sickling.

On your next inhale, bend your left knee about 30 degrees and begin to hinge at the waist. Rise up onto the ball of your left foot and bring both hands to the ground, about a foot in front of you. Shift your gaze so that you're looking at your mat, about three feet out in front of you. Rise higher onto the ball of your left foot and bring your right hand to your heart. Slowly bring your left hand to meet the right in prayer position.

The trick to this pose is to push into the ball of your left foot. Keep your left leg active, as if you're about to stand up on one leg. When you do this, you avoid dumping the weight in your knee, which may irritate your knee and cause you to fall over more easily. Breathe fully and deeply for three to seven breaths before switching sides.

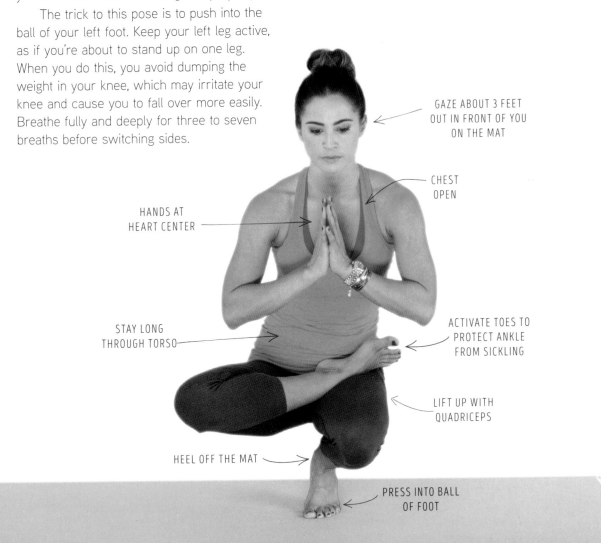

GAZE ABOUT 3 FEET OUT IN FRONT OF YOU ON THE MAT

CHEST OPEN

HANDS AT HEART CENTER

STAY LONG THROUGH TORSO

ACTIVATE TOES TO PROTECT ANKLE FROM SICKLING

LIFT UP WITH QUADRICEPS

HEEL OFF THE MAT

PRESS INTO BALL OF FOOT

SVARGA DVIDASANA bird of paradise pose

If you ever need a pose that makes you feel like a total badass, this one should probably be your pick, because hello, if you can balance on one foot while essentially doing a split with your arms wrapped around your body, then you deserve Badass Status.

To begin, stand in mountain pose (page 106) and find a spot out in front of you that is at eye level and not moving. Focus your gaze softly here. Inhale and lift your toes, spread them as wide as you can, and set them down for a stable foundation in this balancing pose. Then begin to shift your weight to your left foot. On your next inhale, lift your right leg as you distribute your weight evenly across all four corners of your left foot. As you lift the right leg, come slightly forward with your torso so that you can wrap your right arm in front of your right leg as you send your hand back behind the leg. Wrap your left arm around your back and continue to reach through the hands until they clasp. If your hands don't clasp, use a yoga strap to connect them.

If you're prone to hyperextension, be mindful to either micro-bend your standing leg or straighten your leg and lift your kneecap to engage your leg muscles. As you breathe, imagine that air is entering your body through the bottom of your left foot, and follow the breath all the way up through your body, noticing that you grow taller with each inhale. This visualization can help you stay stable and strong in the pose. Breathe for three to seven breaths before taking it to the other side.

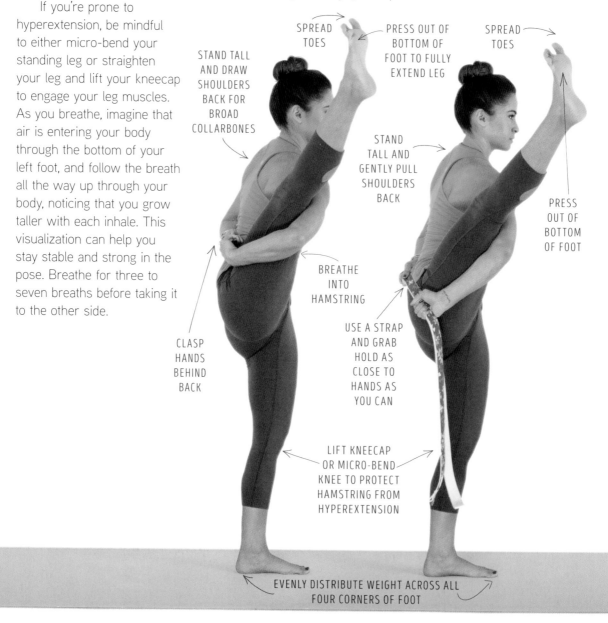

SPREAD TOES

PRESS OUT OF BOTTOM OF FOOT TO FULLY EXTEND LEG

SPREAD TOES

STAND TALL AND DRAW SHOULDERS BACK FOR BROAD COLLARBONES

STAND TALL AND GENTLY PULL SHOULDERS BACK

PRESS OUT OF BOTTOM OF FOOT

BREATHE INTO HAMSTRING

CLASP HANDS BEHIND BACK

USE A STRAP AND GRAB HOLD AS CLOSE TO HANDS AS YOU CAN

LIFT KNEECAP OR MICRO-BEND KNEE TO PROTECT HAMSTRING FROM HYPEREXTENSION

EVENLY DISTRIBUTE WEIGHT ACROSS ALL FOUR CORNERS OF FOOT

DHANURASANA bow pose

Bow pose is a fantastic front-body opener that feels particularly great through the chest. If you spend the majority of the day hunched over a computer or if you're an athlete, I highly recommend adding this pose to your yoga practice.

Begin by lying facedown on your mat. Take a deep breath in. As you exhale, bend both legs and spread the toes. As you inhale, reach back and take hold of the tops of your feet, reaching around the outer edges. If your knees have opened up, bring them back into line with your hips; place a yoga block between your thighs if you struggle to keep your knees in line. As you inhale, peel your chest and legs off the mat. Gaze about three feet out in front of you, on the ground. You have the option of rocking forward and backward with your breath. If you choose to do this, inhale and rock forward, then exhale and rock back. Just be sure to do it on an empty stomach!

Regardless of whether you rock and roll or stay still, breathe length through your spine so as not to compress your low back. Keep your toes active, which will encourage your hamstrings to remain engaged. Breathe into any areas of tightness, particularly in the fronts of your shoulders, and relax your shoulders away from your ears. Take three to seven full, deep breaths in this position before gently releasing.

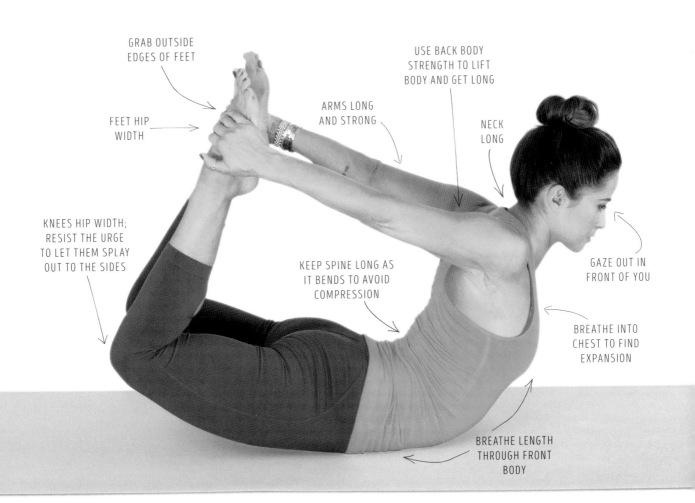

GRAB OUTSIDE EDGES OF FEET

USE BACK BODY STRENGTH TO LIFT BODY AND GET LONG

ARMS LONG AND STRONG

FEET HIP WIDTH

NECK LONG

KNEES HIP WIDTH; RESIST THE URGE TO LET THEM SPLAY OUT TO THE SIDES

KEEP SPINE LONG AS IT BENDS TO AVOID COMPRESSION

GAZE OUT IN FRONT OF YOU

BREATHE INTO CHEST TO FIND EXPANSION

BREATHE LENGTH THROUGH FRONT BODY

PADANGUSTHA DHANURASANA big toe bow pose

This incredibly deep backbend requires a lot of flexibility through the front body. Believe me, you're going to want to warm up like crazy before you attempt this pose. Also be sure that you're comfortable with poses like camel (page 258) and wheel (page 236) before you give this one a try.

Begin in bow pose (page 271). You're going to need to flip your grip in order to get into this pose. I like to do it one hand at a time. Start by sliding your right hand over the top of your right foot, then send your elbow out to the right and up toward the sky. Follow suit with your left arm, lifting your gaze to the sky if it feels okay for your neck. Lengthen from your elbows to your knees. Visualize length between the vertebrae in your spine to prevent compression in your low back. Keep your knees magnetized so that they don't open wider than your hips. Relax your shoulders away from your ears and take three to seven breaths in this pose before releasing.

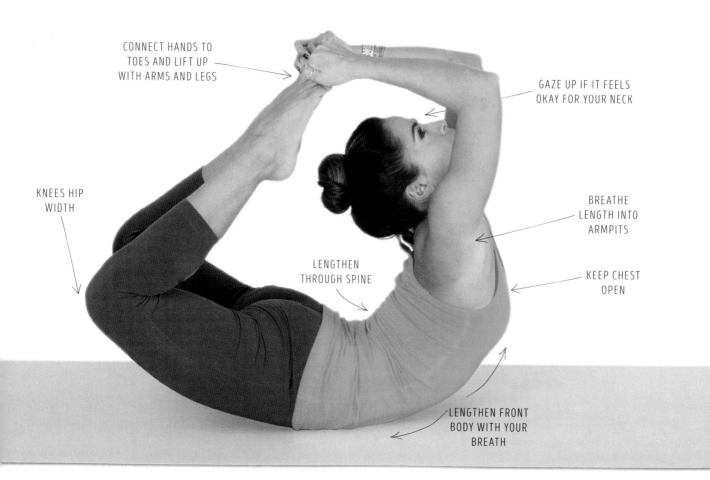

CONNECT HANDS TO TOES AND LIFT UP WITH ARMS AND LEGS

GAZE UP IF IT FEELS OKAY FOR YOUR NECK

KNEES HIP WIDTH

BREATHE LENGTH INTO ARMPITS

LENGTHEN THROUGH SPINE

KEEP CHEST OPEN

LENGTHEN FRONT BODY WITH YOUR BREATH

PINCHA MAYURASANA forearm stand

Forearm stand was a big milestone for me because it requires a lot of upper-body strength, and upper-body strength was something I seriously lacked. It also requires major openness in the armpits and shoulders. Keep those two things in mind as you approach this pose.

The traditional way to do this pose is with the forearms parallel and the palms flat on the ground. This doesn't feel great for my shoulders, so I do it with my palms in prayer position and my elbows underneath my shoulders. Either way is fine; I suggest that you try both to see which works better for you.

Regardless of what you plan to do with your palms, begin by kneeling on the ground. Place your elbows on the mat and grab hold of your opposite biceps with your hands. Be sure that you're actually grabbing the biceps rather than the elbows; grabbing the elbows makes your position just a little too wide, which creates an unstable foundation.

Keep your elbows in place as you bring your palms into position, whether they are flat on the ground with forearms parallel or in prayer position out in front of you. From here, begin to push into your forearms to engage your shoulder girdle. Push so hard that you feel a slight round between your shoulder blades. That's how hard you need to continuously push once you're in the pose.

From here, curl your toes and lift your hips, coming into dolphin pose (page 197). Slowly walk your feet in toward your body, getting them as close to your pelvis as you can. Then lift one leg and spread the toes. Push the mat away with your forearms and use your back-body strength to lift your hips higher until the other leg comes off the mat. If you need to do a little hop off the bottom leg, that's okay. Just avoid kicking up with your top leg because the momentum may project you too far and cause you to flip over, bringing you into a very deep backbend. Move with as much control and strength as you can.

Once both legs are off the ground, aim to get them into a V-shape. This way, they function as a seesaw and you can use them for leverage to find balance and bring your pelvis into a neutral position. Continue to spread your toes and push the mat away with your forearms. Slowly begin to bring your big toe mounds together and breathe length through your entire body. Stay in this position for three to five breaths before slowly lowering one leg and then the other.

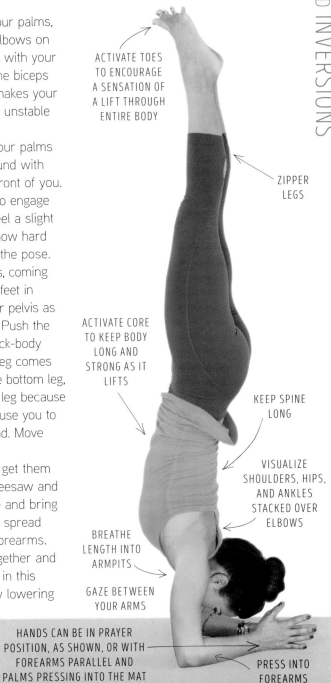

ACTIVATE TOES TO ENCOURAGE A SENSATION OF A LIFT THROUGH ENTIRE BODY

ZIPPER LEGS

ACTIVATE CORE TO KEEP BODY LONG AND STRONG AS IT LIFTS

KEEP SPINE LONG

VISUALIZE SHOULDERS, HIPS, AND ANKLES STACKED OVER ELBOWS

BREATHE LENGTH INTO ARMPITS

GAZE BETWEEN YOUR ARMS

HANDS CAN BE IN PRAYER POSITION, AS SHOWN, OR WITH FOREARMS PARALLEL AND PALMS PRESSING INTO THE MAT

PRESS INTO FOREARMS

PINCHA MAYURASANA (forearm stand) hollow back variation

If you've built significant upper-body strength and are looking to develop flexibility in your upper back and chest, you'll definitely want to start incorporating this hollow back variation of the forearm stand into your practice.

Begin in forearm stand (page 273). Take a few breaths to solidify your foundation, then slowly exhale and send your pelvis past your head as your legs come toward the ground at a slight angle. Keep your kneecaps lifted to engage your quadriceps, and press out of the balls of your feet with the toes spread and active. All this keeps your leg muscles engaged and helps create the sensation of a lift throughout your body rather than dumping your weight into your shoulders and forearms. Keep pressing the mat away from you with your forearms and breathe fully and deeply for three to seven breaths before releasing to child's pose (page 93).

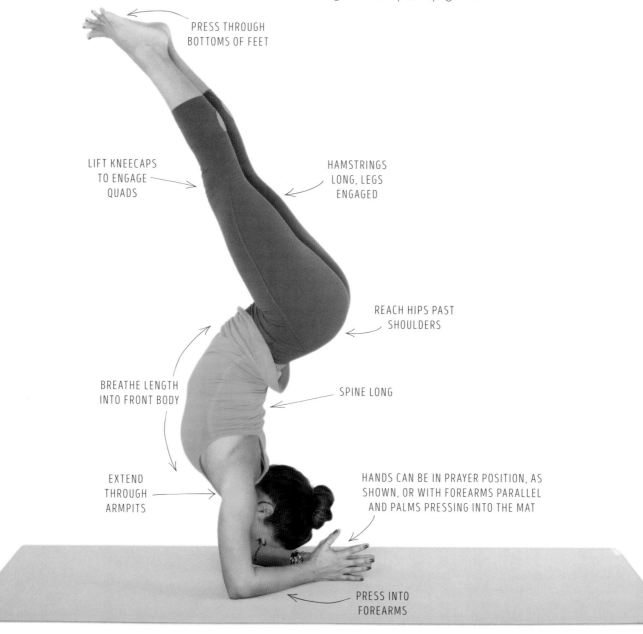

PRESS THROUGH
BOTTOMS OF FEET

LIFT KNEECAPS
TO ENGAGE
QUADS

HAMSTRINGS
LONG, LEGS
ENGAGED

REACH HIPS PAST
SHOULDERS

BREATHE LENGTH
INTO FRONT BODY

SPINE LONG

EXTEND
THROUGH
ARMPITS

HANDS CAN BE IN PRAYER POSITION, AS
SHOWN, OR WITH FOREARMS PARALLEL
AND PALMS PRESSING INTO THE MAT

PRESS INTO
FOREARMS

EKA PADA KOUNDINYASANA 1 one-footed sage pose

Remember when I said that crow pose is kind of like the first step in learning how to fly? This pose helps explain that theory. Once you have crow pose and begin to learn others, like side crow, you can start playing with funky transitions from one amazing pose to the next. One of my favorite transitions is going from side crow pose to this one-footed sage pose. Once you're there, you can bring your top leg back into side crow and then decide where to go next—maybe to tripod headstand or a jump back to chaturanga. The options are endless!

Begin in the full, traditional side crow pose (page 224) with your legs extended to the right. Take a few breaths and find your balance. When you're ready, begin to reach your right leg back behind you. Keep pressing out of the bottoms of both feet and keep your toes spread and engaged to help keep the leg muscles active. You may need to tip forward ever so slightly as you reach your right leg back; just be careful to keep your arms in "wax on, wax off" position and avoid letting your shoulders round. Instead, push into the mat with your hands and imagine that someone is lifting you up by a string tied around your upper back. This sensation of a lift will help keep your pose strong and stable and encourage your intercostal muscles to activate and hold you up. Take three to seven breaths here, keeping your gaze steadily out in front of you. When you're ready, switch sides.

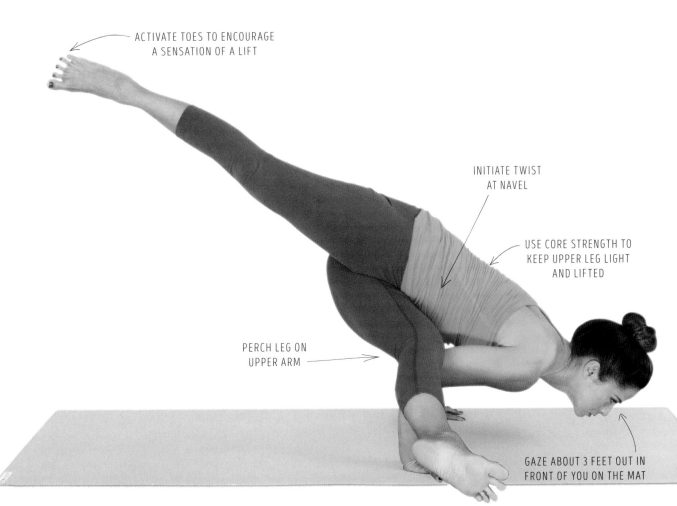

ACTIVATE TOES TO ENCOURAGE
A SENSATION OF A LIFT

INITIATE TWIST
AT NAVEL

USE CORE STRENGTH TO
KEEP UPPER LEG LIGHT
AND LIFTED

PERCH LEG ON
UPPER ARM

GAZE ABOUT 3 FEET OUT IN
FRONT OF YOU ON THE MAT

arm balances and inversions   275

URDHVA DHANURASANA (wheel pose) variation

If wheel pose (page 236) is starting to feel easy-breezy and you're ready to take it a step further, you can lift one leg up to the sky. Try to keep your weight evenly distributed between both hands and your other foot. Spread your toes and straighten your lifted leg as much as you can. Take a few breaths here. When you're ready to release the pose, gently lower your body all the way down to the mat, then switch sides.

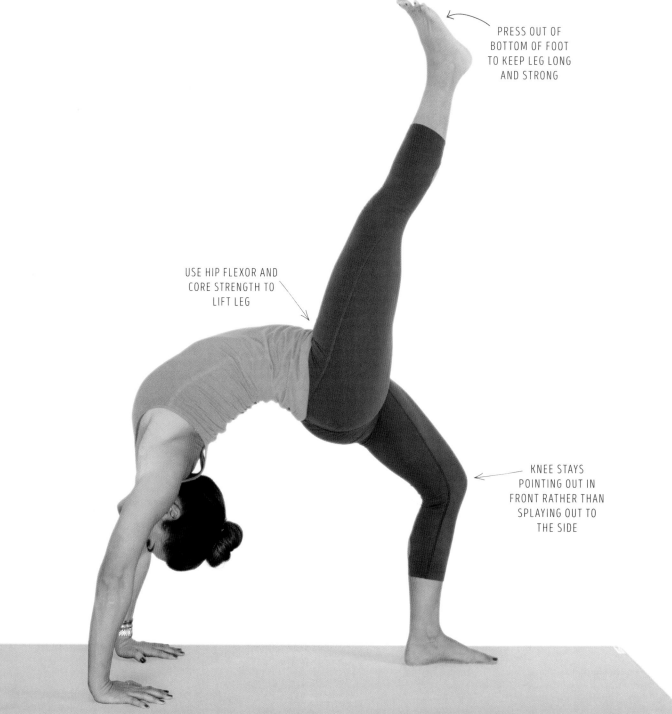

PRESS OUT OF BOTTOM OF FOOT TO KEEP LEG LONG AND STRONG

USE HIP FLEXOR AND CORE STRENGTH TO LIFT LEG

KNEE STAYS POINTING OUT IN FRONT RATHER THAN SPLAYING OUT TO THE SIDE

EKA PADA GALAVASANA flying pigeon pose

Flying pigeon pose is the next step after baby pigeon—adult pigeon, if you will. It requires major core and back-body strength, so keep that in mind if you're struggling with the full expression.

Begin in baby flying pigeon pose (page 228) with your left shin crossed over your arms and your right foot lifted. As you inhale, spread your right toes and use your back-body strength to extend your right leg behind you. Keep using your hamstring strength to keep the right leg long and strong. Imagine that your leg is so strong that if someone walked by and tried to push it, it wouldn't budge.

You may find that your left foot has a tough time staying up on your right arm. In this case, see if you can use your left toes like fingers and flex them so that they grip into your right arm. Breathe fully and deeply in this position before you return to baby flying pigeon, then exit the pose and take it to the other side.

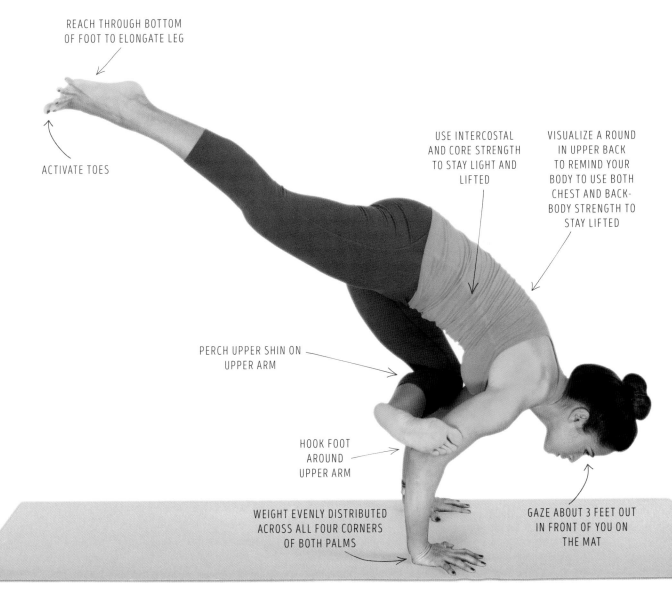

REACH THROUGH BOTTOM OF FOOT TO ELONGATE LEG

ACTIVATE TOES

USE INTERCOSTAL AND CORE STRENGTH TO STAY LIGHT AND LIFTED

VISUALIZE A ROUND IN UPPER BACK TO REMIND YOUR BODY TO USE BOTH CHEST AND BACK-BODY STRENGTH TO STAY LIFTED

PERCH UPPER SHIN ON UPPER ARM

HOOK FOOT AROUND UPPER ARM

WEIGHT EVENLY DISTRIBUTED ACROSS ALL FOUR CORNERS OF BOTH PALMS

GAZE ABOUT 3 FEET OUT IN FRONT OF YOU ON THE MAT

ADHO MUKHA VRKSASANA handstand

If you're on social media and even halfway interested in yoga, there's no doubt that you're quite familiar with handstand. It seems to be the holy grail pose for so many people, and I get it. I mean, this pose looks so fun! You're turning your world upside down with how funky it is! But it also requires a lot of balance, strength through the upper body and core, and flexibility in the armpit and shoulder areas. If you're working on this pose, my best advice is to stay consistent with your practice and don't give up. You will get there eventually.

building strength for handstand

To start building strength for handstand and to understand what it feels like to have your pelvis over your head, I suggest working with a partner rather than a wall. A wall is, in my opinion, a false sense of security. You know that it will be there, so you're more likely to kick up using your momentum and rely on it to be there for you, rather than lift up using your strength or hop up off the bottom leg using a combination of momentum and strength. So find a partner. Have her stand behind you with her dominant leg out in front and the other leg behind so that she's in an athletic stance. Then take downward-facing dog facing your partner. From here, rise up onto the balls of your feet, look between your thumbs, and jump forward, intending to push the mat away and bring your pelvis over your head. This is going to feel awkward and scary, but your friend is going to put her hands on the backs of your hips and push your hips down so that you don't tip over. As soon as you're up, let her push you down and then immediately jump up again. This is a great way to build shoulder strength. Take a rest after three to seven repetitions before practicing again.

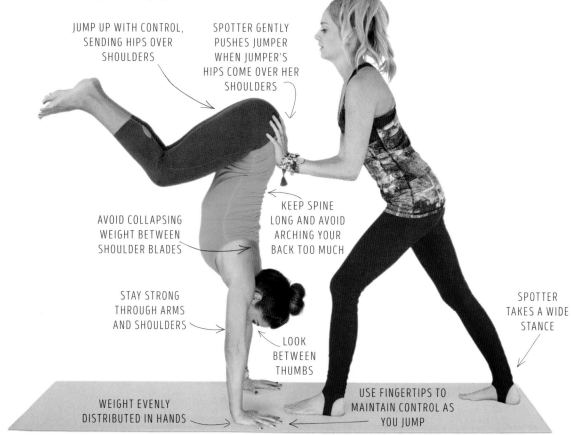

JUMP UP WITH CONTROL, SENDING HIPS OVER SHOULDERS

SPOTTER GENTLY PUSHES JUMPER WHEN JUMPER'S HIPS COME OVER HER SHOULDERS

AVOID COLLAPSING WEIGHT BETWEEN SHOULDER BLADES

KEEP SPINE LONG AND AVOID ARCHING YOUR BACK TOO MUCH

STAY STRONG THROUGH ARMS AND SHOULDERS

SPOTTER TAKES A WIDE STANCE

LOOK BETWEEN THUMBS

WEIGHT EVENLY DISTRIBUTED IN HANDS

USE FINGERTIPS TO MAINTAIN CONTROL AS YOU JUMP

coming into full handstand

Begin by bringing your hands down onto the mat, placing them shoulder width apart. Spread your fingers and grip into the mat like you're a rock climber, plugging the bases of your fingers into the mat—especially the index fingers and thumbs. Imagine that there's suction in the center of your palm, and visualize a long line of energy rising up through that suction. You want to be fully rooted into the mat but also have the sensation that you are lifting up through your entire body. Look between your thumbs and walk your feet as far forward as you can. Press your hands into the mat until you feel a round happening between your shoulder blades. Then lift one leg and spread your toes. Use your back-body strength to lift that leg as high as you possibly can. Perhaps you have so much strength that your leg just floats up, bringing the other leg with it. Or perhaps you need to do a little hop off the bottom foot. That's fine; just make sure to use your strength and control to come into the posture. Avoid kicking over with your top leg, because the momentum may send you over into a deep backbend. Once your legs are up, bring them into a V-shape, keeping the toes spread. Use your legs like a seesaw to find balance in the middle and allow your pelvis to come into a neutral position. Once your pelvis is neutral and you feel balanced, slowly scissor your legs together and press your big toe mounds together as you continue to lift up through the balls of your feet. Take three to seven breaths here before slowly coming out of the pose with strength and control.

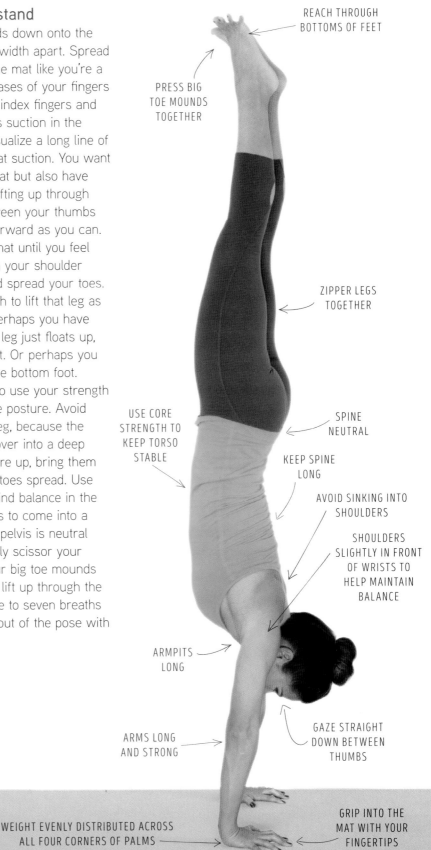

REACH THROUGH BOTTOMS OF FEET

PRESS BIG TOE MOUNDS TOGETHER

ZIPPER LEGS TOGETHER

USE CORE STRENGTH TO KEEP TORSO STABLE

SPINE NEUTRAL

KEEP SPINE LONG

AVOID SINKING INTO SHOULDERS

SHOULDERS SLIGHTLY IN FRONT OF WRISTS TO HELP MAINTAIN BALANCE

ARMPITS LONG

GAZE STRAIGHT DOWN BETWEEN THUMBS

ARMS LONG AND STRONG

WEIGHT EVENLY DISTRIBUTED ACROSS ALL FOUR CORNERS OF PALMS

GRIP INTO THE MAT WITH YOUR FINGERTIPS

GANDA BHERUNDASANA chin stand pose

Confession: Chin stand pose used to scare me because it looks like it puts the neck in a precarious position. But the truth is, the majority of your weight should be in your arms. You can think of the chin as a kickstand—there to help you balance, but not necessarily what you want to rely on. My advice is to be sure that you have solid upper-body strength and feel comfortable in positions like headstand (pages 229 and 232) and forearm stand (page 273) before giving this pose a try.

Begin in low plank (page 110). Bend your arms about 90 degrees, use your toes to send yourself forward so that your elbows are directly over your wrists, and gently place your chin on the ground. Lift one leg and use both back-body and core strength to get your leg perpendicular to the ground. Follow with the other leg. Spread your toes and reach your legs toward the sky. Continue to push the mat away with your hands, keeping the majority of your weight in your upper body. Breathe length through your spine and squeeze your legs together as you feel a long line of energy running through the crown of your head all the way up through your toes. Take three to seven deep breaths here before slowly lowering one leg, then the other.

KEEP TOES ACTIVE TO ENCOURAGE A LONG LINE OF ENERGY FROM HEAD TO FEET

LIFT LOWER LEGS TO THE SKY OR BEND THEM, BRINGING FEET TOWARD HEAD

VISUALIZE LENGTH THROUGH SPINE

USE CORE STRENGTH TO KEEP TORSO AND LEGS LIGHT AND LIFTED

MAJORITY OF WEIGHT IN HANDS

GRIP INTO THE MAT WITH YOUR FINGERTIPS

CHIN ACTS AS A KICKSTAND AND BEARS VERY LITTLE WEIGHT

GANDA BHERUNDASANA (chin stand pose) variation
scorpion pose chin stand

If you're feeling solid in your chin stand, you can take it a step further by moving into the scorpion pose variation.

Start in chin stand (opposite) and slowly bend your left knee, reaching the toes toward your head. Continue to push the mat away with your hands, breathing length through your spine so that you don't compress your low back. When you feel secure, come into the full expression of the pose by bending your right leg as well. Breathe for three to seven breaths before slowly releasing one leg, then the other.

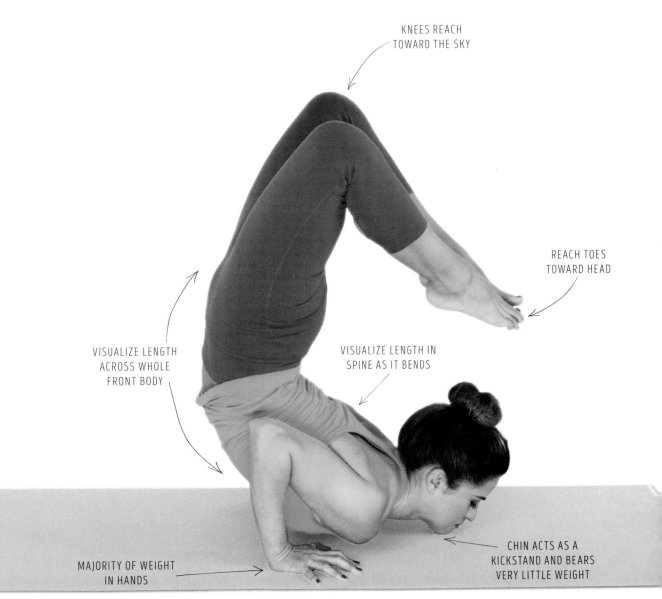

KNEES REACH TOWARD THE SKY

REACH TOES TOWARD HEAD

VISUALIZE LENGTH ACROSS WHOLE FRONT BODY

VISUALIZE LENGTH IN SPINE AS IT BENDS

CHIN ACTS AS A KICKSTAND AND BEARS VERY LITTLE WEIGHT

MAJORITY OF WEIGHT IN HANDS

VRSCHIKASANA PINCHA MAYURASANA
scorpion pose forearm stand

Scorpion pose from forearm stand is a beautiful pose that brings together all the elements of what we work on in the yoga practice: strength, balance, flexibility, and focus. I suggest attempting this pose only after you have a solid forearm stand and wheel pose (page 236).

Begin by coming into forearm stand (page 273). Press the mat away from you, and when you're ready, start to bend your legs with active feet. As you do this, arch your back and visualize length through your entire spine. Take your gaze forward. The farther you look out in front of you, the deeper your upper back will bend, and it's important to get a deep bend in the upper back because it'll help protect your low back. Breathe length through your entire front body from your knees through your shoulders. After three to seven breaths, slowly release the pose the same way you went in.

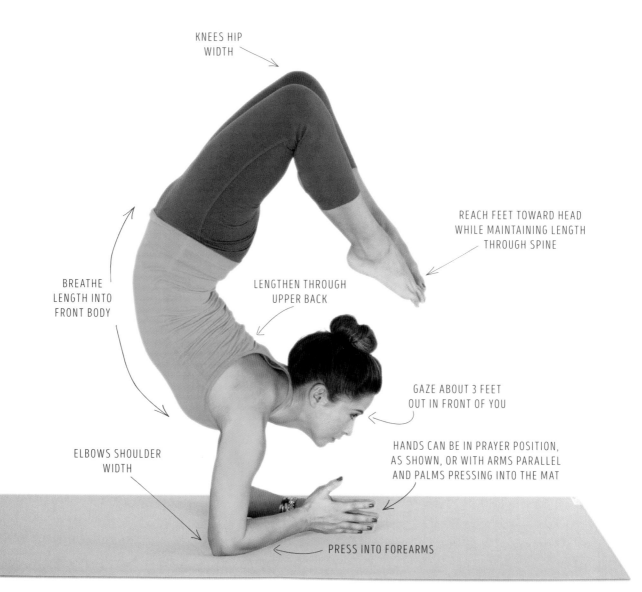

KNEES HIP WIDTH

REACH FEET TOWARD HEAD WHILE MAINTAINING LENGTH THROUGH SPINE

BREATHE LENGTH INTO FRONT BODY

LENGTHEN THROUGH UPPER BACK

GAZE ABOUT 3 FEET OUT IN FRONT OF YOU

ELBOWS SHOULDER WIDTH

HANDS CAN BE IN PRAYER POSITION, AS SHOWN, OR WITH ARMS PARALLEL AND PALMS PRESSING INTO THE MAT

PRESS INTO FOREARMS

VRSCHIKASANA scorpion pose handstand

Want to know a secret? I find this pose far more accessible than handstand. Something about the belly being out on one side and the shins being out on the other creates what feels like an effortless balance provided that you remember to lift your gaze, which arches your back evenly.

Begin in handstand (page 278) with your legs in a V-shape and your toes spread. Slowly bend your left leg, reaching the toes toward your head. As you do this, lift your gaze out in front of you. Doing this will help you arch your back and create a beautiful, space-filled backbend. Keep pressing the mat away from you, being mindful to micro-bend your elbows if you are prone to hyperextending in the arms. Use your fingertips to maintain your balance, and when you've found that balancing sweet spot, slowly begin to bend your right leg back as well, keeping the toes spread. Imagine that if you were able to look to your right into a mirror, your body would be making the shape of a capital P. Elongate through your back and breathe fully and deeply for three to seven breaths, then slowly release with control.

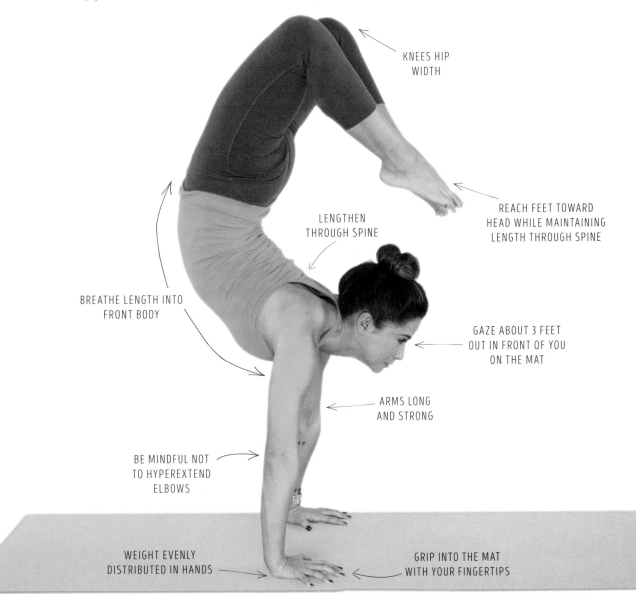

KNEES HIP WIDTH

REACH FEET TOWARD HEAD WHILE MAINTAINING LENGTH THROUGH SPINE

LENGTHEN THROUGH SPINE

BREATHE LENGTH INTO FRONT BODY

GAZE ABOUT 3 FEET OUT IN FRONT OF YOU ON THE MAT

ARMS LONG AND STRONG

BE MINDFUL NOT TO HYPEREXTEND ELBOWS

WEIGHT EVENLY DISTRIBUTED IN HANDS

GRIP INTO THE MAT WITH YOUR FINGERTIPS

EKA PADA KOUNDINYASANA 2 one-legged sage pose

This is a really cool arm balance that makes a great base for funky transitions. I love going from this pose to chin stand (page 280) using strength from the posterior chain. It's beautiful, but it's also just plain fun.

Begin in lizard pose (page 191). On your next inhale, bring your right arm underneath your right leg so that your right hamstring rests on your right triceps. Then press into the mat with your hands and use your left toes to send your entire body slightly forward. Lift your right leg, spread the toes, and lift your left leg using your back-body strength. Firm your core and get as long as you can from head to toes. Make sure that your legs stay engaged, which will help you stay long, strong, and lifted in the pose. Breathe for three to seven breaths before releasing and taking it to the other side.

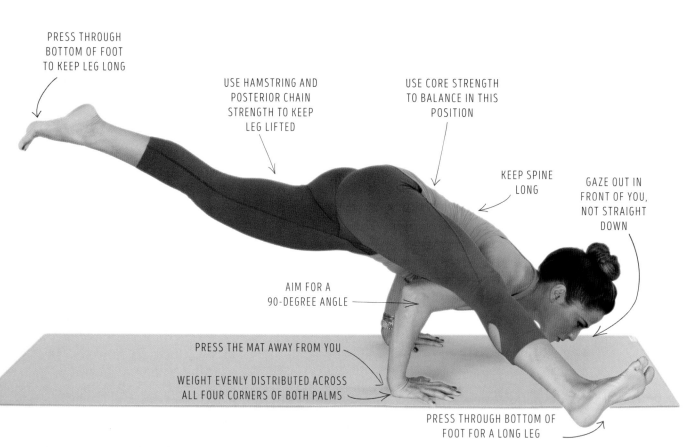

PRESS THROUGH
BOTTOM OF FOOT
TO KEEP LEG LONG

USE HAMSTRING AND
POSTERIOR CHAIN
STRENGTH TO KEEP
LEG LIFTED

USE CORE STRENGTH
TO BALANCE IN THIS
POSITION

KEEP SPINE
LONG

GAZE OUT IN
FRONT OF YOU,
NOT STRAIGHT
DOWN

AIM FOR A
90-DEGREE ANGLE

PRESS THE MAT AWAY FROM YOU

WEIGHT EVENLY DISTRIBUTED ACROSS
ALL FOUR CORNERS OF BOTH PALMS

PRESS THROUGH BOTTOM OF
FOOT FOR A LONG LEG

TITIBHASANA firefly pose

Saying the Sanskrit name for firefly pose in class always gets me a few laughs. This super-fun pose requires a good amount of hip flexibility, core strength, and upper-body strength.

There are two ways to enter the pose. The first (which I prefer) is to sit on the ground with your legs bent. Then lift your right leg and set the back of your right knee as high up on the back of your right arm as you can. Balance here as you do the same thing on the left side. Then rock forward, placing your hands on the ground, shoulder width apart, and use your core strength and the momentum from your rock forward to lift yourself up. Press out of the bottoms of your feet and spread your toes. Use your core strength to lift your hips high and gaze forward as you breathe fully and deeply.

The other way to enter the pose is to stand with your feet a little wider than hip width apart. Bend over, thread your arms through your legs, and set your hands down on the ground slightly behind you, shoulder width apart. Then bend your knees deeply and press into your hands as you transfer your weight from your feet to your hands. Lift your feet off the ground and use your core strength to lift your hips high. Use your intercostal muscles and core strength to keep yourself lifted. Press out of the bottoms of your feet and spread your toes to keep your legs engaged. Look out in front of you and breathe for three to seven breaths. When you're ready, release the pose.

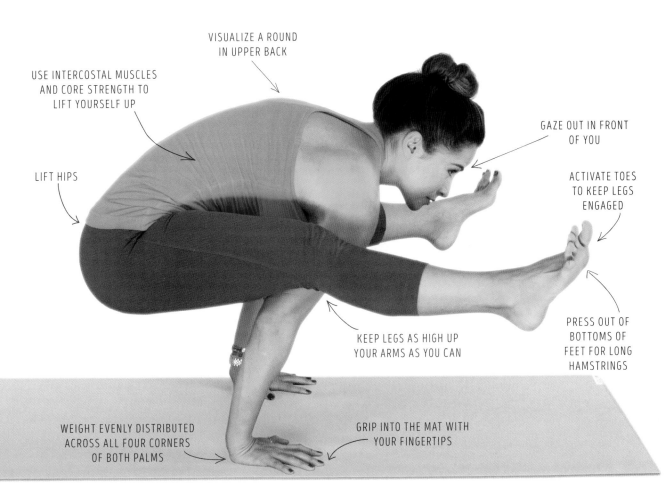

VISUALIZE A ROUND IN UPPER BACK

USE INTERCOSTAL MUSCLES AND CORE STRENGTH TO LIFT YOURSELF UP

GAZE OUT IN FRONT OF YOU

LIFT HIPS

ACTIVATE TOES TO KEEP LEGS ENGAGED

KEEP LEGS AS HIGH UP YOUR ARMS AS YOU CAN

PRESS OUT OF BOTTOMS OF FEET FOR LONG HAMSTRINGS

WEIGHT EVENLY DISTRIBUTED ACROSS ALL FOUR CORNERS OF BOTH PALMS

GRIP INTO THE MAT WITH YOUR FINGERTIPS

URDHVA DHANURASANA (wheel pose) variation

This very deep backbend is best approached after you feel quite comfortable in wheel pose. It requires a lot of flexibility through the shoulders and upper back, so keep that in mind if you're working toward this pose.

Begin in wheel pose (page 236). When you're ready, slowly bring your right forearm to the ground, followed by your left forearm. Your elbows should be directly underneath your shoulders, and your hands can be either flat on the ground or in prayer position. Gaze between your elbows and lift your hips. Keep your knees pointing forward and avoid letting your toes splay out to the sides. Breathe fully and deeply for three to seven breaths before returning to wheel pose and releasing.

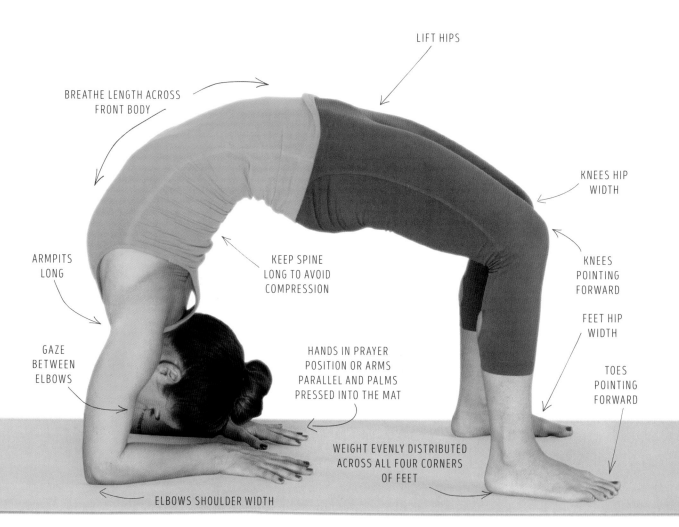

LIFT HIPS

BREATHE LENGTH ACROSS FRONT BODY

KNEES HIP WIDTH

ARMPITS LONG

KEEP SPINE LONG TO AVOID COMPRESSION

KNEES POINTING FORWARD

FEET HIP WIDTH

GAZE BETWEEN ELBOWS

HANDS IN PRAYER POSITION OR ARMS PARALLEL AND PALMS PRESSED INTO THE MAT

TOES POINTING FORWARD

WEIGHT EVENLY DISTRIBUTED ACROSS ALL FOUR CORNERS OF FEET

ELBOWS SHOULDER WIDTH

KAPOTASANA pigeon pose

This extremely deep backbend is best reserved for when you feel very comfortable in wheel pose (page 236) and bow pose (page 271) and can flip the grip like in dancer's pose (page 179).

    Begin kneeling on the mat with your knees and ankles hip width apart. Lift your hips and bring your hands into prayer position at your heart. Tuck your tailbone slightly as you press your hips forward, lift your chest, and lean back. Reach your arms overhead as you continue to lean back and lift your chest so that your spine makes the shape of an upside-down U. Bring your hands down to the mat. Walk your fingers to the outsides of your feet and place your hands on the backs of your feet. Then, as you exhale, spiral your elbows in so that they're in line with your shoulders and bring your forearms down. Gaze between your forearms with your head off the mat. Keep your spine light and lifted and breathe length from your knees through your elbows. Take three to seven breaths in this position. When you're ready to release, walk your hands underneath your shoulders and press into the mat to lift up and come out of the pose.

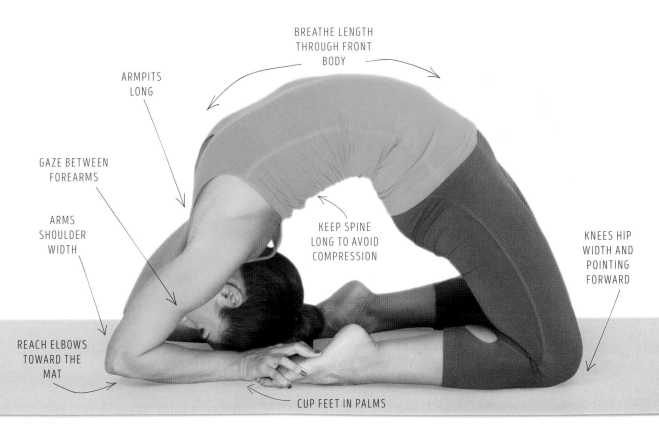

BREATHE LENGTH THROUGH FRONT BODY

ARMPITS LONG

GAZE BETWEEN FOREARMS

ARMS SHOULDER WIDTH

KEEP SPINE LONG TO AVOID COMPRESSION

KNEES HIP WIDTH AND POINTING FORWARD

REACH ELBOWS TOWARD THE MAT

CUP FEET IN PALMS

sequence 1

1. GARLAND POSE
(page 182)

2. CROW POSE (page 222)
A)

B)

3. HALF VINYASA

4. to WARRIOR 3 (page 194)
A)

B)

C)

5. STANDING PIGEON POSE
variation (page 201)

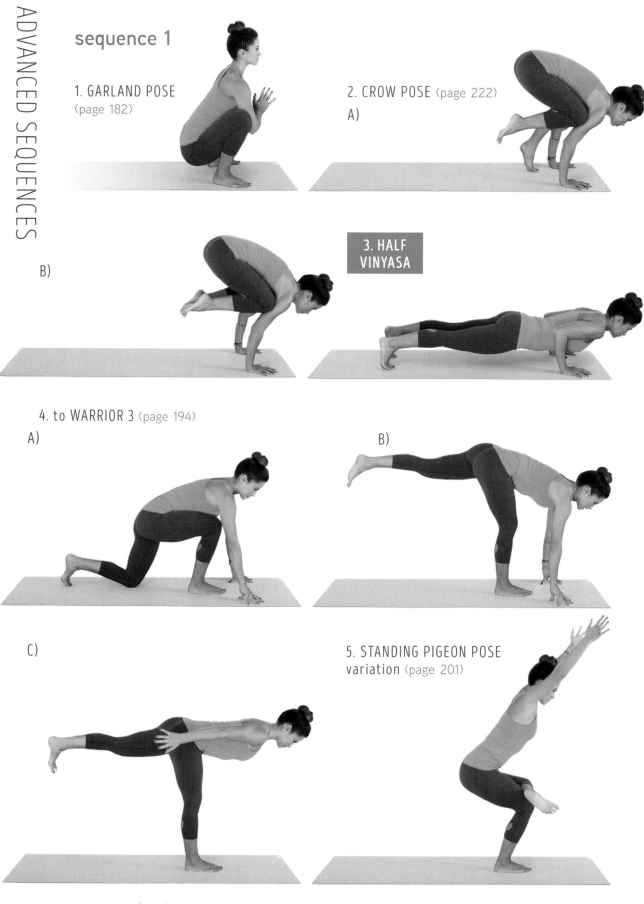

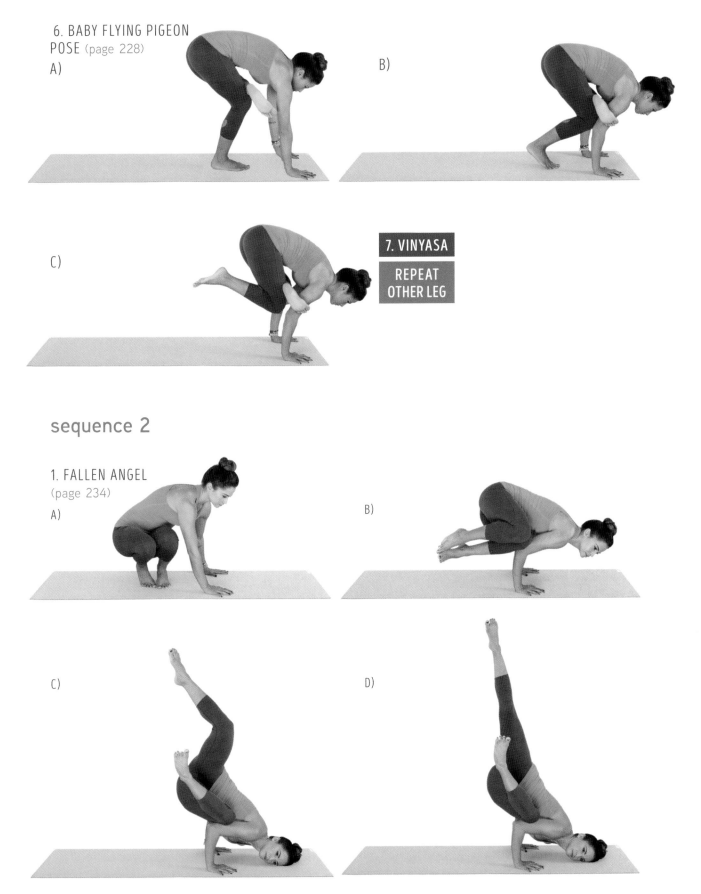

6. BABY FLYING PIGEON POSE (page 228)

A)

B)

C)

7. VINYASA

REPEAT OTHER LEG

sequence 2

1. FALLEN ANGEL
(page 234)

A)

B)

C)

D)

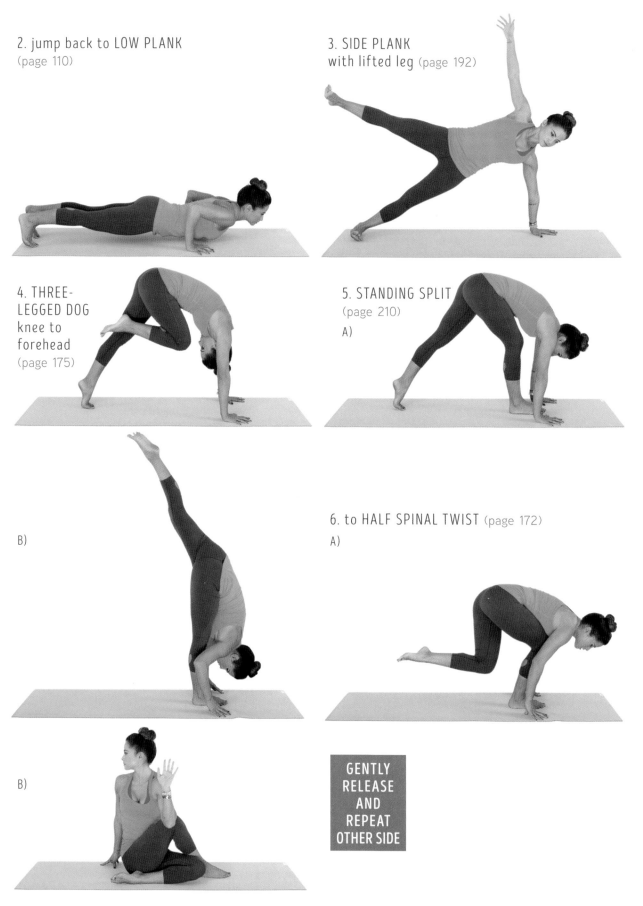

2. jump back to LOW PLANK
(page 110)

3. SIDE PLANK
with lifted leg (page 192)

4. THREE-LEGGED DOG
knee to forehead
(page 175)

5. STANDING SPLIT
(page 210)
A)

B)

6. to HALF SPINAL TWIST (page 172)
A)

B)

GENTLY
RELEASE
AND
REPEAT
OTHER SIDE

sequence 3

1. EAGLE POSE (page 204)

2. WARRIOR 1
(page 113)

3. PIGEON POSE (page 97)

4. MERMAID POSE (page 164)
A)

B)

5. KING PIGEON POSE (page 263)
A)

B)

6. CAMEL POSE (page 258)

7. VINYASA

REPEAT OTHER LEG

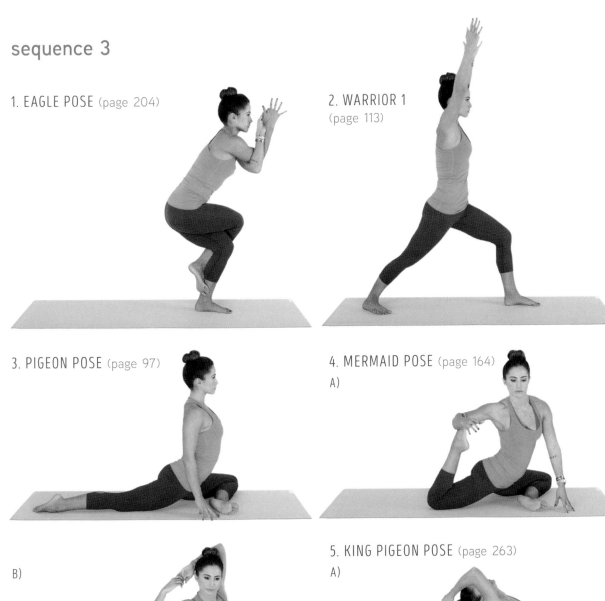
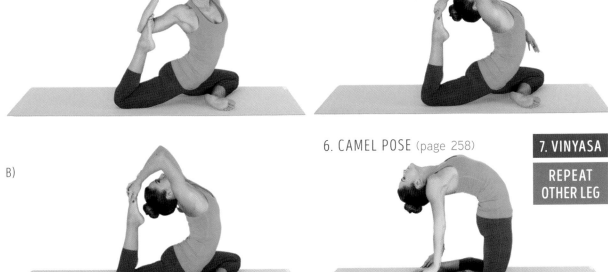

sequence 4

1. GARLAND POSE
(page 182)

2. TRIPOD HEADSTAND
(page 232)

A)

B)

C)

D)

E)

F)

3. CROW POSE (page 222)

A)

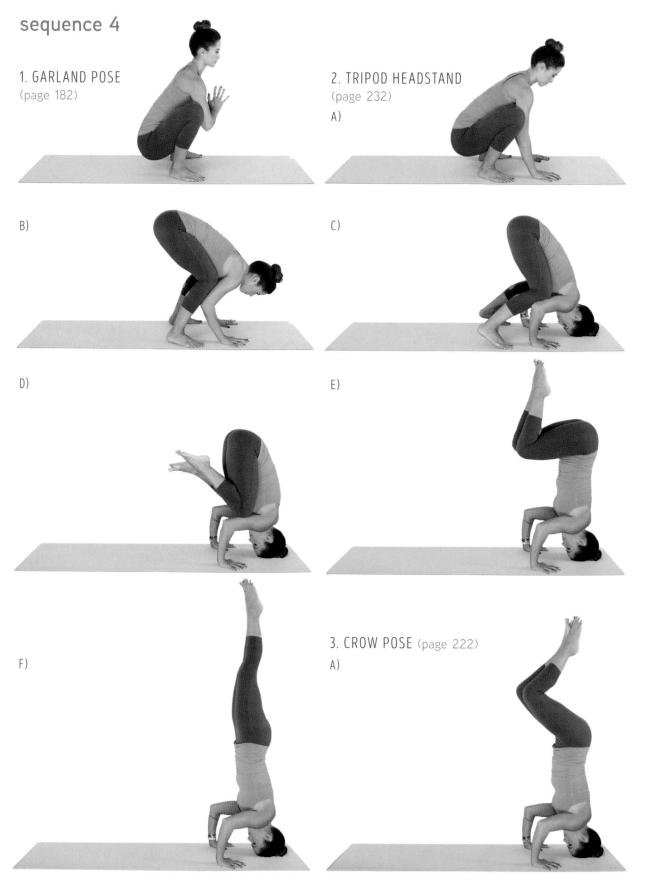

B) 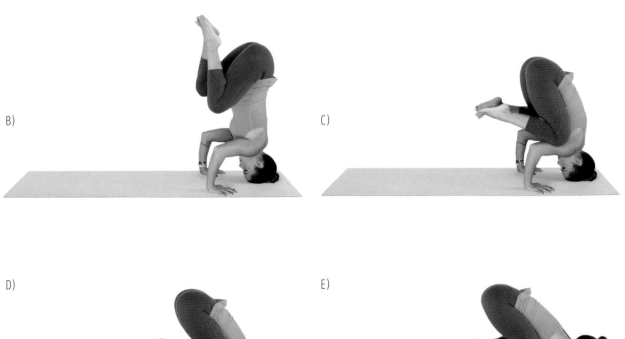 C)

D) 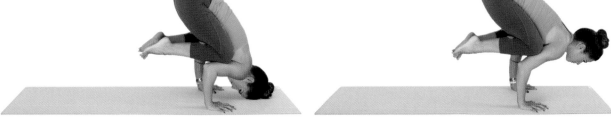 E)

4. LOW PLANK (page 110)

F)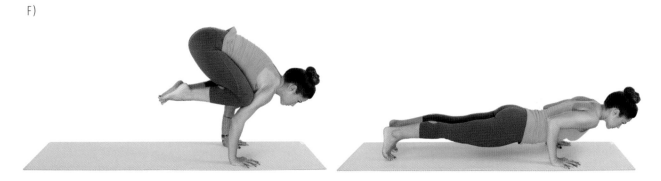

5. BOW POSE (page 271)

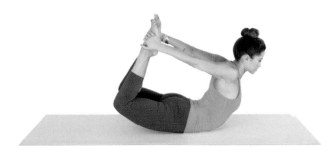

6. BIG TOE BOW POSE (page 272)

A)
B)

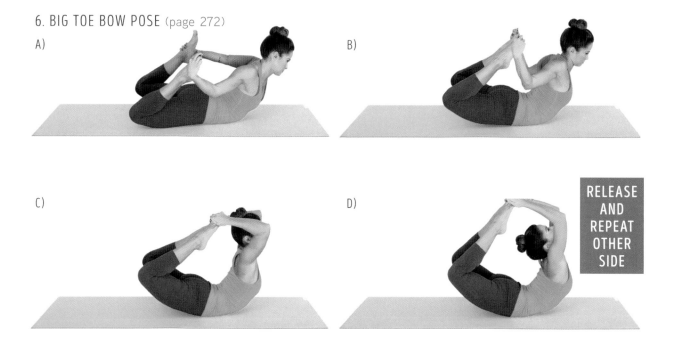

C)
D)

RELEASE
AND
REPEAT
OTHER
SIDE

sequence 5

1. VINYASA

2. ONE-LEGGED SAGE POSE
(page 284)

A)
B)

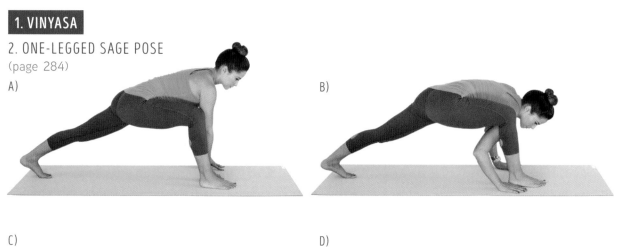

C)
D)

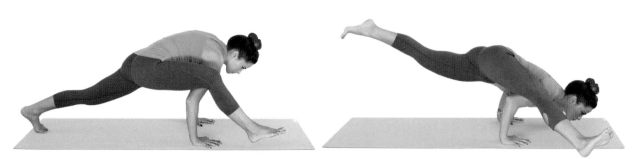

3. SCORPION POSE CHIN STAND (page 281)

A)

B)

4. VINYASA

REPEAT OTHER SIDE

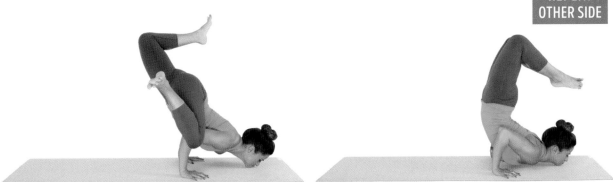

5. MOUNTAIN POSE
(page 106)

6. FIREFLY POSE (page 285)

A)

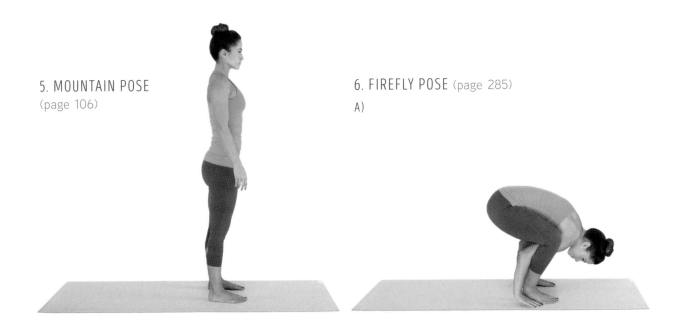

B)

C)

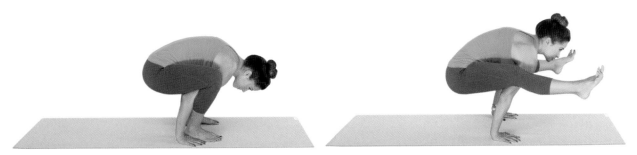

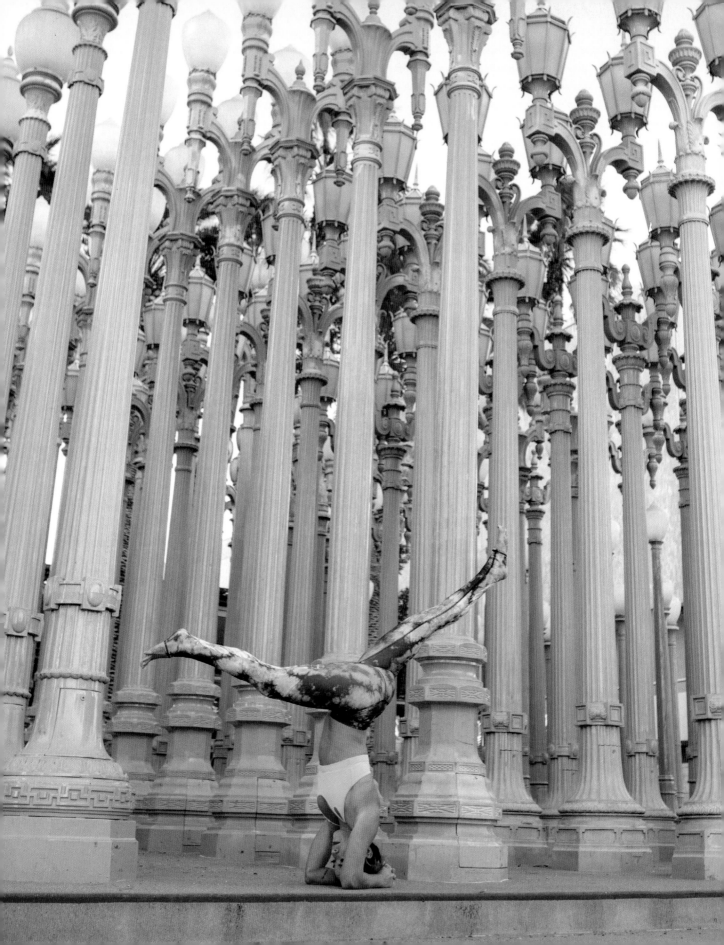

you can do anything but not everything

The problem with being so sick for such a painfully long time is that when you finally get better, you're off and running the second your feet hit the ground. This might not seem like a problem, but when you haven't been going full speed for years and then you suddenly put the pedal to the metal, well, you might just realize that you could've used a learner's permit before hopping onto the racetrack.

Greg has to retire from hockey for reasons I legally can't talk about because we may or may not have been blackmailed into signing a nondisclosure agreement. My unofficial recommendation to anyone considering playing hockey in a corrupt third-world country? Reconsider. (This was not Germany; we loved it there.)

We return to the U.S., and I have never been so grateful to be home. After years of moving around, I am excited to settle down for a bit. We crash with my parents while we hunt for a place to live.

I picture a loft-style, converted warehouse–type space with bright natural light, exposed beams, and hardwood flooring. I envision a dedicated office space for my business and a studio space for shooting my YouTube videos. I can see it so clearly in my head that when we walk into the first place we tour, I can't believe my eyes: it's like seeing a dream come true. This building is a restored factory. There are thirteen-foot windows and nineteen-foot ceilings. It is the perfect place to set up YogaByCandace, LLC.

The same week we move in, we head to Costa Rica, where I lead a retreat. It is the biggest retreat I've done, and I earn more money from that one retreat than I've made in months. It's not about the money, but I feel so happy to be healthy enough to be working and traveling and doing what I want to do with my life. I understand what a gift that is, and my heart is full as I do my work with pride and love.

I've recently hired Lauren as my marketing director, and she holds down the fort back home while I teach. She lines up sponsored posts with small businesses whose missions are in line with ours and helps bring my second dream to life: a discovery box service.

I got the idea for the quarterly YBC Mantra Box after getting pitch after pitch from small businesses that wanted to send us goods but didn't have the money to pay for exposure.

I thought, *Why not make a small amount available for purchase, do some blogger outreach, and feature the businesses on our blog? It would be a win-win for everyone involved. The small businesses that don't have the inventory to participate in large-scale subscription services like Birchbox would get exposure within our niche community. The people who order the boxes would be surprised with products from small businesses in the health and wellness industry that they hadn't heard of, and their sharing them on social media would be great PR for those businesses. And we would get paid for our efforts in putting it all together.*

Lauren's job is to explain all this to potential partners and get them on board. When we have everything squared away with the businesses, we promote the idea on the blog. It completely sells out.

After we get back from Costa Rica, I tell Greg that I need a car. We go to the dealership, and I use money I've earned to get my shiny new car. It's our money, of course, but it makes me feel good knowing that my hard work has earned the money we're spending. To this day, every time I get in that car, I feel a sense of gratitude. The car is beautiful, with heated seats and a great sound system (which is a must-have because I can't *not* sing along to the radio when I drive—you should try it; it's the best stress reliever). But the gratitude is not about the car. The gratitude is about having my health back, and about all I've been able to do since I've been back on my feet. Much like the handstand in the yoga practice, the car is not the thing I celebrate. I celebrate the hard work it took to get there—the hard work I was excited to do after fighting through the worst years of my life.

A week after I get my car, I head to New York City for a yoga conference. At the end of a fully scheduled Friday, I'm walking back to my hotel. It's rush hour and, having just left a PR meet-and-greet, I'm lugging a new yoga mat, three swag bags, and all my gear from the day. I've got my headphones on and I am walking with a pepper in my stepper. The sidewalk is my runway! The world is my oyster! The sun is shining, and there is nothing I can't do!

I step off the curb when the walk light comes on, and I immediately fall. I feel a sharp, searing pain, and I try to get up but can't.

In case you're wondering whether there's a preferred time and place to sprain your ankle, there is. And it's not in the middle of rush hour on Fifth Avenue in New York City.

A good Samaritan helps me up and walks me over to a bench. She goes back out to the road to hail me a cab, which takes over fifteen minutes. I am in so much pain that I cannot put any weight on my foot.

The cab whisks me to my hotel, where the concierge all but carries me to my room. He brings me ice and helps pack my bag. I call Greg, who hops in his car to come get me.

Suddenly, I panic. I'm supposed to leave for a three-week European retreat tour in ten days. We have two retreats lined up in Greece with Sophie, a weekend in Italy, and then a long weekend retreat that I've coordinated myself in Morocco (Africa has always been on my bucket list). How am I supposed to travel? Teach? Give all these people a week to remember?

NAMASLAY COMMANDMENT #9:
DEFY YOUR LIMITS.

When I get home, I get crutches. Because we're still waiting for the health insurance forms to go through, a sports therapist who follows me on Instagram offers to come look at my ankle. I am wary because who knows, this person could be the next Craigslist Killer, but I'm desperate and have no insurance. As it turns out, though, she's an extremely knowledgeable therapist who's worked with a number of sports teams and has seen hundreds of ankle injuries. She diagnoses it as a classic sprain, not a break, and teaches me how to use a piece of foam to compress the ankle and reduce the swelling. I thank her profusely, and she laughs it off and says, "It's the least I can do—your yoga videos on YouTube have helped me so much!" I am blown away. The power of social media, my friends.

A week later, I am on a flight to London, then to Athens, and then on a ferry to Sifnos, a beautiful Greek island. A couple who are attending this retreat were students of mine when I first started teaching yoga in Germany, and I hug them with so much joy in my heart because it feels like one of those Oprah a-ha full-circle moments.

Our retreat venue is a whitewashed boutique hotel on an organic olive farm. It is perched on the side of a steep mountain that overlooks the Aegean Sea, which is the deepest, most vibrant blue color I've ever seen. The students are a cool, laid-back bunch from all over the world.

I hobble into my first yoga class and tell myself that it's time to figure it out. No more woe-is-me nonsense. These people have paid a lot of money for a great yoga program, and it's time to roll up my sleeves and get creative. Unable to demonstrate the majority of the poses, I do my best. And what do you know?

My best is enough.

I realize that my best has *always* been enough.

A week later, Greg arrives, and soon we head to Italy, where we spend a few days touring Rome. I am exhausted but happy. My ankle hurts, but it's getting better. As a result of being the default photographer for my blog, Greg has developed a great eye, and we spend our time in Rome looking for inspiring shots that we can blow up and use to decorate our new home.

A few days later, we're on a flight to Marrakesh. I'm nervous because I've booked a private riad. The photographs show a large clay-colored venue with brightly tiled flooring and a pool in the back. But who knows if the venue will actually look like the photos?

To our relief, the venue is as beautiful as it was in the photos. The woman who runs the riad is a young, divorced Muslim woman. She is breathtakingly beautiful with dark-rimmed eyes and olive skin. Her kindness and warmth make her even more beautiful, and over the week we talk about struggles and triumph.

"It is not easy to be a Muslim woman who is divorced. But I have to live the best life I can. And I have to take care of myself first," she says. "People think it's selfish to take care of yourself, but it's not. It is a necessity."

She is so, so right.

Our students are the funniest, most loving, laid-back bunch of women from Singapore, Australia, the U.K., and France. At dinners we laugh until we cry, and during the day they set out and explore the surrounding area. We have yoga every morning and evening, and I am filled to the brim with gratitude for how lucky I am to have these women here. And how lucky I've been at all my retreats, to connect with such incredible people. I know they've booked a retreat to take care of themselves and I am supposed to be the one delivering a great experience, but I always finish the week feeling inspired by them, their courage, their kindness, and their good vibes. They are always strong, smart, funny, and above all kind.

And I realize that this is not a mistake. Your vibe attracts your tribe. Through being authentically yourself, you attract the right people into your world.

*****

Once we are home, I set up my office space. I feverishly write blog posts, film videos, and negotiate sponsored post details with companies. Lauren and I work tirelessly from morning to night, never stopping. I rarely take a lunch break; I just go, go, go. We are so excited about this little business that is thriving and growing, and I don't see a glass ceiling for us. This is the start of something big, I can feel it. I dream up all the things we will accomplish. Retreats all over the world, maybe with a humanitarian aspect. Video bundles to help increase the steady revenue stream. A book. An app. A line of clothing. Props. Teacher trainings. The options are endless.

I feel like there is never enough time in the day for all the things I want to do, though. I work all the time. I don't hang out with friends. I don't take time to do anything for myself. I feel like my life was on pause due to my health issues, and, now healthy, I am feverishly working to make up for lost time. I wake up at 4:45 a.m., eat breakfast, go to the gym, and am at my desk by 7:00 a.m., where I work until 11:00 p.m. with few breaks in between.

A few weeks later, Greg and I head to a long weekend retreat in upstate New York. I've rented a large home on sprawling grounds. It is the first retreat I've done that filled up so quickly that we had to start a waiting list in case of cancellations.

The group of women are lovely. We laugh and share stories about the scariest things ever to happen to us. We realize that we are out in the middle of nowhere, and there are two escaped fugitives at large somewhere around us. After we share our stories, we make Greg go around and check all the rooms. It feels like a big family, and it's a wonderful weekend, but at the end I am exhausted.

When we return home, I crash and burn. It's been too much activity for me. I can feel pain and inflammation rearing their ugly heads. I feel overwhelmed and stressed, like I've got way too much on my plate. We have two more retreats scheduled this summer, and the thought of trying to put them on when I still haven't

fully unpacked and settled into our new place makes me want to cry. I start to feel depressed, and all the subconscious clenching I've been doing lately has my jaw in so much pain that it's waking me in the middle of the night.

I wake up in the morning, go to the gym, and sit down at my desk for another day of work. I have over 200 new emails. I head to YouTube to work on the comments. I pride myself in trying to respond to every comment I get.

Do you have a yoga video for back pain?

I'm a total beginner, how do you suggest people get started with yoga?

Can you do longer meditation videos?

I can't hear you, the audio sucks.

You're so fuckable.

This video sux! You don't tell me where to breathe!

You forgot the left side.

You're too big.

You're too thin.

What do you eat?

You eat meat?! What kind of yogi are you?!

Why isn't there any music?

I love that you don't have any music.

The pace is too fast.

I am a soldier serving overseas, and I want to thank you for this video. We do it every morning and it has helped me so much with my back pain. Thank you, from the other side of the world.

I break down in tears. The pain in my jaw is so bad that I worry I might have an abscess or infection, so I go to the dentist.

"So what's been going on?" she says as I settle into the chair.

"My jaw really hurts," I say and open my mouth.

She pokes. She prods.

"There's nothing wrong with your teeth. Are you stressed out?"

My lower lip quivers as I try to keep my emotions in check. But I burst into tears. The hygienist takes my hand in hers and offers me a tissue.

"Tell me about this past year," she says.

"Well, since last summer, I've moved from LA to the Czech Republic. I went to Costa Rica to lead a yoga retreat. I went back to Europe. My husband lost his job, and we flew back home to the U.S. We went to a wedding in Florida. The day we flew back north, we got a call from Germany with a job offer for my husband. The only stipulation was that we had to be on a flight the next day. We got on that flight and moved back to Europe. Then I traveled to Dubai for a site visit for work, and then my husband's contract was up, so we went back to the U.S., where we crashed with our parents while looking for a place to live. I traveled to Miami for a retreat. We finally found a place to live but didn't have any furniture, not even a bed, and before we could get ourselves situated it was time to travel back to Costa Rica for another retreat. Shortly after that, I went to Greece, Italy, and Morocco for work. Afterward, I came back to the U.S. to fully move in, then led a retreat in upstate New York, and now here I am." I'm exhausted just telling her about my year.

"Candace," the dentist says. "I see cases like this at least twice a week. There's nothing physically wrong with you. You people are stressed out! You've got to lower your stress levels. It's not worth it to keep up this pace if you're feeling this bad."

I leave feeling relieved but defeated. I feel so sad that I couldn't keep up with everything I wanted to do. After years of dealing with health issues, I have my health back and I just want to go, go, go. But I can't. All this running around has caught up with me, and I feel miserable. I lack a work/life balance.

And I am embarrassed, because let's be honest, I blog for a living. I teach yoga for a living. I ship out discovery boxes for a living. I film YouTube videos for a living. I'm not curing cancer over here. I'm not a rocket scientist. But all this work, it's *work* for me. Retreats, while I love them, are not vacations for me. All that traveling, all those time changes, they take their toll on my body. Inflammation and pain are key indicators. It is time to seek out a balance.

I cancel my remaining two retreats. I write a blog post saying that I am overwhelmed and need a break. I feel like a failure, even though I know better. Then the comments on the post start rolling in. Every single one of them is uplifting.

It takes strength to realize when you need a break and even more strength to act on it. You are an inspiration.

Take care of you and have no guilt about doing so! It takes a strong person to admit you need time.

Don't set a deadline for feeling better. Please take good care. Don't give when you don't have the capacity to give— that is something I am also working on for myself, so thanks for setting a good example for everyone!

You are braver and stronger than you think, just by opening up to us. I am grateful to have stumbled upon your Instagram account and started reading your blog. It has

opened my eyes and taught me so much! You have the YBC community's support.

Each comment fills my heart and makes me feel like we truly are in this together. Yoga. Union. I love this little corner of the Internet so much. I log out, shut down my computer, and don't feel guilty about not responding to each comment like I normally do. I know they understand. They're my people.

I put Buckles in the car and we head to my hometown. The Appalachian Trail runs through it, and we go for a hike, something I haven't done in years. I let him off leash and he runs like the wind up and over the hills, jumping into streams and swimming in the Housatonic River. He loves life so much. I smile, realizing that I can learn a lot from him. His ability to stay in the moment, every moment, is inspiring.

Being outdoors, away from the noise of the city, makes me feel like I'm in a different world. When I'm working, I'm so *connected*. With the click of a button I can post a photo and have full conversations with YBCers from anywhere from Portugal to Panama. On one hand, it's beautiful to feel so connected, to show up at retreats feeling like I already know the people attending. It makes me feel like my work matters. And that's all anyone really wants, right? To matter. To make a difference. To help and connect. But on the other hand, while out on my hike, I am alone. And it feels so nice. So refreshing. So beautifully, peacefully quiet. I'm so deep in the forest that the air actually smells like pine, and all I hear as I walk down the trodden path is the hollow sound of my footsteps.

The next day I pack up my car and go to the beach. I read. I swim. I close my eyes and feel the sun soak into my skin. I feel so happy and nourished and grateful to be in this moment.

When I return to work a week later, I update the blog with my newly set, self-imposed rules. I am on a mission to find balance.

• **Shut down social media.** I turn off all notifications for my social media accounts. When I have the time and energy to respond to comments, I will log in and do my best to answer them. With a large following and people constantly asking for tips, I acknowledge that it probably isn't likely that I'll get to every comment, but I will do my best and let that be enough.

• **Be more thankful.** Period, end of story. Thankful for everything. For getting up in the morning, for the water that runs from the tap with which I brush my teeth. For my Wi-Fi connection, for all the work I have, for my dog, for my health, for everything. Having an attitude of gratitude makes the day far better than suffering from a case of the Poor Me's.

• **Stop the negative self-talk.** I noticed that every time I did something great, I would take maybe half a second to feel good about it, and then I'd think, 'Well, if I had done *this*, it would be *that* much better.' I'm sick of that. I just want to do my best and let that be enough. No more second-guessing myself, no more beating myself up. Life is too short for that.

By the end of the summer, I am feeling so much better. I have what feels like a solid work/life balance. Work is thriving, and my life is at a place where I feel like a normal person. A lot of those inspirational quotes will tell you that normal is boring and encourage you to do everything in your power not to be normal. But when you've been sick for years, normal is cause for celebration.

NAMASLAY COMMANDMENT #5:
DO THE LITTLE THINGS.

In August, there is much to be celebrated. Like the beautiful normalcy that has become my life, and also the phone call I am currently on. But first, let me back up a second.

Blogging is weird in that you "meet" a lot of people online, and sometimes you feel closer to them than you do to your friends in real life. Hayley Mason from *Primal Palate,* a Paleo blog, has become a friend, and I've reached out to her because a small publishing house has asked us if we can pen a book about yoga and cats.

Now, I don't know anything about a connection between yoga and cats. Because I'm allergic to them, I don't even care for cats that much. Plus, my Husky would kill me if he knew that I wrote a book on cats. But I would love the opportunity to bring my book idea to life, that one I had way back when in yoga teacher training. So I want to get in touch with this publishing house, and since Hayley has published three incredible Paleo books, I ask her opinion.

She talks to me about publishing. She tells me what I should look for and talks about what makes a great book. These are things I have not even considered. For example, feel how smooth the page of this book is to the touch. The paper is thicker than, say, a textbook page, which is notoriously thin like a magazine, but it isn't so thick that it's hard to turn the page. Look at the binding. See how secure it is? How easily the pages move as you flip through the book? Feel the texture of the front cover. Notice the flaps on the cover for easy bookmarking. Bookmaking is an art. And none of these elements are things I was aware of until Hayley points them out to me.

After talking with Hayley, I go to my local bookstore. There are a few yoga books. There are some fitness books. I pull them all and sit at the café inside the store. The bindings aren't great. The pages feel like construction paper. The photographs are dull and lackluster. The content is okay, but they're not the beautiful, visual learning tools I envision.

I look at the samples that the publishing house has sent to me. The pages look like they were bound together with Elmer's Glue. The photos are grainy and too dark. The books are crap. I sigh, and Hayley and I talk again.

"I could reach out and see if my publisher would take a call with you," Hayley offers.

Two weeks later, I am on a conference call with Hayley's publisher. And now I hold my breath.

"Yeah, I took a look at your proposal," says Erich, the president of Victory Belt Publishing.

There's a pause, and I think I can hear my heartbeat.

"We'd love to publish your book."

Silent tears of joy roll down my cheeks as Lauren jumps in to ask questions about the contract.

In first grade, we had to write our autobiographies. Looking back, that seems like a curious project for first graders, since we hadn't really lived that long, but whatever. In our "about me" section on the author page, we wrote our aspirations.

Candace, I wrote, *wants to be an author one day.*

The most popular girl in the class said, "You want to be an author? I want to be a model!" And all the other girls, myself included, changed their bios to say that they wanted to be models, too. Hey, when you're in first grade, you're just trying to fit in. Or at least I was.

My teacher tried her best to persuade me to go back to wanting to be an author. "But that's what you wanted to do first," she said.

"Yes, but I want to be a model more," I stubbornly lied.

In this phone call, I smile, realizing that since I'll be posing for *Namaslay,* I will be doing both.

Dreams do come true, again and again.

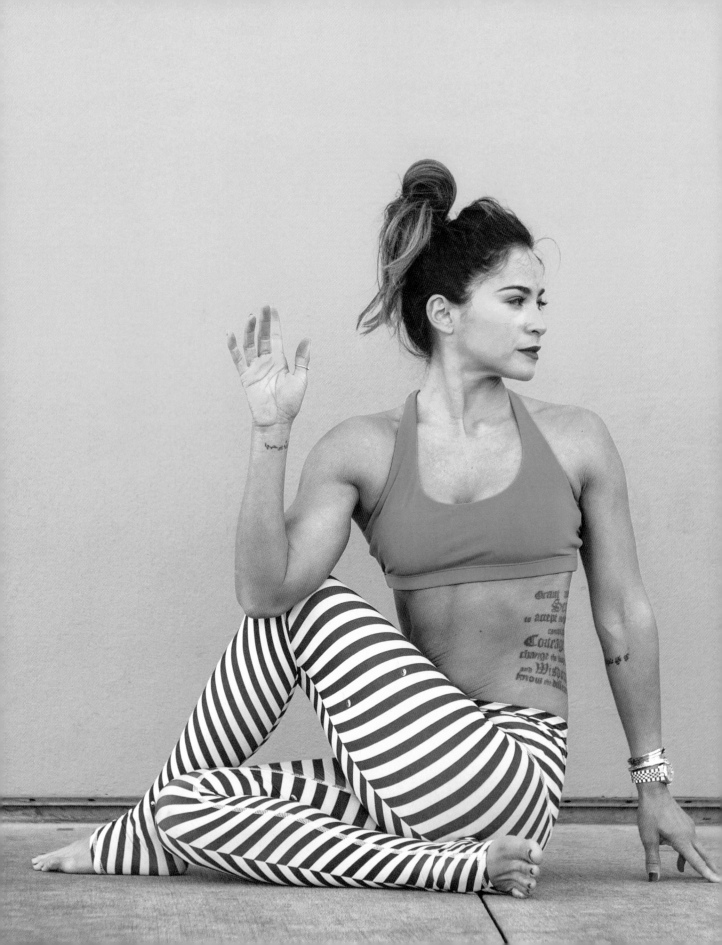

CHAPTER 6:

the restorative practice

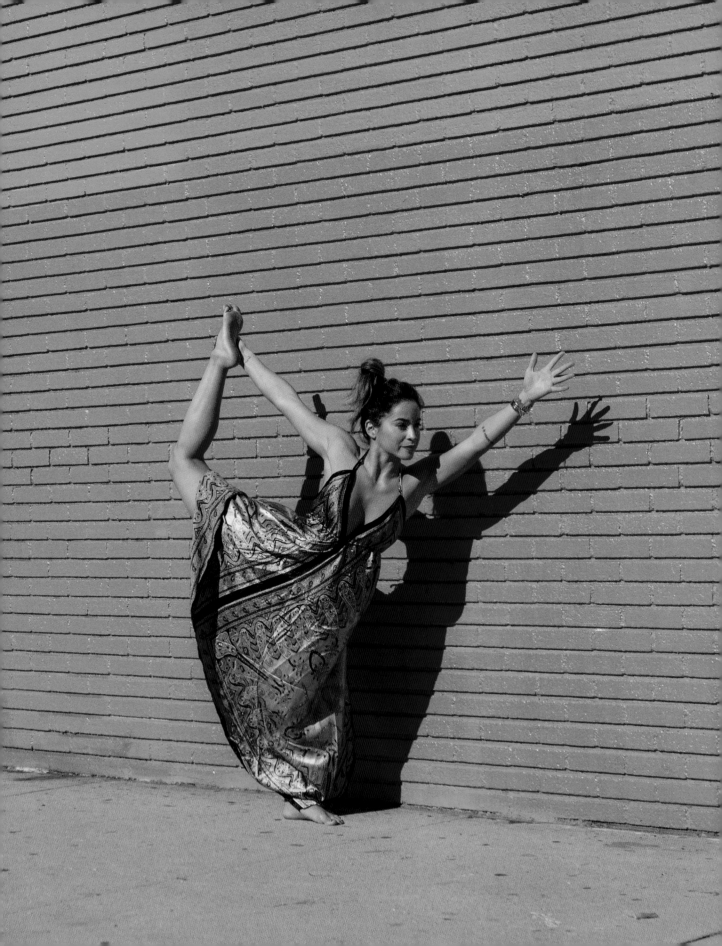

perseverance

November 2014

When I was sixteen, my mom kept me from getting into too much trouble by talking me into going to Costa Rica to do a study abroad program. I lived with a host family in a small town where only a handful of people spoke English, aside from my six fellow exchange students.

I was fearless back then. Remember, this was a time before Facebook and Instagram. Forget smartphones—no one I knew even had a cell phone, really! I communicated with my family and friends back home through the ancient art of the handwritten letter (to this day, one of my favorite ways to communicate) and through emails, when the Internet connection at the local Internet café wasn't slower than a sloth (which was rare).

I attended the local high school and my host family's gatherings, and even went to church with my host mom a few times. I said yes to everything and went for it full steam ahead. It didn't occur to me to feel embarrassed by my lack of Spanish. I just did my best. I spoke barely any Spanish when I arrived, and six months later I left nearly fluent.

In the years since, I've returned to Costa Rica over fifteen times. A few of the other exchange students and I are still quite close, more than fifteen years later. One of them, Benthe, is German, and we took a spontaneous girls' trip to Istanbul together when I was living in Germany. Another, Bethany, from Maine, came to my wedding and remains one of my dearest friends.

I'm telling you all this because I'm on a plane back to Costa Rica, on my way to lead my first solo retreat. I'm exhausted but also fueled by a rekindled fearlessness. I've led retreats before, but often with Sophie as the logistics coordinator. This time, I'm doing it myself. And I don't really know how I pulled it off.

Actually, I do.

I promoted the retreat on my blog. I wrote about it on Instagram. And somehow, miraculously, people signed up. I'm expecting five students from all over— two Swedes, a Swiss guy, a French woman, and a Canadian. I've rented a mansion in the jungle, and I'm anxious about whether it'll live up to its gorgeous online photos, but I don't have time to worry about that now. I'm too tired.

I woke up at 2:45 a.m. in a small town outside of Prague. Greg drove me to the airport, where I caught a flight to Brussels. From there I flew to New Jersey, and from there to Miami, where I have an old friend named James, who graciously let me ship a bunch of swag-bag stuff to his apartment.

This has been another perk of growing my blog. Businesses in the health and wellness industries want to send me stuff! I take organic beauty products, coconut oil, and a bunch of new fitness gear. Then, a few hours later, I hop on a flight from Miami to Costa Rica.

I arrive at the car rental desk thirty-six hours after leaving Prague, sticky and stinky and so jet-lagged that I almost don't know what century it is, but I am powering through because I am feeling invincible.

I insist that the car rental associate speak to me in Spanish. When I respond, he looks taken aback.

"Did you hear her?!" he asks the associate next to him. "What an accent! Where did you learn Spanish?"

I beam. I am good with language. I always have been good with language. It's one of my things. I can hear a word or phrase in another language and, more often than not, replicate it perfectly. I tell them about my study abroad in Tilarán, the small town about two hours away.

"I'm a little nervous about navigating my way to this mansion, though," I say. "It's in the middle of nowhere!"

He points to the map. "Don't be. You have the map, and besides, you're nearly Tica [Costa Rican], so you can stop and ask for directions. You'll be fine."

"Well, I'll have my friend Alejandra with me, too," I say and look at my watch, wondering where she is.

Alejandra and I met when I was sixteen, during the aforementioned study abroad. She is petite like me, and brunette, with kind eyes and a fabulous smile. She's agreed to cook typical Costa Rican food for our group and to help with the housecleaning. As she's currently out of work, the week-long job will help her out a great deal. She's grateful for that, and I am grateful to have someone I know and trust to help me. Plus, it doesn't hurt that she's one of my oldest friends, and we get to spend time together!

Alejandra was supposed to have met me at the rental car place an hour ago. I take a seat and pick up my Kindle as I wait for her.

An hour later, an associate calls me to his desk. "The phone is for you," he says.

It's Alejandra.

"Candace!" she exclaims. "I'm so sorry! My phone died, and I had to ask someone to use theirs. Listen," she says breathlessly, "I was taking the bus to meet you and we've been detained. The police came on board and searched all the bags, and someone had a box filled to the brim with tuna fish cans. The police opened it, and each can was filled with cocaine. Of course no one is claiming the box, and now they are interrogating everyone. I'm so sorry, but there is nothing I can do. The second I'm allowed to go, I will take a taxi and meet you!"

The thing about Costa Ricans is that they are very *tranquilo*. Laid-back. No rush. Nothing to be worried about. Ever. It's a good lesson for me.

I'm hungry, I'm tired, and I'm jet-lagged. But I say, "*Tranquila,* I'll see you when I see you," and hang up.

Three hours later, she arrives and we're off.

When we arrive at the mansion, I am relieved to note that it is every bit as beautiful as it appeared online. The white exterior with honey brown trim contrasts sharply against the lush green jungle backdrop. The gray granite infinity pool has a waterfall at one end and is flanked by a hammock that overlooks the jungle and, just beyond, the ocean.

Alejandra and I race around town getting groceries for the week and setting up the rooms for the students. I am in a panic because two of the bedrooms are joined by a Jack-and-Jill bathroom. That's fine—the students knew that when they chose their rooms— but surprise! The door to the bathroom is glass! It's frosted glass, so you can't make out every detail, but you can *definitely* see through it. I say a silent prayer that the students will be chill.

The next afternoon, the students begin arriving. They are tired from traveling and just want to rest. Our last student arrives at 8:00 p.m., exhausted. "I can't wait to go to sleep," she says. "But I'm so excited about this week. I have been so stressed out, and it will be nice to just relax."

After I show her to her room, I draw a bath. My heart is full, and I am in great spirits despite feeling jet-lagged. Alejandra has been an incredible help and is great with the students even though they don't share a common language. The students seem really laid-back and easygoing, and I am sure we'll all get along great and have a wonderful week together.

As I sink into the tub, I hear a knock outside my bedroom door. "*Si!*" I call, thinking it is Alejandra. No one comes in.

Another knock.

"*Ale, entra!*" I say.

Nothing.

I get out of the tub, wrap a towel around myself, and rush to the bedroom door. It's the Canadian woman who just arrived.

"I'm so sorry to bother you," she exclaims. "But . . . there is a scorpion under my bed!"

OMG.

I am not someone who is easily freaked out by bugs. With the exception of spiders, I can handle nearly anything. But scorpions? I've never even seen one, and I have no idea what to expect. How big is this sucker? What do I do with it? Can we just let it go? Is it poisonous?! I have so many questions, none of which I will ask because my Canadian student certainly doesn't know, and besides, I'm supposed to be the leader. The one with everything under control.

"Okay," I say calmly and tighten the towel around me.

We walk quickly to the other wing of the mansion, where I knock on Alejandra's door. She opens the door and looks me up and down, as I'm sopping wet and wrapped in a towel.

"Don't ask," I smile. "Listen, we have a situation." I explain the rogue scorpion, and she looks at us very calmly and reaches down to pick up her sneaker.

"Listen, I'm very sorry to have to say this," she says carefully in Spanish, "but we are going to have to kill it. Scorpions can be very dangerous, and we are at least forty-five minutes from a hospital. If one of us got stung, it would be very bad. If it weren't a scorpion, I would let it go free, but we can't."

I nod solemnly and translate for my student, and the three of us continue to her room. When she opens the door, we quickly scan the floor. Nothing. I look down at my feet, wishing I had put on sneakers instead of flip-flops. The bathwater continues to drip from my hair, creating a puddle on the floor.

"It was under the bed," the student says and backs out of the room. Ale and I look at each other. I tighten the towel around me again and tell her to go around to the other side of the bed. I look around my side and squat low to grip the base of the box spring, and together we move it about three feet.

As we move the bed, a big brown scorpion scurries across the floor. It is the size of a TV remote control and just as thick. Its curled tail looks like a fat braid and tapers at the end in the same way. I am awestruck and horrified and thank my lucky stars that Alejandra is here.

Killing this poor thing is going to be like killing a rat, and I ask Alejandra if she sees it.

"Yep," she says and moves closer with her sneaker raised overhead.

I have to step out of the room because I feel so bad about the poor scorpion's impending doom.

There's a loud whack.

"It's done," Alejandra says. She picks up the dead scorpion and takes it outside. The student thanks us profusely and we leave.

"I don't know what I would do without you here!" I say to Alejandra as I walk her back to her room.

"Oh, please, it's nothing. I hate that I had to kill it, but we are so far from everything up here in the jungle that it just wouldn't have been safe for us," she sighs.

"No, I understand," I say, and thank her again before returning to my bath.

* * * * *

I am still jet-lagged, on Czech time, and the next morning I am up before everyone else. I go out to the kitchen and boil some water. I cut up a lemon and some ginger and pour the water into my cup.

I quietly slide the glass door open and walk out onto my private patio. I sit in the chair and take a slow, deep breath as I take in the sight. The expansive jungle canopy sways gently before me, looking much like the parachute that we played with in gym class when I was in elementary school—big and billowy. The birds squawk at each other, howler monkeys make these prehistoric dinosaur sounds, and for a second I feel like I'm in a scene from *Jurassic Park*. I look up at the sky, blue, not a cloud to be seen, and out in the distance I see the ocean—calm and quiet, with soft rolling waves. I feel an overwhelming sense of gratitude and pride. I did this. I created this opportunity for myself and for others. The idea that I am so much more powerful than I give myself credit for is underscored in this moment. I have come so far from that day in the bathtub when I was in so much pain that I wanted to disappear. Life is so, so good.

NAMASLAY COMMANDMENT #6:
MANIFEST GRATITUDE.

To me, the restorative practice is like eating a delicious warm chocolate lava cake that's actually good for you. It's so good that you might audibly moan, and no one around you will care because they are all experiencing the same incredible flavors and they get it.

The restorative practice is my favorite because it's slow, gentle, and nourishing. It's the opposite of the fast-paced power vinyasa classes that are so popular. For the most part, these poses are effortless. You relax into them, surrendering all effort. They are not meant to be done with an athletic, push-yourself mentality. The restorative practice is about turning off strain and exertion and the need to go further and do more. It is about being grounded and open, letting gravity work its magic as you gently stretch deeper and deeper into each posture.

Restorative yoga is excellent for developing flexibility. It's also a wonderful way to calm the mind and de-stress, and it may help lower anxiety, tension, and mild depression.

The restorative poses I'm featuring in this book are mostly yin poses. They're meant to be held for one to five minutes or longer. It's important to be very mindful to move slowly as you enter into and release each pose. Because of the nature of the postures and how deep you're stretched, moving in or out too quickly can put you at risk for injury.

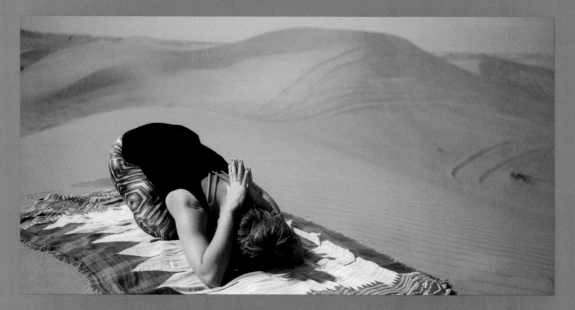

props for the restorative practice

You will need a number of props for the restorative practice. Feel free to get creative if you don't currently own these props. Don't let a lack of props prevent you from doing this practice.

- BOLSTERS: Bolsters are vital to the practice. There are a couple of different types. I recommend a rectangular bolster if you're a beginner because it gives you two options. If you lay your rectangular bolster flat, it is lower, and you can do a smaller backbend over it. If you turn it on its side, it is much higher, giving you the option to take your backbend much deeper. A round bolster is just one height no matter which way you turn it and therefore is best, in my opinion, for a more advanced student. Look for a bolster that offers medium cushioning. If it's too soft, it won't offer much support. If it's too firm, it may feel uncomfortable. I also like a bolster with a removable cover that you can wash now and then.

- BLOCKS: Block material is a personal choice. Foam blocks are usually somewhat soft, which is nice for the restorative practice because more often than not you'll be draping your body over the blocks. Another great option is something ergonomic like a Bhoga Block, which is made of wood but has such a unique shape that you can place it underneath your body and melt right into it without pain. Cork blocks are okay—they offer a tiny bit of give, which makes them moderately comfortable. I don't recommend rectangular wooden blocks, as I personally find them uncomfortable.

- BLANKETS: I recommend a thick, heavy blanket made of a wool or cotton blend. Avoid synthetics and any material that is too thin. A heavy blanket offers more support when folded.

- STRAP: A belted yoga strap can be used in a number of different ways for the restorative practice. It's especially helpful for people with tight hips in poses like reclined bound angle (page 135) because it adds extra support and security.

- CHAIR: A chair is a unique prop that isn't often used in the regular practice but can add another dimension to the restorative practice. A folding chair is ideal because it doesn't slide around like a computer chair—although a computer chair can be kind of nice because it may give you the luxury of customizing the height of the seat to suit your needs.

supported bridge pose

You'll need: a yoga block, rolled blanket, or bolster

Find the ridges of the backs of your hip bones and place your prop underneath. Slowly lower your body, resting your weight fully on the prop. Keep your feet hip width apart with your knees bent. You can bring your hands to your belly as shown or place them down at your sides— whichever feels more comfortable for you. Then close your eyes and totally relax into the pose, feeling gravity pull you down with each exhale.

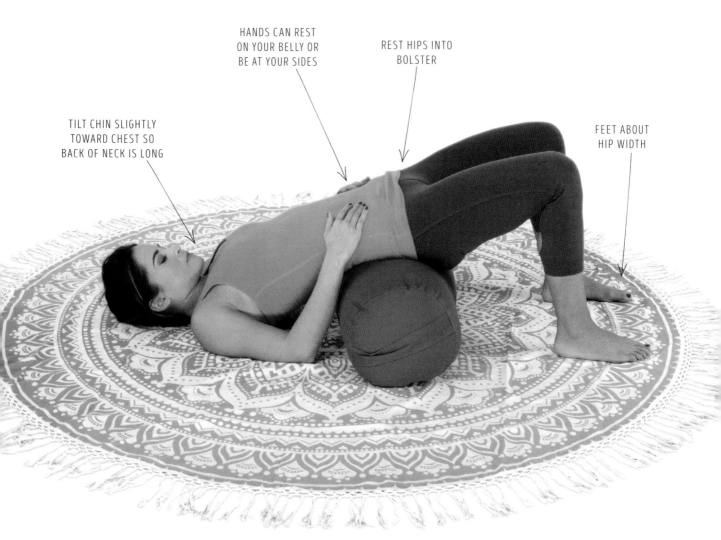

HANDS CAN REST
ON YOUR BELLY OR
BE AT YOUR SIDES

REST HIPS INTO
BOLSTER

TILT CHIN SLIGHTLY
TOWARD CHEST SO
BACK OF NECK IS LONG

FEET ABOUT
HIP WIDTH

supported caterpillar pose

You'll need: two bolsters and a blanket

This delicious pose is excellent for opening up tight hips and hamstrings. Begin seated with your legs a little wider than hip width apart. Place a folded blanket underneath your sitting bones. Then place one bolster between your legs, as close to your pelvis as you can. Place the second bolster on top and slide it about one-fourth of the way away from you. Place your forearms on the top bolster and rest your left cheek on your arms. Stay here for one to three minutes before turning your head to the other side for another one to three minutes.

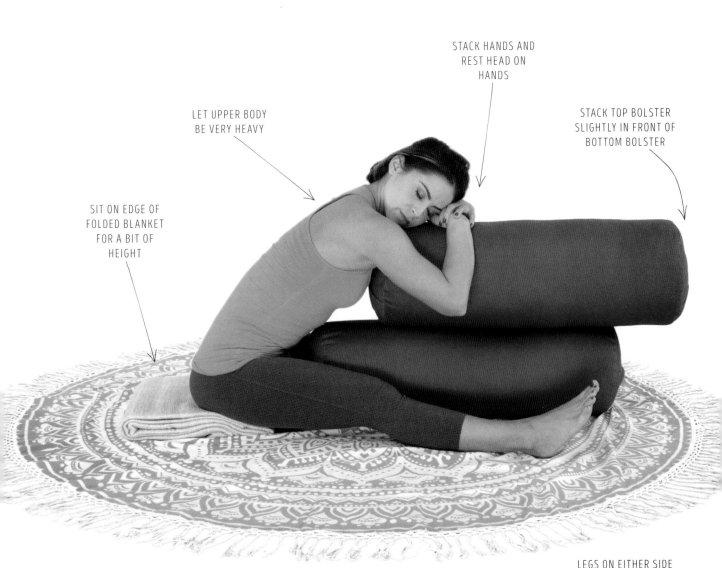

STACK HANDS AND
REST HEAD ON
HANDS

LET UPPER BODY
BE VERY HEAVY

STACK TOP BOLSTER
SLIGHTLY IN FRONT OF
BOTTOM BOLSTER

SIT ON EDGE OF
FOLDED BLANKET
FOR A BIT OF
HEIGHT

LEGS ON EITHER SIDE
OF BOLSTERS

supported reclined bound angle pose

You'll need: two bolsters, blankets, or yoga blocks

This pose is a wonderful way to open up the groin and inner thighs. Begin seated on your mat with your legs straight out in front of you. Bend your knees and bring your feet halfway back. Place your feet on the ground, keeping your feet and knees together. Open up your knees so that the bottoms of your feet touch and slide one prop under each knee. Slowly lower your torso so that you're lying on the mat. You can place your hands at your sides, up overhead, or on your stomach as shown—whatever feels best for you. Close your eyes and relax into the pose, breathing space into any areas of tightness you feel. Stay here for one to five minutes before slowly making your way out of the pose.

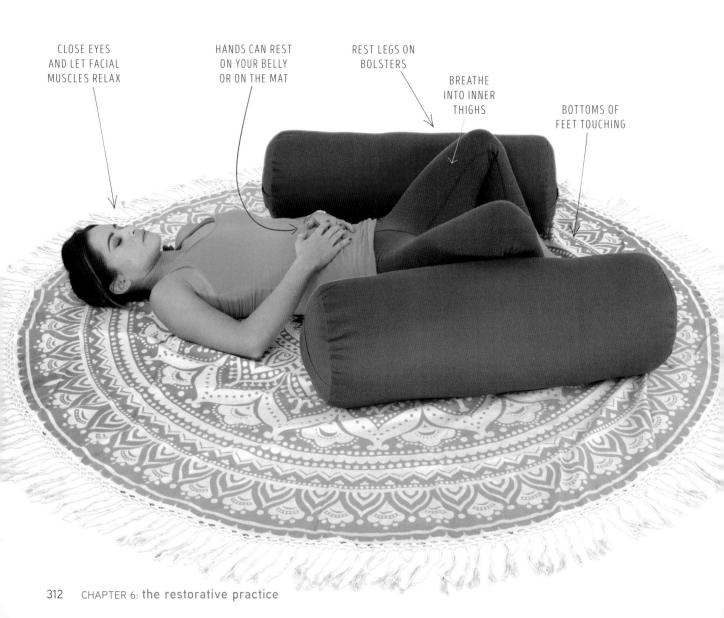

CLOSE EYES AND LET FACIAL MUSCLES RELAX

HANDS CAN REST ON YOUR BELLY OR ON THE MAT

REST LEGS ON BOLSTERS

BREATHE INTO INNER THIGHS

BOTTOMS OF FEET TOUCHING

supported pigeon pose

You'll need: a block, a bolster, and a folded blanket

This is the pose to do if you're dealing with tightness in the backs of your hips. Begin in pigeon pose (page 97) with your left leg behind you. Slide a folded blanket under your shin so that the knee rests comfortably on the mat. Then slide a yoga block under your right sitting bone. (You may not need the block if you're quite open in the hips and your hips easily face forward with your right thigh coming down onto the mat.) Bring the bolster in toward your pelvis and melt your upper body over the top of it. Rest your hands over the bolster and place your left temple on top of your hands. Breathe here for one to three minutes, then turn your head and breathe for another one to three minutes before gently releasing.

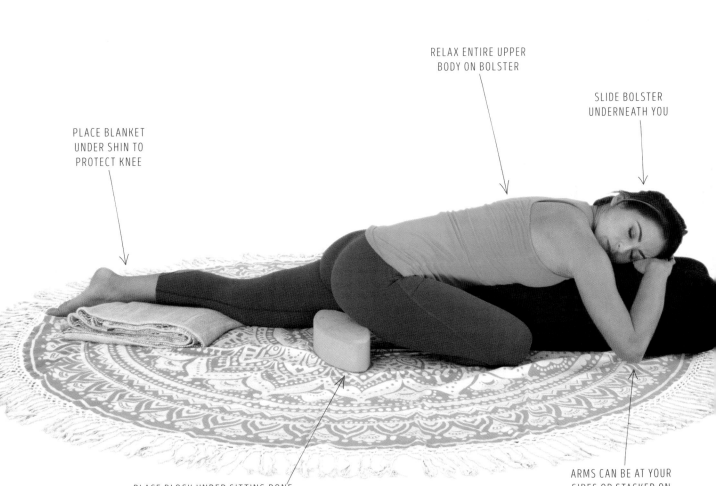

RELAX ENTIRE UPPER
BODY ON BOLSTER

SLIDE BOLSTER
UNDERNEATH YOU

PLACE BLANKET
UNDER SHIN TO
PROTECT KNEE

PLACE BLOCK UNDER SITTING BONE
TO KEEP HIPS EVEN

ARMS CAN BE AT YOUR
SIDES OR STACKED ON
THE BOLSTER

supported fish pose with blocks

You'll need: two yoga blocks

Supported fish pose is hands-down my favorite yin pose. It feels incredible on the chest and helps relieve tightness in the back. I recommend cork or foam blocks for this pose. Unless they have an ergonomic design that molds to your body, wooden blocks will be too hard.

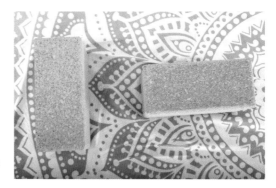

Place the blocks as shown in the photo to the right. Position the back of your head on the top block (the one on the left in the photo). Then lower your back so that the second (vertical) block is between your shoulder blades. You should feel very comfortable in this position; if you don't, make any needed adjustments. Once the blocks are in position, extend your legs and open them about mat width apart. Let your feet splay out to the sides as you fully relax into the pose. If you want a very deep stretch through your chest, you can take your arms out to the sides, bending them about 90 degrees. Alternatively, you can keep your arms at your sides or place your hands on your stomach—whatever feels best for you. Close your eyes and breathe deeply for three to five minutes.

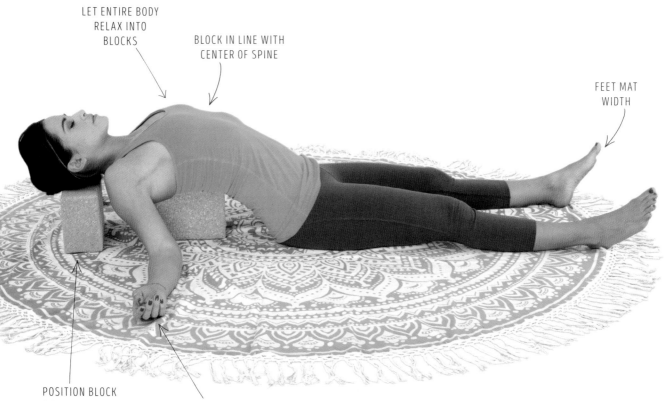

LET ENTIRE BODY RELAX INTO BLOCKS

BLOCK IN LINE WITH CENTER OF SPINE

FEET MAT WIDTH

POSITION BLOCK SO IT SUPPORTS BACK OF HEAD

FOR A DEEPER CHEST STRETCH, OPEN ARMS AS SHOWN. IF THAT FEELS TOO INTENSE, BRING HANDS TO STOMACH.

supported fish pose with a bolster

You'll need: a bolster

More often than not, bolsters are thicker than blocks, which means a deeper stretch for your chest when you're in this pose. For this reason, I suggest doing supported fish pose with a bolster only when you feel very comfortable doing the pose with blocks. A rectangular bolster will give you more options: if you lay it the long way on one side, it'll be shorter (meaning less of a backbend for you), and if you lay it the other long way, it'll be taller (meaning a deeper backbend for you). A round bolster just has one height (usually quite high), which will offer a deeper backbend.

   Begin seated with your legs straight out in front of you. Bring the bolster behind you, lining it up with your spine and having it end about 4 to 6 inches from your low back. Gently lay your upper body over the bolster. You should feel very comfortable in this position; if you don't, rearrange the bolster until you do—play around with pushing it farther away or pulling it closer to find that perfect sweet spot. Your arms can be at your sides as shown, or you can place your hands on your stomach. Take your legs about mat width apart and close your eyes. Breathe here for three to five minutes before slowly coming out of the pose.

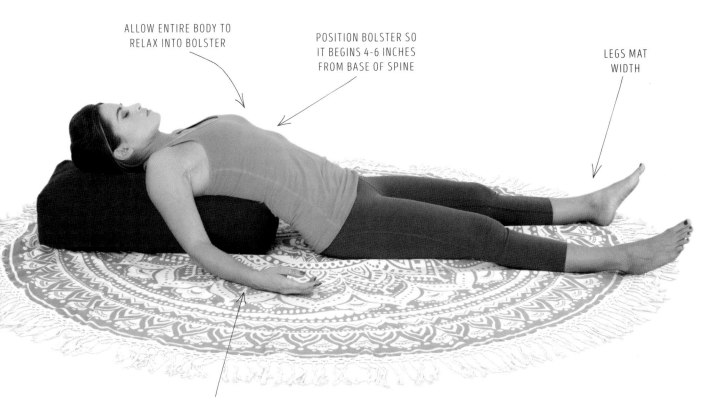

ALLOW ENTIRE BODY TO
RELAX INTO BOLSTER

POSITION BOLSTER SO
IT BEGINS 4-6 INCHES
FROM BASE OF SPINE

LEGS MAT
WIDTH

FOR MODIFIED CHEST OPENING, TAKE ARMS TO SIDES OR HANDS TO BELLY.
FOR DEEPER CHEST OPENING, BEND ARMS TO 90-110 DEGREES AND REST
ON THE GROUND WITH PALMS FACING UP.

supported fish pose with cobbler's pose legs

You'll need: four blocks

This pose kills two birds with one stone, as it opens up both the chest and the hips. Begin seated with your knees bent and your knees and feet together. Slowly open your knees so that the bottoms of your feet come to touch. Place a block underneath each knee (you could also use bolsters or rolled blankets), then position two blocks behind you for support and lie over the top of them. Make any adjustments you need to in order to feel completely comfortable in the pose. Your hands can be on your stomach or at your sides—whichever feels better for you. Close your eyes and totally relax into the position. With each exhale, let go of any tension you feel, allowing your body to open up. Stay here for one to five minutes before slowly releasing the pose.

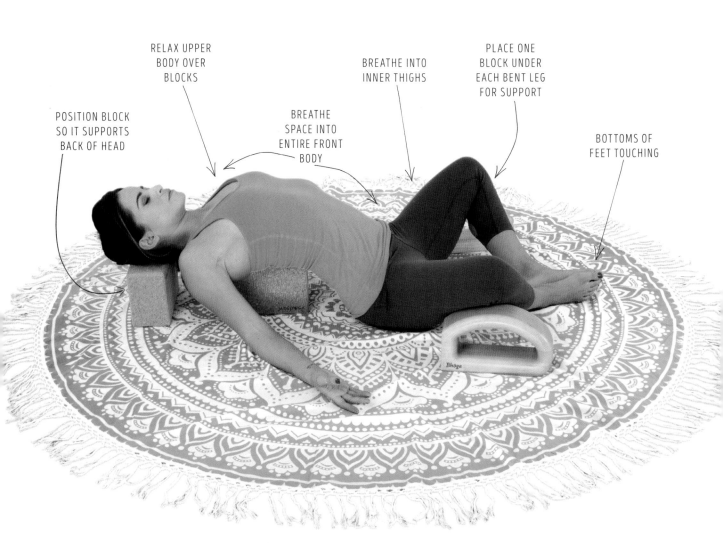

RELAX UPPER BODY OVER BLOCKS

BREATHE INTO INNER THIGHS

PLACE ONE BLOCK UNDER EACH BENT LEG FOR SUPPORT

POSITION BLOCK SO IT SUPPORTS BACK OF HEAD

BREATHE SPACE INTO ENTIRE FRONT BODY

BOTTOMS OF FEET TOUCHING

supported supine spinal twist

You'll need: one bolster

This detoxifying pose is excellent for relieving overall tightness through the hips, back, and chest. Begin by lying on your mat with a bolster placed to your right, about 8 inches away from you, in line with your right leg. Bend your left leg and bring it up and over your body until it comes down onto the bolster. Aim to have your knee in line with your hip. As you breathe, feel the twist through your torso, then decide what you will do with your hands, as you have a few options. You can place your right hand on the outside of your left knee and open your left arm perpendicular to your body, or, if you want a deeper stretch through your chest, you can bend both arms 90 degrees. With each exhale, focus on each part of your body getting heavier and heavier, as if gravity is pulling you deeper into the posture. Stay here for one to five minutes before slowly switching sides.

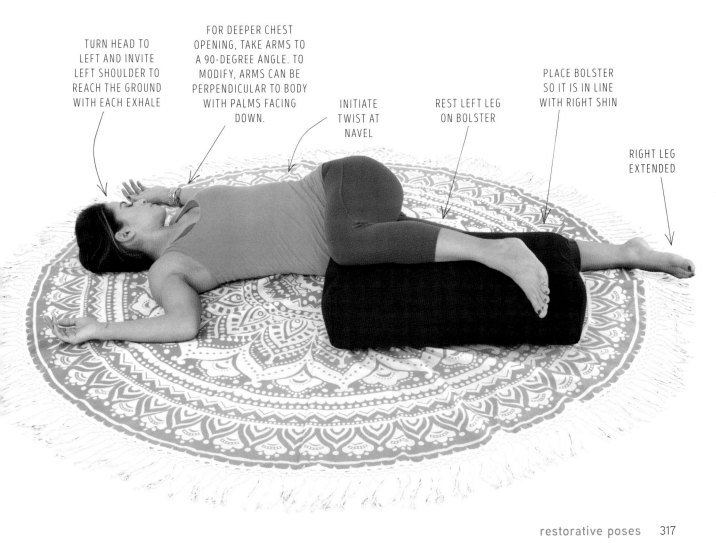

TURN HEAD TO LEFT AND INVITE LEFT SHOULDER TO REACH THE GROUND WITH EACH EXHALE

FOR DEEPER CHEST OPENING, TAKE ARMS TO A 90-DEGREE ANGLE. TO MODIFY, ARMS CAN BE PERPENDICULAR TO BODY WITH PALMS FACING DOWN.

INITIATE TWIST AT NAVEL

REST LEFT LEG ON BOLSTER

PLACE BOLSTER SO IT IS IN LINE WITH RIGHT SHIN

RIGHT LEG EXTENDED

downward-facing rest

You'll need: a bolster and a folded blanket

This calming pose is wonderful for reducing stress and anxiety. Begin by placing a folded blanket on your mat, where your pelvis will go. The blanket will provide padding for the tops of your hips and your pelvis. Then place a bolster horizontally on the mat where your shins will go. With both props in place, lie down with your shins resting on the bolster and your pelvis over the blanket. Your arms can be at your sides, or you can position one hand in front of the other, making a little pillow for your temple, as shown. Rest on one side of your face for one to three minutes before turning your head and switching sides for another one to three minutes.

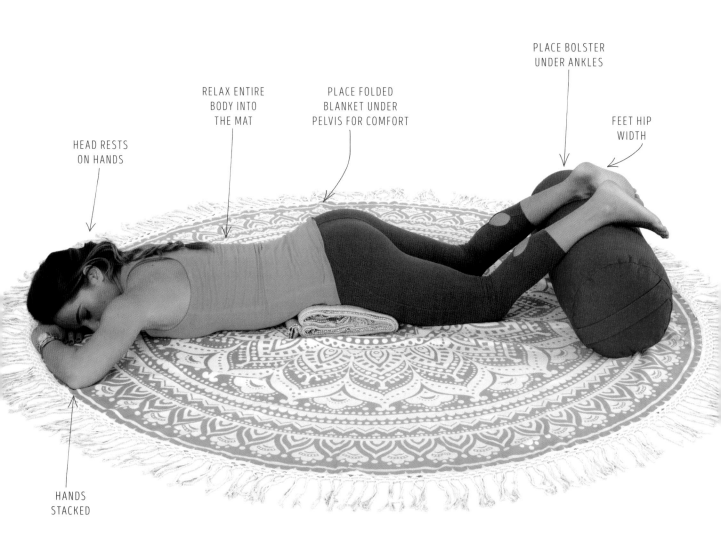

PLACE BOLSTER
UNDER ANKLES

RELAX ENTIRE
BODY INTO
THE MAT

PLACE FOLDED
BLANKET UNDER
PELVIS FOR COMFORT

FEET HIP
WIDTH

HEAD RESTS
ON HANDS

HANDS
STACKED

supported child's pose

You'll need: a bolster and a rolled blanket

People with very tight hips often find regular child's pose to be really tough. If that's the case for you, give this supported version a try. The props make the pose quite comfortable and effectively help open up the backs of the hips. Begin by kneeling on your mat. Place a thick rolled blanket on top of your calves. Then open your knees and place a bolster vertically in front of you, as close to your pelvis as you can. Sit your hips back onto the blanket and lay your torso over the top of the bolster. Place your hands on the bolster and relax your left temple on your hands. Stay here for one to three minutes before turning your face to the other side for another one to three minutes, then release the pose.

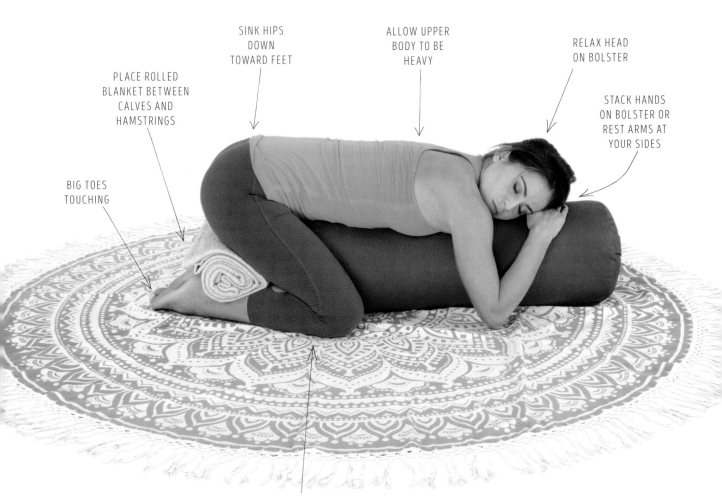

SINK HIPS DOWN TOWARD FEET

ALLOW UPPER BODY TO BE HEAVY

RELAX HEAD ON BOLSTER

PLACE ROLLED BLANKET BETWEEN CALVES AND HAMSTRINGS

STACK HANDS ON BOLSTER OR REST ARMS AT YOUR SIDES

BIG TOES TOUCHING

KNEES WIDE TO ACCOMMODATE BOLSTER

supported prone hip opener

You'll need: a bolster

If you deal with tightness through the inner thighs, I highly recommend adding this supported prone hip opener to your practice. Begin by lying facedown on your mat. Place a bolster vertically next to your right leg so that the top of the bolster is in line with the top of your right hip bone. Then bend your right knee and open your hip so that you can rest your lower leg on the bolster. Keep your right ankle in line with your right knee and totally relax into the position. You can stack your hands, making a little pillow for your left temple, as shown, or your arms can be at your sides. Stay in this position for one to three minutes before switching sides.

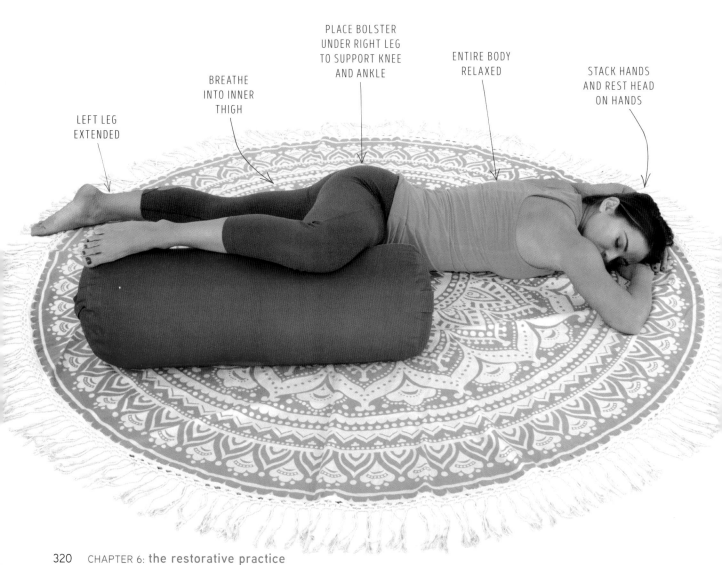

LEFT LEG
EXTENDED

BREATHE
INTO INNER
THIGH

PLACE BOLSTER
UNDER RIGHT LEG
TO SUPPORT KNEE
AND ANKLE

ENTIRE BODY
RELAXED

STACK HANDS
AND REST HEAD
ON HANDS

supported reclined bound angle pose variation

You'll need: a yoga strap and a bolster

This pose is a deep hip and chest opener, and the strap offers a tremendous amount of support that helps you really sink into the pose and find openness. Begin seated with the bottoms of your feet together and your knees open. Then wrap a yoga strap around your waist, bringing the ends in front of you. Hook the strap through the buckles and tighten securely. Then bring the strap around the outsides of your feet. You may need to adjust the strap a few times to find the right length and tension. From here, bring the bolster behind you, in line with your spine, about 4 to 6 inches from the base of your spine. Slowly lie back over the bolster, feeling fully supported by both props. Adjust the props if you need to—it's important that you feel very comfortable and secure in the posture. Once your props are in position, either place your hands on your stomach or open up your arms as shown for a very deep stretch through the chest. Close your eyes and breathe deeply for one to five minutes.

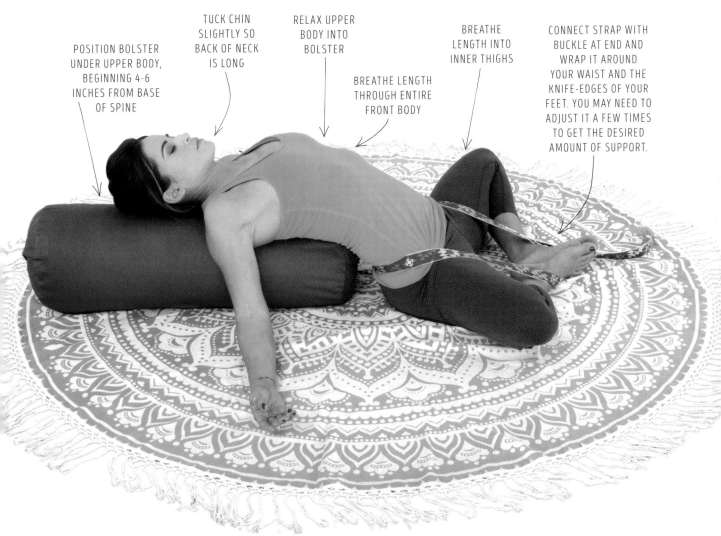

POSITION BOLSTER UNDER UPPER BODY, BEGINNING 4-6 INCHES FROM BASE OF SPINE

TUCK CHIN SLIGHTLY SO BACK OF NECK IS LONG

RELAX UPPER BODY INTO BOLSTER

BREATHE LENGTH THROUGH ENTIRE FRONT BODY

BREATHE LENGTH INTO INNER THIGHS

CONNECT STRAP WITH BUCKLE AT END AND WRAP IT AROUND YOUR WAIST AND THE KNIFE-EDGES OF YOUR FEET. YOU MAY NEED TO ADJUST IT A FEW TIMES TO GET THE DESIRED AMOUNT OF SUPPORT.

legs on a chair pose

You'll need: a chair and a folded blanket

This grounding pose helps realign the back, effectively relieving low-back pain. It's also good for reducing stress and anxiety. Begin by placing a folded blanket on the mat where you'll position your hips. Then place a chair a short distance away so that your calves can rest on the seat of the chair. Lie down with your hips supported by the blanket and your calves on the seat. Your hands can be on your stomach, or you can open your arms out to the sides. Close your eyes and breathe for one to five minutes.

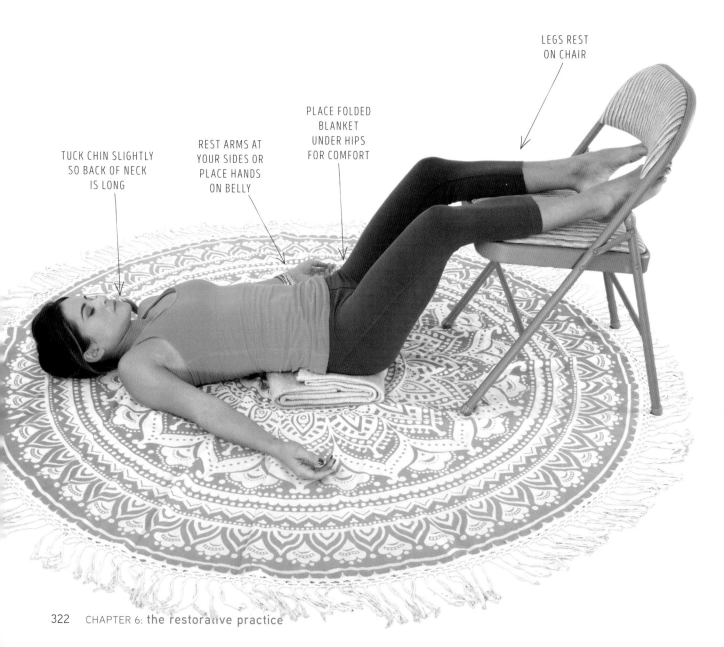

LEGS REST
ON CHAIR

PLACE FOLDED
BLANKET
UNDER HIPS
FOR COMFORT

REST ARMS AT
YOUR SIDES OR
PLACE HANDS
ON BELLY

TUCK CHIN SLIGHTLY
SO BACK OF NECK
IS LONG

side-lying savasana

You'll need: two folded blankets

This side-lying savasana is always an option for people who find regular corpse pose (page 136) to be too much pressure on the low back. Position yourself on your left side with your knees bent between 45 and 90 degrees. Place a folded blanket between your knees. Place another folded blanket underneath your head so that your left cheek rests comfortably. Bend your arms 90 degrees and stack your forearms in front of you. Close your eyes and breathe deeply for one to five minutes before switching sides.

PLACE FOLDED BLANKET
UNDER HEAD TO KEEP
SPINE NEUTRAL

PLACE FOLDED BLANKET
BETWEEN LEGS FOR
COMFORT AND KNEE
SUPPORT

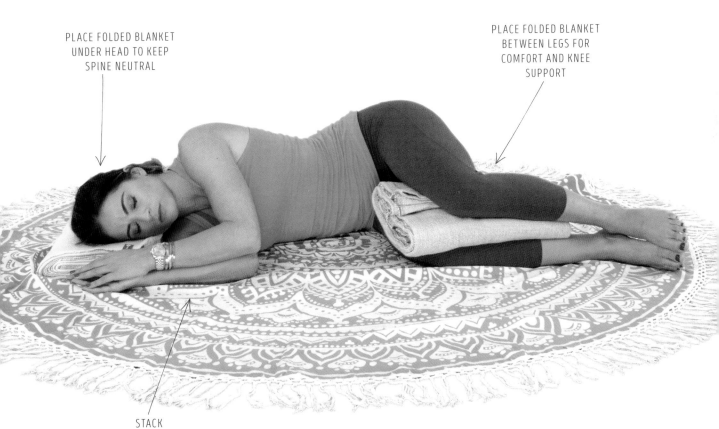

STACK
FOREARMS

supported corpse pose

You'll need: an eye mask, a folded blanket, and a bolster

For a deeply relaxing corpse pose, an eye mask, folded blanket, and bolster certainly help. The eye mask encourages tired eyes to sink deep into the sockets, the folded blanket supports the head and brings it into alignment with the spine, and the bolster helps alleviate low-back pressure. Begin by placing the bolster horizontally on your mat so that the backs of your knees can rest comfortably on top of it. Then place the folded blanket underneath your head, making sure that the edge of the blanket is in line with the base of your neck (but not underneath your shoulders). Then slip the eye mask on, lie back, and relax. Breathe for one to ten minutes in this posture before slowly coming out.

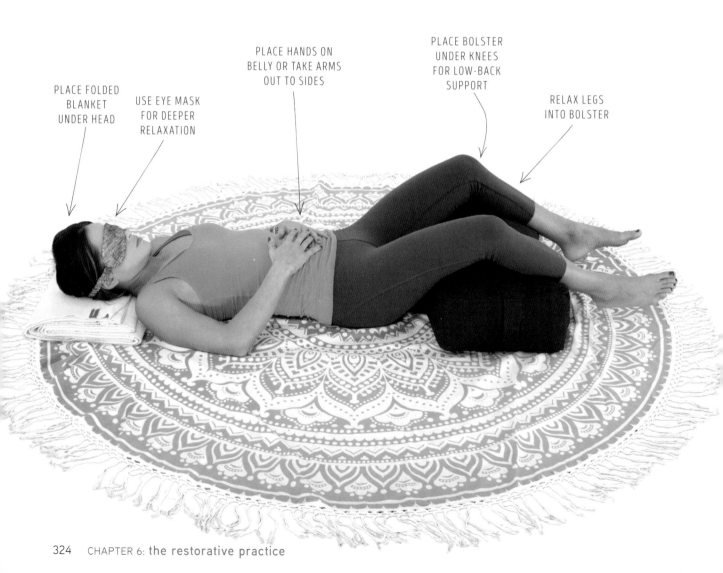

PLACE FOLDED
BLANKET
UNDER HEAD

USE EYE MASK
FOR DEEPER
RELAXATION

PLACE HANDS ON
BELLY OR TAKE ARMS
OUT TO SIDES

PLACE BOLSTER
UNDER KNEES
FOR LOW-BACK
SUPPORT

RELAX LEGS
INTO BOLSTER

supported reclining hero pose

You'll need: two blocks and four bolsters

This pose is ideal for opening up the front body and gently stretching the quads and areas around the knees. Begin by coming up onto your shins in a kneeling position. With your thighs perpendicular to the floor, touch your inner knees together. Slide your feet slightly wider than hip width apart, with the tops of the feet on the floor. Position two blocks side by side between your shins, underneath your hips. As you exhale, sit back onto the blocks. Then stack two bolsters behind you with the edge of the bottom bolster touching the edge of the blocks. Finally, place a bolster to your left for your left arm to rest and another bolster to your right for your right arm to rest. Lie back, relaxing your upper body onto the two stacked bolsters. Close your eyes and breathe for one to five minutes.

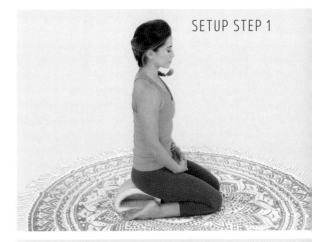

SETUP STEP 1

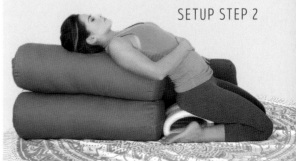

SETUP STEP 2

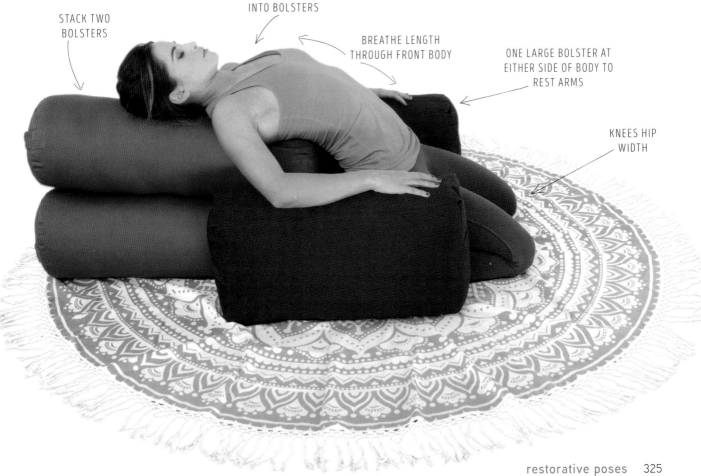

STACK TWO BOLSTERS

MELT UPPER BODY INTO BOLSTERS

BREATHE LENGTH THROUGH FRONT BODY

ONE LARGE BOLSTER AT EITHER SIDE OF BODY TO REST ARMS

KNEES HIP WIDTH

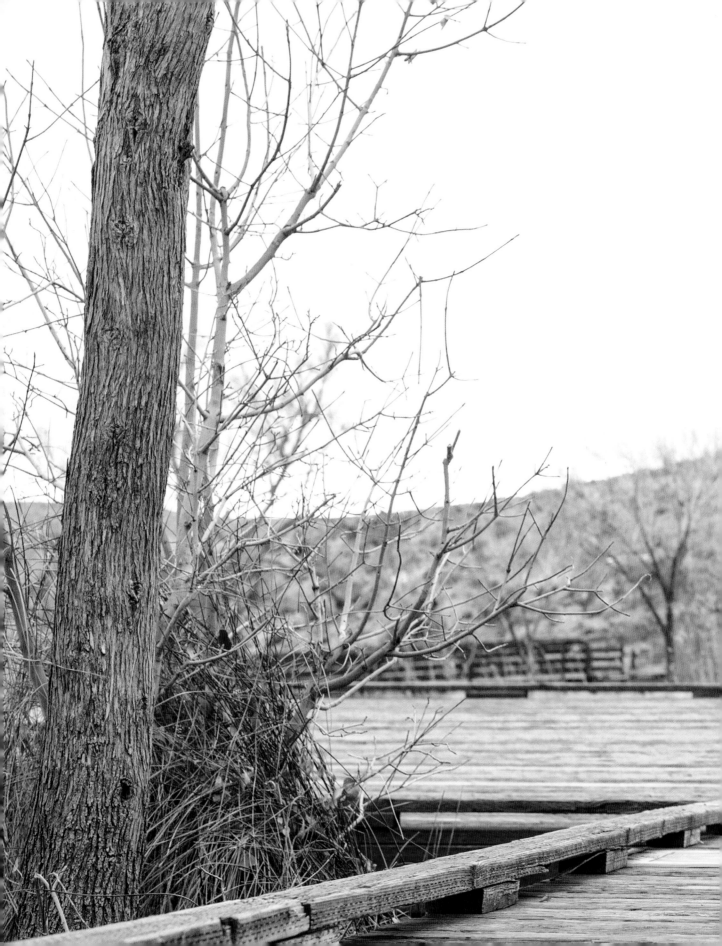

sequences

With yoga, as with most things, change and transformation are gradual: they come with dedication to a consistent practice. So I put together the following sequences to supplement those found at the ends of the beginner, intermediate, and advanced chapters. When you're just starting out, it can be tricky to create sequences in your head, so these routines will serve as guides that you can follow until you're ready to piece together your own. Keep in mind that they are just suggestions. If you come across a pose that you don't care for or that doesn't feel entirely right for your body, feel free to swap it out for something else. And remember to work within a pain-free range as you pick and choose what works for you.

warm-up sequences

It's imperative to warm up before you jump into a practice. Choose one or two of the following sequences for your warm-up and move slowly and with intention. Take a few breaths in each pose before moving on.

warm-up 1

1. CAT/COW POSE (page 83)

2. EASY POSE chin to chest
(page 90)

A)   B)

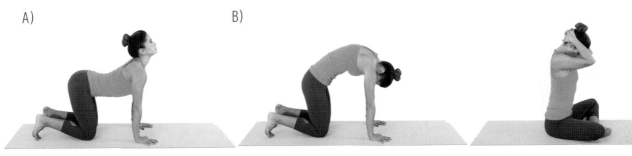

3. SEATED SIDE-BODY STRETCH (each side) (page 91)

4. EASY POSE forward fold

5. DOWNWARD DOG
(page 100)

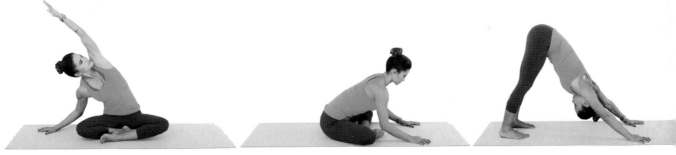

6. STANDING FORWARD FOLD
(page 107)

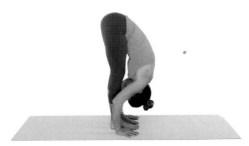

warm-up 2

1. RECLINED BOUND ANGLE POSE
(page 135)

2. SUPINE ROLLING KNEES

A)

B)

C)

D)

E)

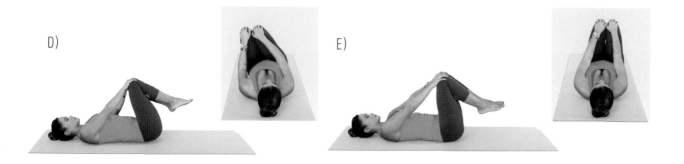

3. ROCK & ROLL with round back x5

A)

B)

4. RAG DOLL POSE
(page 124)

5. STANDING FORWARD FOLD
with bent knees (page 107)

6. MOUNTAIN POSE
(page 106)

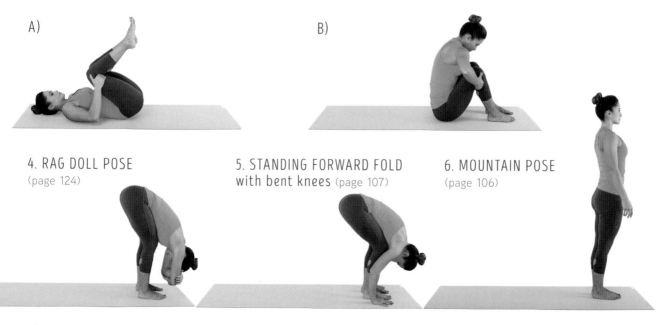

warm-up 3

1. MOUNTAIN POSE
(page 106)

2. GARLAND POSE
(page 182)

3. HERO POSE
(page 94)

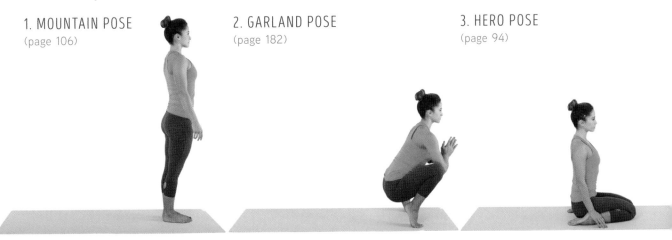

4. LOW LUNGE (each side)
(page 117)

5. COBRA POSE
(page 129)

6. CHILD'S POSE
(page 93)

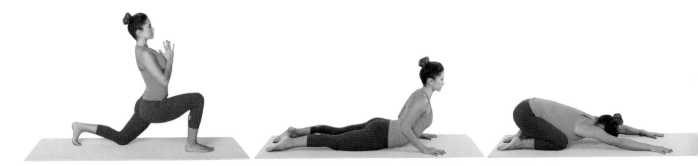

warm-up 4

1. COBBLER'S POSE (page 88)

2. GODDESS POSE (page 181)

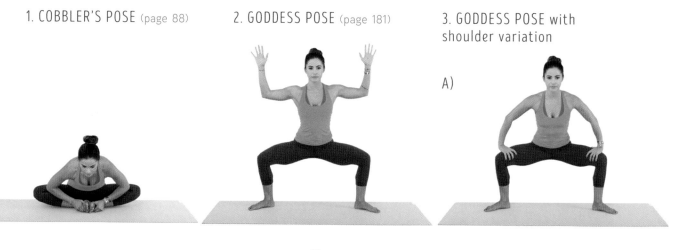

3. GODDESS POSE with shoulder variation

A)

B) C) D)

4. DEEP INNER-THIGH STRETCH (each side)

5. WIDE-LEG FORWARD FOLD D (page 123)

6. FROG POSE (page 212)

A)

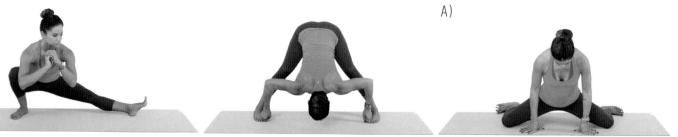

B) C)

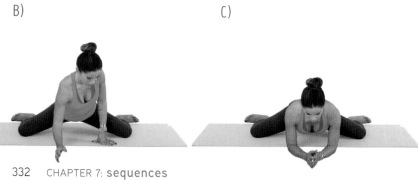

warm-up 5

1. EASY POSE chin to chest
(page 90)

2. EASY POSE elbows to sky

A)

B)

3. DOWNWARD DOG (page 100)

A)

B)

C)

4. HIGH LUNGE (each side) (page 112)

5. STANDING PIGEON POSE (each side) (page 201)

A)

B)

6. MOUNTAIN POSE side-body stretch (each side) (page 106)

A)

B)

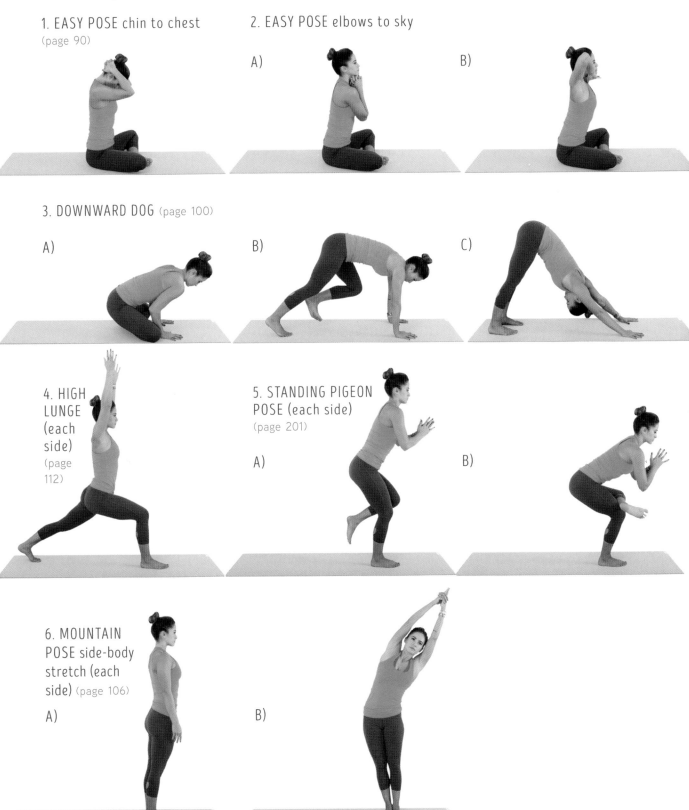

thirty-day program to de-stress

I'm going to come right out and say it: stress is a silent killer. It's one of those things that we all know is bad for us, yet it's tough to just quit it. It's like junk food—theoretically it's easy to stop eating junk food if we stop buying it and bringing it into our homes, but how can we stop bringing stress into our lives since we don't actively bring it in?

Drumroll, please.

Yoga.

Now, just like with nearly everything else, yoga isn't a quick fix for stress. Yes, it will help in times of chaos, but yoga is far more effective when it is a consistent practice. This Thirty-Day Program to De-stress offers a no-brainer way to start implementing the practice into your life. The sequences are intentionally short so that super-busy people like you and me will be able to squeeze them into our days. If you find yourself with more time on your hands, add in some of your favorite poses. If you find yourself with less time on your hands, feel free to take out a few poses. Make the program work for you. The idea is to begin a consistent yoga practice to help decrease stress. Therefore, the emphasis is on the yoga practice itself rather than on the actual poses. Always move within a pain-free range, and honor how you feel each day.

DAY 1:

RESTORATIVE FLOW (3 minutes in each pose):

1. SUPPORTED CATERPILLAR POSE
(page 311)

2. SUPPORTED PIGEON POSE
(each side) (page 313)

3. SUPPORTED FISH POSE
(page 315)

4. SUPPORTED RECLINED BOUND ANGLE POSE
(page 312)

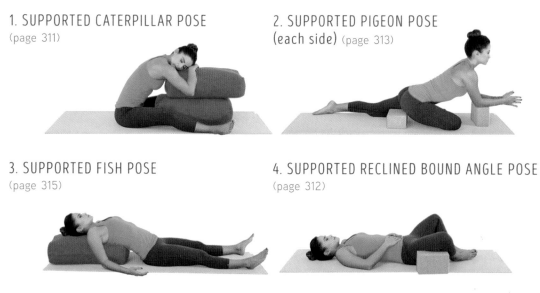

DAY 2:

1. 5-minute BODY SCAN MEDITATION (page 61)

2. CAT/COW POSE
(page 83)

A)

B)

3. DOWNWARD DOG
(page 100)

4. COBRA POSE
(page 129)

5. INTENSE SHOULDER STRETCH (each side)

A)

B)

C)

D)

6. HALF VINYASA TO SEATED

7. STAFF POSE
(page 98)

8. COBBLER'S POSE
(page 88)

9. HALF SPINAL TWIST (each side)
(page 172)

10. HAPPY BABY POSE
(page 130)

11. CORPSE POSE
(page 136)

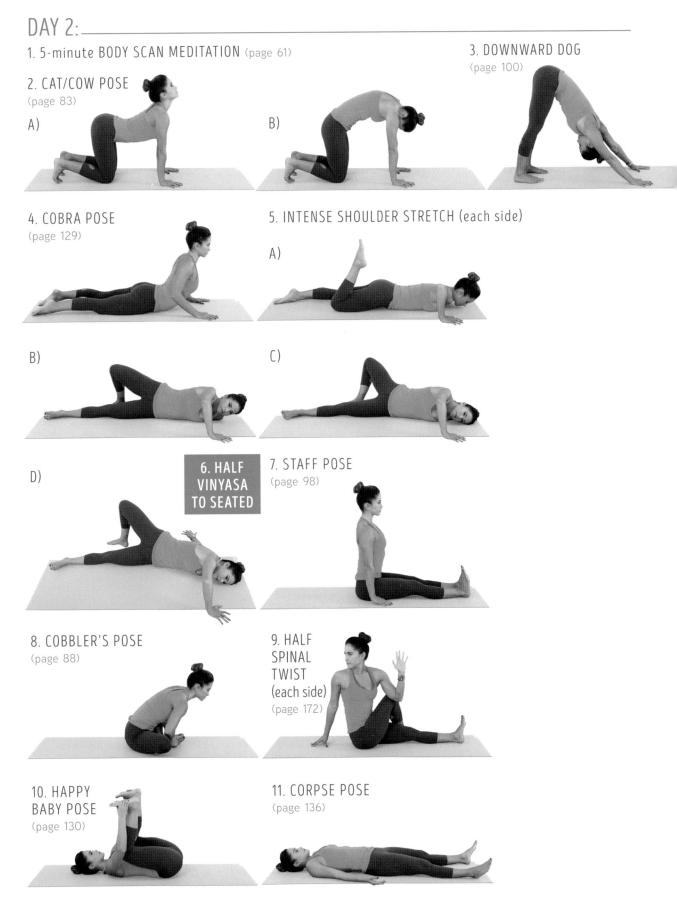

DAY 3: _____

1. 5-minute MANTRA MEDITATION (page 62). WARM-UP of choice.   **2. VINYASA**

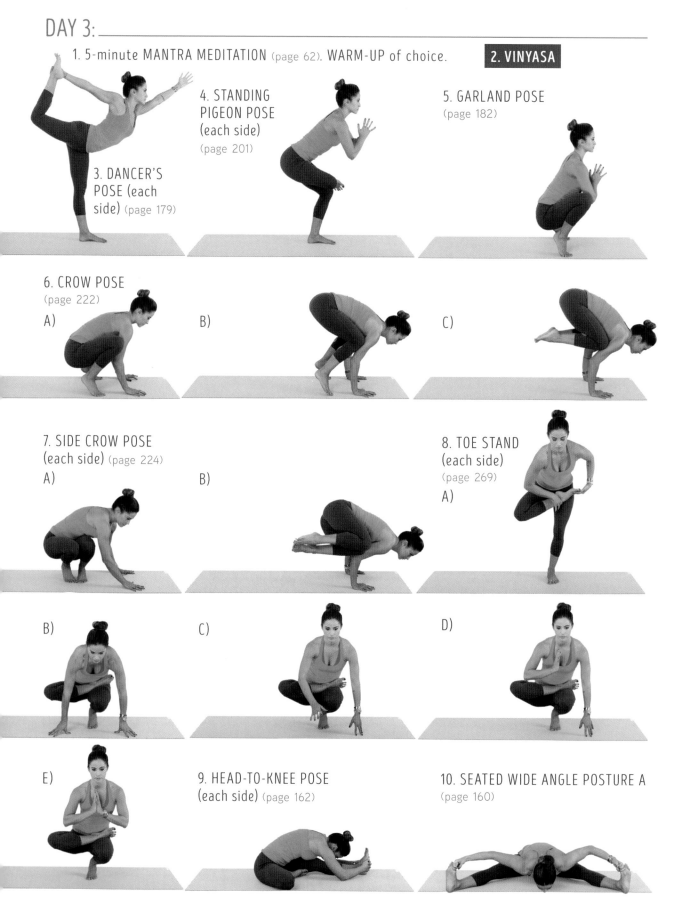

3. DANCER'S POSE (each side) (page 179)

4. STANDING PIGEON POSE (each side) (page 201)

5. GARLAND POSE (page 182)

6. CROW POSE (page 222)
A)   B)   C)

7. SIDE CROW POSE (each side) (page 224)
A)   B)

8. TOE STAND (each side) (page 269)
A)

B)   C)   D)

E)

9. HEAD-TO-KNEE POSE (each side) (page 162)

10. SEATED WIDE ANGLE POSTURE A (page 160)

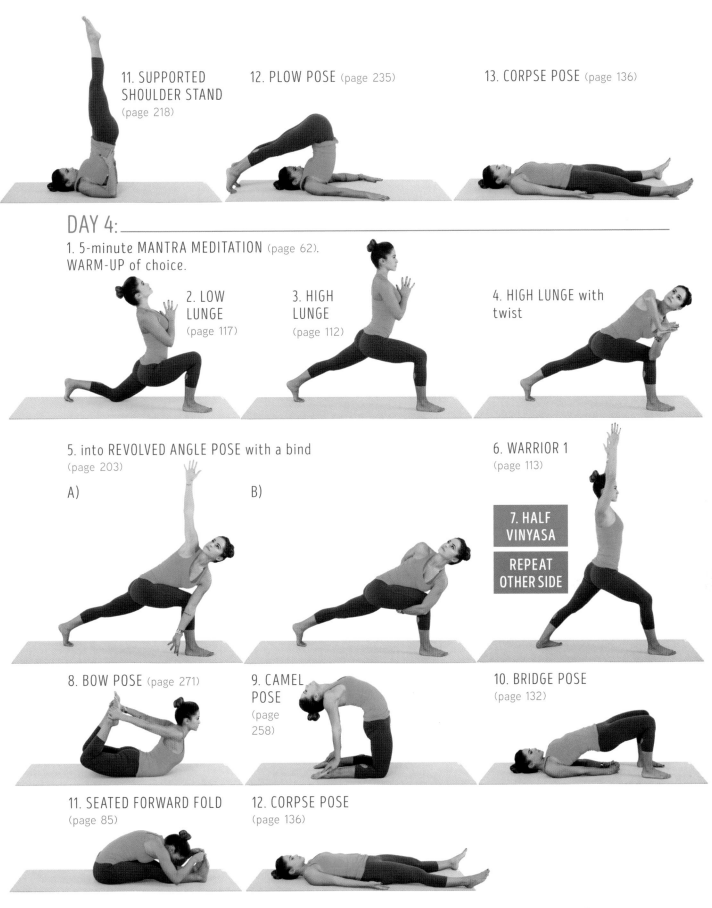

11. SUPPORTED SHOULDER STAND (page 218)

12. PLOW POSE (page 235)

13. CORPSE POSE (page 136)

DAY 4:

1. 5-minute MANTRA MEDITATION (page 62).
WARM-UP of choice.

2. LOW LUNGE (page 117)

3. HIGH LUNGE (page 112)

4. HIGH LUNGE with twist

5. into REVOLVED ANGLE POSE with a bind (page 203)

A)

B)

6. WARRIOR 1 (page 113)

7. HALF VINYASA

REPEAT OTHER SIDE

8. BOW POSE (page 271)

9. CAMEL POSE (page 258)

10. BRIDGE POSE (page 132)

11. SEATED FORWARD FOLD (page 85)

12. CORPSE POSE (page 136)

DAY 5:

YIN YOGA (3 minutes in each pose):

1. SUPPORTED BRIDGE POSE
(page 310)

2. CORPSE POSE with knees in and feet wide (page 136)

3. LEGS ON A CHAIR POSE
(page 322)

DAY 6: REST

DAY 7:

1. 5-minute **PRANAYAMA** of choice (page 73).
WARM-UP of choice.

2. PLANK
(page 109)

3. SIDE PLANK variation
(page 192)

4. PLANK

5. SIDE PLANK VARIATION ON OTHER SIDE

6. KNEE TO ELBOW

7. KNEE TO ARMPIT

8. Slide to WRIST

9. Pop up KNEE TO ARMPIT

REPEAT OTHER SIDE

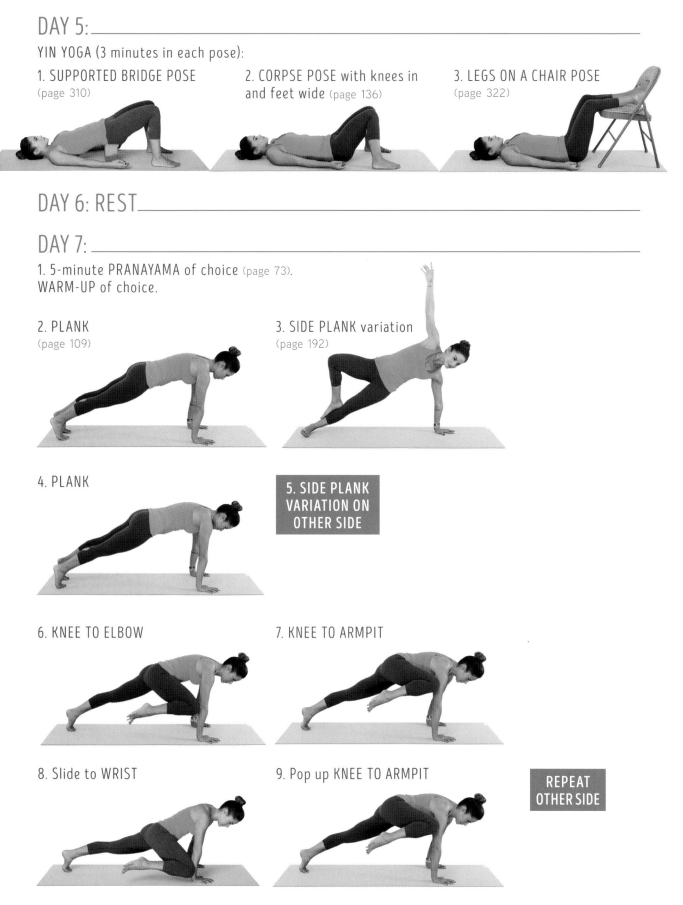

10. CRUNCH with block as prop x10

A)

B)

C)

D)

11. BELLY STRETCH

12. CORPSE POSE (page 136)

DAY 8:

1. 6-minute MANTRA MEDITATION (page 62).

2. DOWNWARD DOG
(page 100)

3. THREE-LEGGED DOG
with bent knee (page 175)

REPEAT OTHER SIDE

4. LOW LUNGE
(page 117)

5. RUNNER'S LUNGE

6. INTENSE STRETCH
(page 206)

7. HALF VINYASA

REPEAT OTHER SIDE

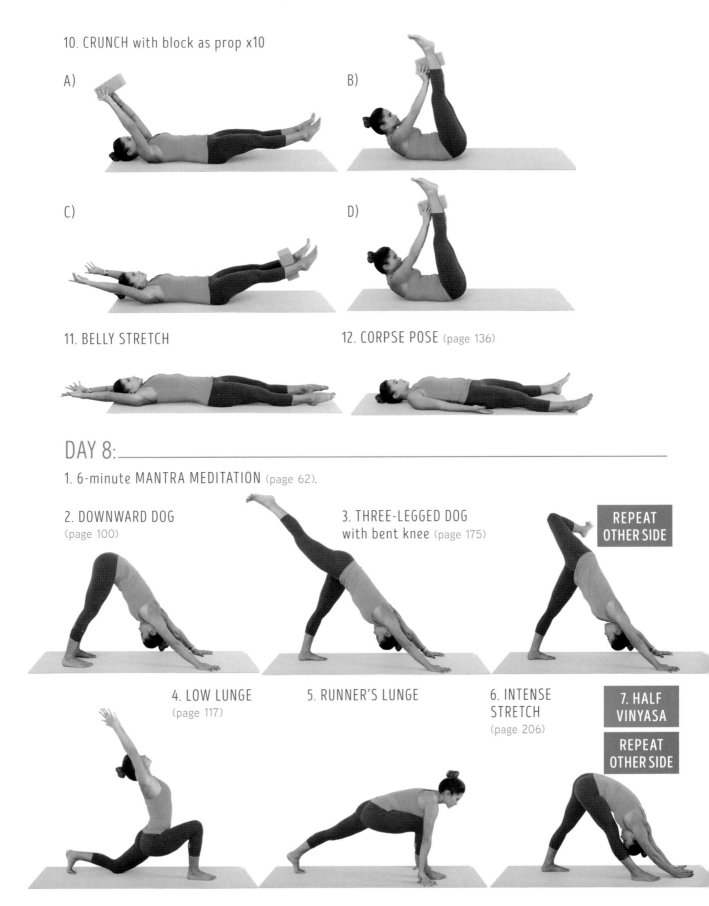

8. STANDING FORWARD FOLD
(page 107)

9. HIGH LUNGE
(page 112)

10. STANDING SPLIT
(page 210)

11. VINYASA
REPEAT OTHER SIDE

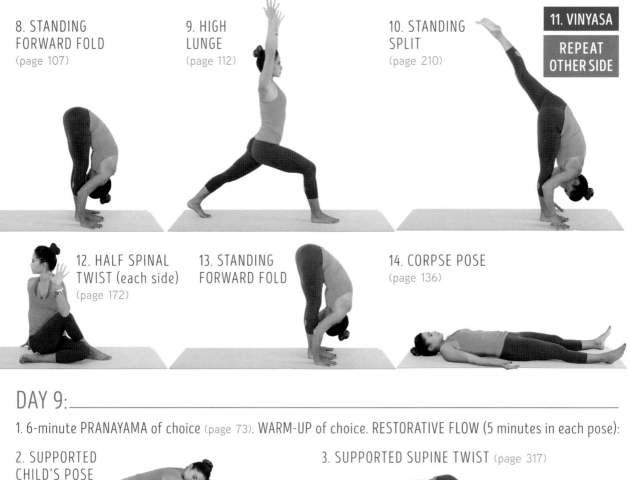

12. HALF SPINAL TWIST (each side)
(page 172)

13. STANDING FORWARD FOLD

14. CORPSE POSE
(page 136)

DAY 9:

1. 6-minute PRANAYAMA of choice (page 73). WARM-UP of choice. RESTORATIVE FLOW (5 minutes in each pose):

2. SUPPORTED CHILD'S POSE
(page 319)

3. SUPPORTED SUPINE TWIST (page 317)

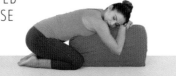

4. DOWNWARD-FACING REST
(page 318)

5. SUPPORTED RECLINED BOUND ANGLE POSE
(page 321)

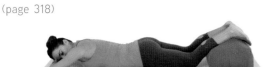

DAY 10:

1. 6-minute BODY SCAN MEDITATION (page 61). WARM-UP of choice.

2. CHAIR POSE
(page 125)

3. CHAIR TWIST
(page 126)

4. STANDING FORWARD FOLD
(page 107)

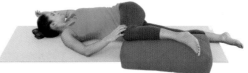

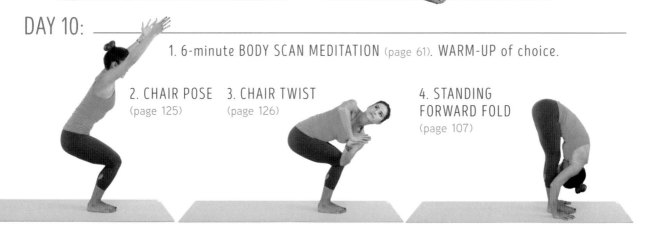

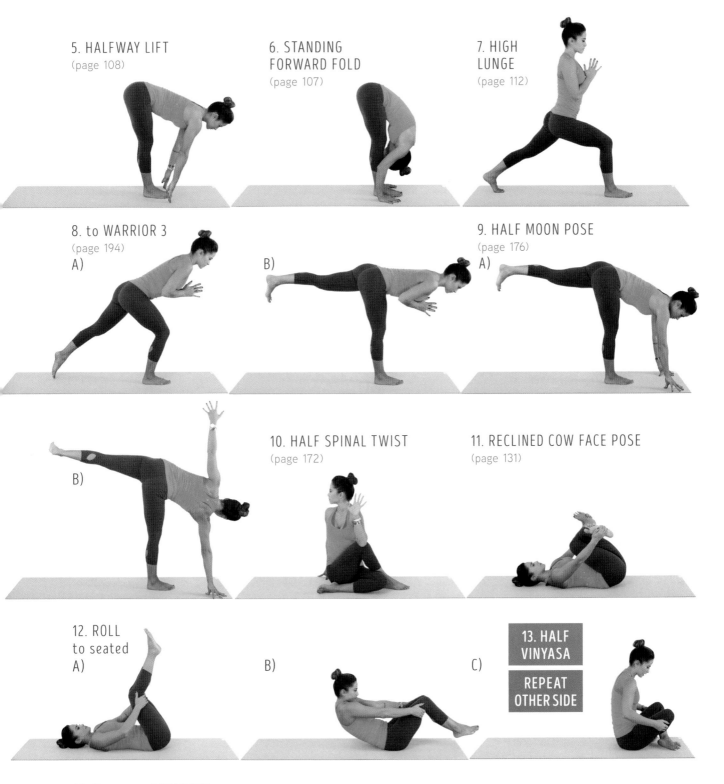

5. HALFWAY LIFT
(page 108)

6. STANDING FORWARD FOLD
(page 107)

7. HIGH LUNGE
(page 112)

8. to WARRIOR 3
(page 194)
A)

B)

9. HALF MOON POSE
(page 176)
A)

B)

10. HALF SPINAL TWIST
(page 172)

11. RECLINED COW FACE POSE
(page 131)

12. ROLL to seated
A)

B)

13. HALF VINYASA

REPEAT OTHER SIDE

C)

14. 5-minute SAVASANA
(page 136)

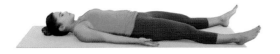

DAY 11: _____

1. 6-minute
SILENT MEDITATION.
WARM-UP
of choice.

TAKE 4-7 BREATHS IN EACH POSE:

2. FIRE
LOG POSE
(each side)
(page 87)

3. HEAD-TO-KNEE POSE
(each side) (page 162)

4. SEATED FORWARD FOLD
(page 85)

5. GATE POSE
(each side)
(page 84)

6. FROG POSE
(page 212)

7. COBBLER'S POSE
(page 88)

8. RECLINED COW FACE POSE
(each side) (page 131)

9. HAPPY BABY POSE
(page 130)

10. RECLINED FROG POSE

11. 5-minute SAVASANA
(page 136)

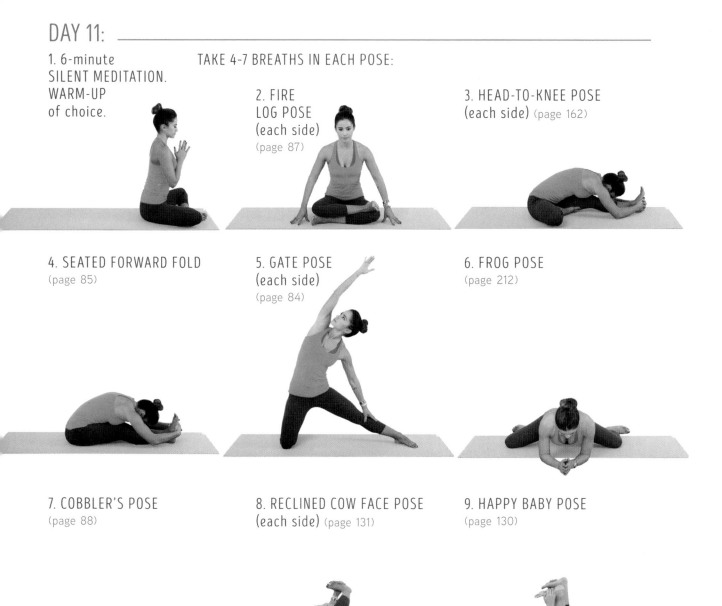

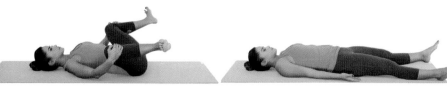

DAY 12:

1. 6-minute MANTRA MEDITATION (page 62).

WARM-UP
of choice.

2. RAG
DOLL POSE
(page 124)

3. WARRIOR 1
(page 113)

4. WARRIOR 1
variation
(page 180)

5. WARRIOR 2
(page 114)

6. TRIANGLE
POSE
(page 185)

7. REVOLVED
TRIANGLE
POSE
(page 205)

8. STANDING
SPLIT
(page 210)

9. CHAIR POSE
(page 125)

10. HALF VINYASA

11. VINYASA TO SEATED

REPEAT OTHER SIDE

12. REVERSE TABLE POSE (page 127)

13. UPWARD PLANK (page 214)

14. RECLINED BOUND ANGLE POSE
(page 135)

15. 5-minute SAVASANA (page 136)

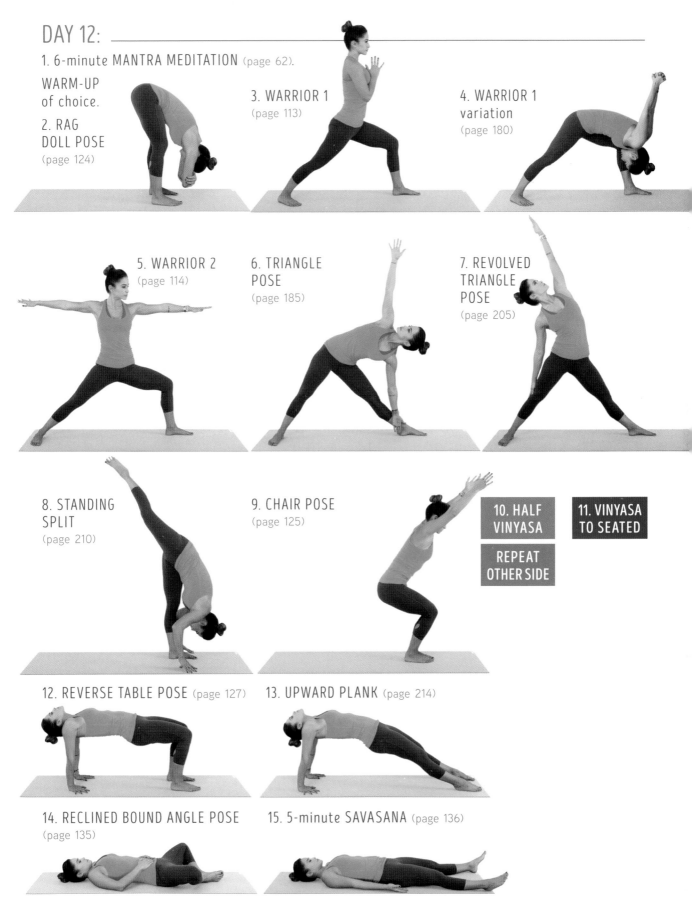

DAY 13:

1. 6-minute MUDRA MEDITATION (page 58). WARM-UP of choice.

2. RUNNER'S LUNGE

3. INTENSE STRETCH (page 206)

4. EXTENDED SIDE ANGLE POSE (page 187)

5. GODDESS POSE (page 181)

6. WIDE-LEG FORWARD FOLD A (page 120)

7. WIDE-LEG FORWARD FOLD B (page 121)

8. WIDE-LEG FORWARD FOLD C (page 122)

9. WIDE-LEG FORWARD FOLD D (page 123)

10. HALF VINYASA

REPEAT OTHER SIDE

11. 5-minute SAVASANA (page 136)

DAY 14: REST

DAY 15:

1. 7-minute MUDRA MEDITATION (page 58). WARM-UP of choice. RESTORATIVE FLOW (5 minutes in each pose):

2. SUPPORTED CATERPILLAR POSE (page 311)

3. SUPPORTED FISH POSE (page 314)

4. SUPPORTED RECLINED BOUND ANGLE POSE (page 312)

5. SUPPORTED BRIDGE POSE (page 310)

6. SUPPORTED BELLY DOWN TWIST (each side)

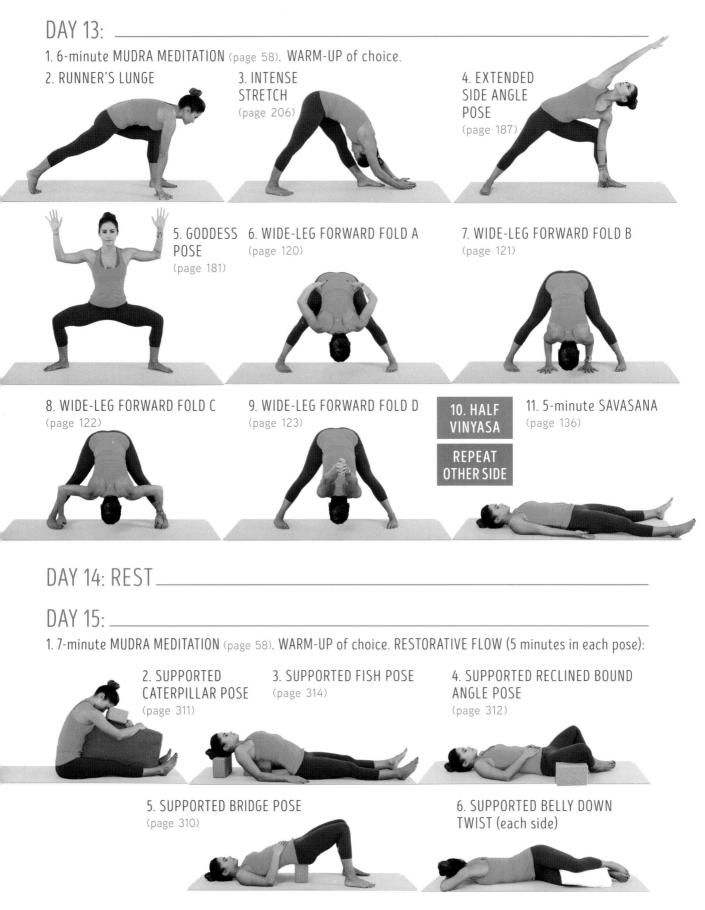

DAY 16:

1. 7-minute MUDRA MEDITATION (page 58). WARM-UP of choice.

2. TREE POSE
(page 105)

3. HALF VINYASA

REPEAT OTHER SIDE

4. DANCER'S POSE
(page 179)

5. HALF VINYASA

REPEAT OTHER SIDE

6. EAGLE POSE
(page 204)

7. HALF VINYASA

REPEAT OTHER SIDE

8. BALANCING STICK POSE

9. HALF VINYASA

REPEAT OTHER SIDE

10. HALF SPINAL TWIST
(each side) (page 172)

11. RECLINED FROG POSE

12. IT BAND STRETCH (each side)

13. 5-minute SAVASANA
(page 136)

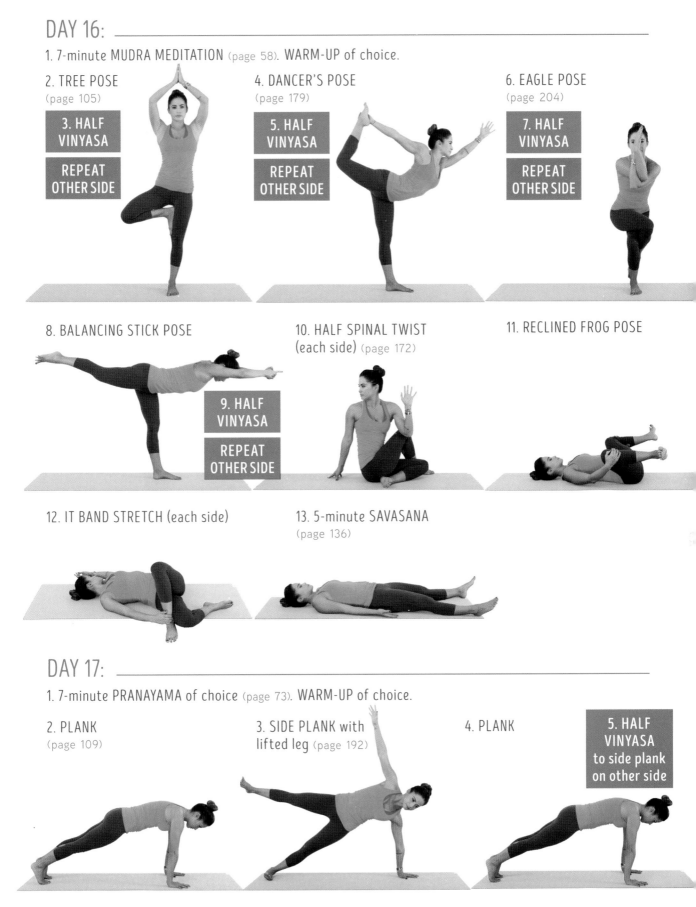

DAY 17:

1. 7-minute PRANAYAMA of choice (page 73). WARM-UP of choice.

2. PLANK
(page 109)

3. SIDE PLANK with
lifted leg (page 192)

4. PLANK

**5. HALF VINYASA
to side plank
on other side**

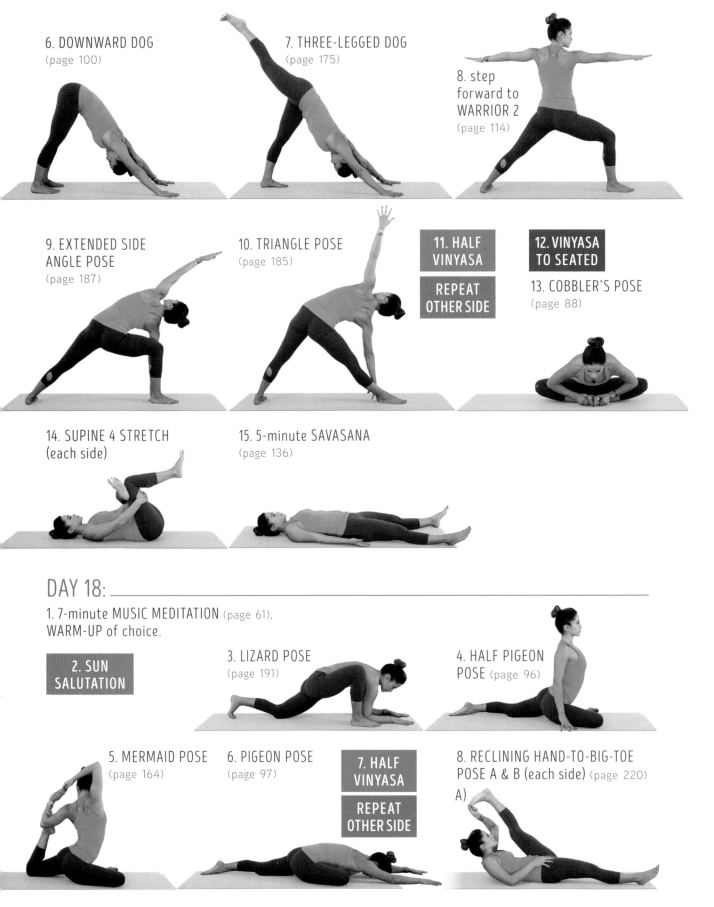

6. DOWNWARD DOG
(page 100)

7. THREE-LEGGED DOG
(page 175)

8. step forward to WARRIOR 2
(page 114)

9. EXTENDED SIDE ANGLE POSE
(page 187)

10. TRIANGLE POSE
(page 185)

11. HALF VINYASA

REPEAT OTHER SIDE

12. VINYASA TO SEATED

13. COBBLER'S POSE
(page 88)

14. SUPINE 4 STRETCH
(each side)

15. 5-minute SAVASANA
(page 136)

DAY 18:

1. 7-minute MUSIC MEDITATION (page 61). WARM-UP of choice.

2. SUN SALUTATION

3. LIZARD POSE
(page 191)

4. HALF PIGEON POSE (page 96)

5. MERMAID POSE
(page 164)

6. PIGEON POSE
(page 97)

7. HALF VINYASA

REPEAT OTHER SIDE

8. RECLINING HAND-TO-BIG-TOE POSE A & B (each side) (page 220)
A)

B)

9. 5-minute SAVASANA
(page 136)

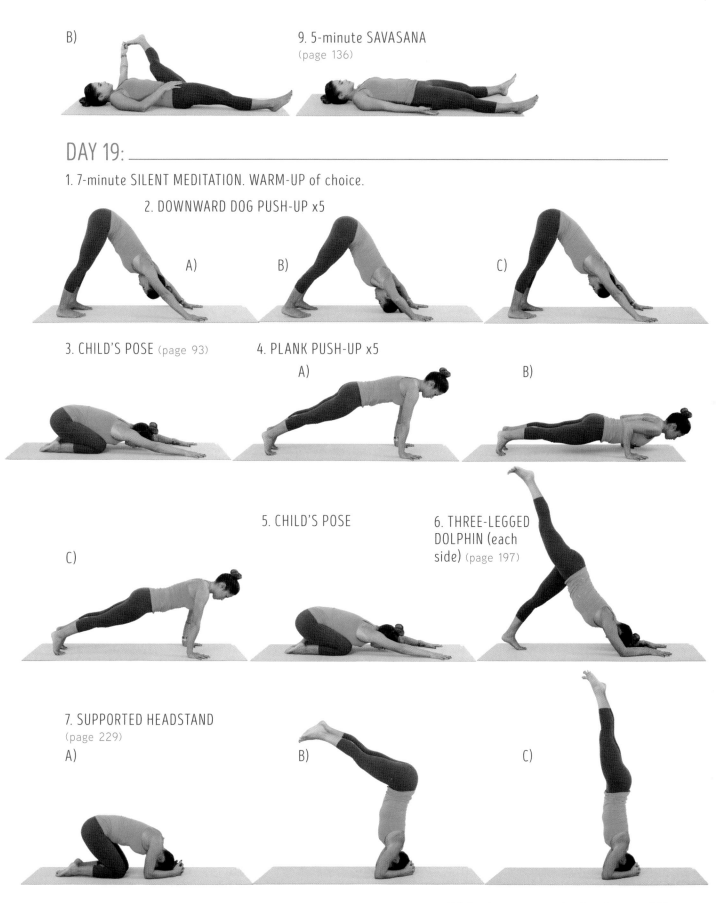

DAY 19: _____

1. 7-minute SILENT MEDITATION. WARM-UP of choice.

2. DOWNWARD DOG PUSH-UP x5

A)

B)

C)

3. CHILD'S POSE (page 93)

4. PLANK PUSH-UP x5

A)

B)

5. CHILD'S POSE

6. THREE-LEGGED DOLPHIN (each side) (page 197)

C)

7. SUPPORTED HEADSTAND
(page 229)

A)

B)

C)

8. HEADSTAND SPLIT (each side)

9. HEADSTAND TWIST (each side)

10. CHILD'S POSE (page 93)

11. SUPPORTED SHOULDER STAND (page 218)

12. PLOW POSE (page 235)

13. 5-minute SAVASANA (page 136)

DAY 20: REST

DAY 21:

1. 7-minute SILENT MEDITATION. WARM-UP of choice.

2. DOWNWARD DOG (page 100)

3. THREE-LEGGED DOG knee to forehead x5 (page 175)

A)

B)

4. GODDESS POSE (page 181)

5. TRIANGLE POSE (page 185)

6. REVOLVED TRIANGLE POSE (page 205)

7. HALF VINYASA

REPEAT OTHER SIDE

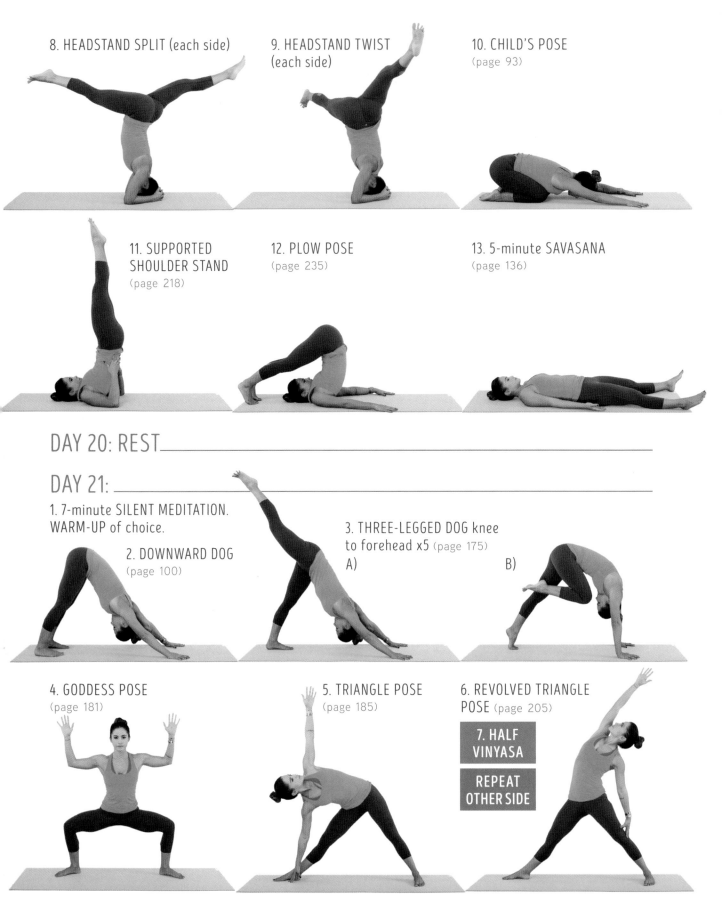

8. RABBIT POSE (page 165)

9. CHILD'S POSE (page 93)

10. 5-minute SAVASANA (page 136)

DAY 22: _____

1. 7-minute SILENT MEDITATION. WARM-UP of choice. RESTORATIVE FLOW (5 minutes in each pose):

2. SUPPORTED RECLINED BOUND ANGLE POSE (page 321)

3. SUPPORTED BRIDGE POSE (page 310)

4. SIDE-LYING CORPSE POSE (page 323)

DAY 23: _____

1. 8-minute MUDRA MEDITATION (page 58). WARM-UP of choice.

2. 30-second FOREARM PLANK (page 109)

3. LIFT LEG (each side)

4. DOWNWARD DOG (page 100)

5. JUMP to front of mat

6. CHAIR POSE (page 125)

7. STANDING FORWARD FOLD (page 107)

8. HALFWAY LIFT (page 108)

9. VINYASA

10. HIGH LUNGE (page 112)

11. BABY GRASSHOPPER POSE (page 190)

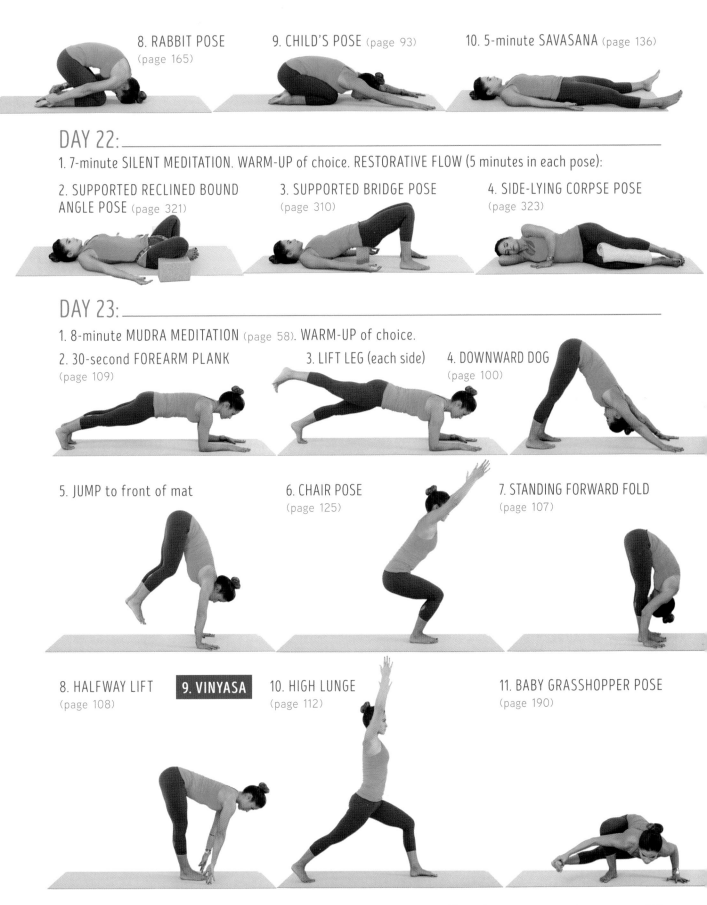

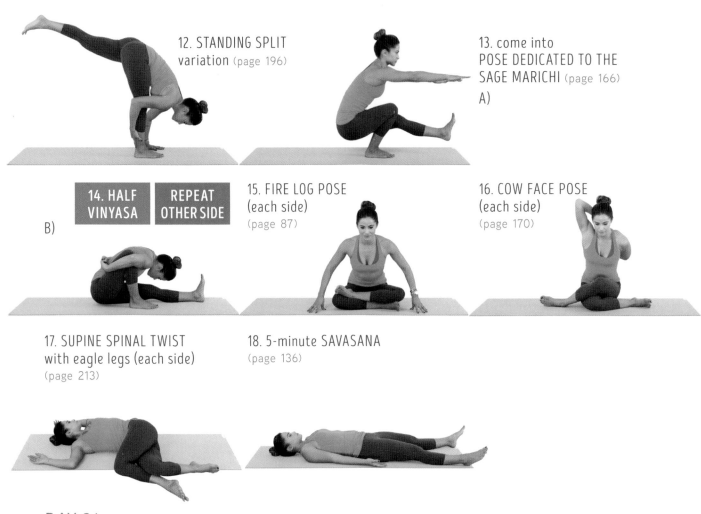

12. STANDING SPLIT variation (page 196)

13. come into POSE DEDICATED TO THE SAGE MARICHI (page 166)
A)

B)

14. HALF VINYASA   **REPEAT OTHER SIDE**

15. FIRE LOG POSE (each side) (page 87)

16. COW FACE POSE (each side) (page 170)

17. SUPINE SPINAL TWIST with eagle legs (each side) (page 213)

18. 5-minute SAVASANA (page 136)

DAY 24: _____

1. 8-minute BODY SCAN MEDITATION (page 61). WARM-UP of choice.

2. SPHINX POSE (page 133)

3. COBRA POSE (page 129)

4. COBRA POSE looking over right shoulder

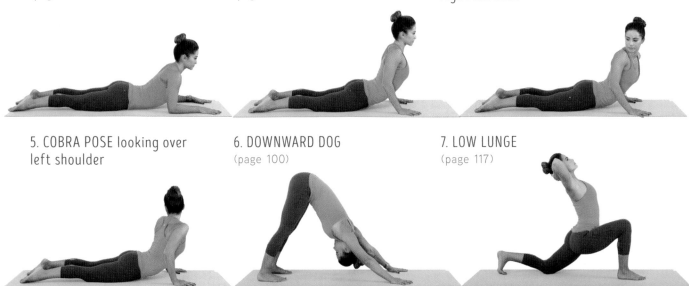

5. COBRA POSE looking over left shoulder

6. DOWNWARD DOG (page 100)

7. LOW LUNGE (page 117)

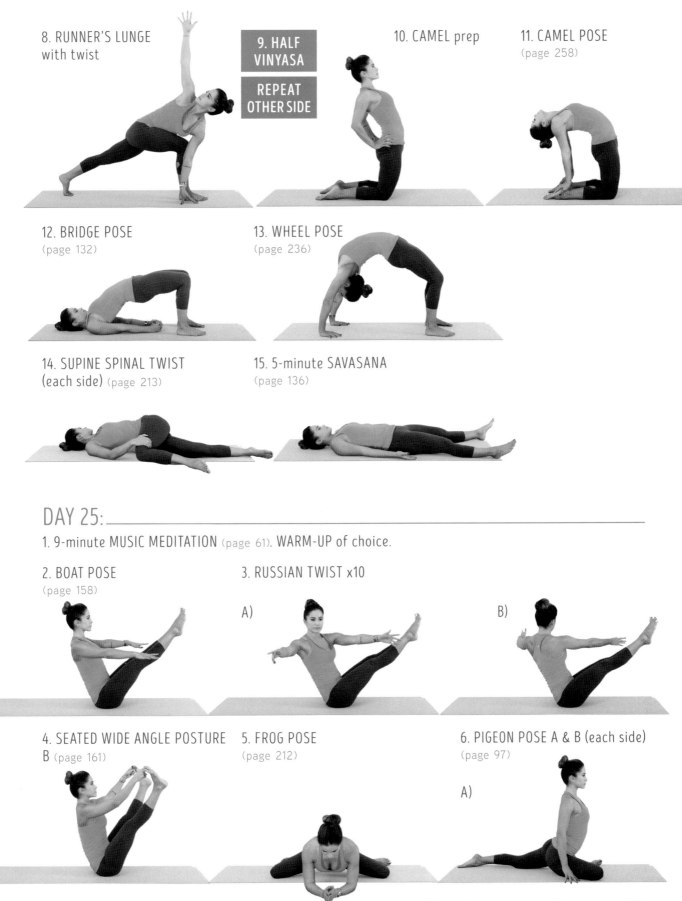

8. RUNNER'S LUNGE
with twist

9. HALF VINYASA

REPEAT OTHER SIDE

10. CAMEL prep

11. CAMEL POSE
(page 258)

12. BRIDGE POSE
(page 132)

13. WHEEL POSE
(page 236)

14. SUPINE SPINAL TWIST
(each side) (page 213)

15. 5-minute SAVASANA
(page 136)

DAY 25:

1. 9-minute MUSIC MEDITATION (page 61). WARM-UP of choice.

2. BOAT POSE
(page 158)

3. RUSSIAN TWIST x10

A)

B)

4. SEATED WIDE ANGLE POSTURE
B (page 161)

5. FROG POSE
(page 212)

6. PIGEON POSE A & B (each side)
(page 97)

A)

B)

7. FIREFLY POSE
(page 285)

8. CHILD'S POSE
(page 93)

9. BRIDGE POSE
(page 132)

10. 5-minute SAVASANA
(page 136)

DAY 26:

1. 9-minute MUDRA MEDITATION (page 58). WARM-UP of choice.

2. EXTENDED PUPPY DOG POSE
(page 99)

3. COBRA POSE
(page 129)

4. UPWARD-FACING DOG
(page 198)

5. THREE-LEGGED DOG
(page 175)

6. WARRIOR 1
(page 113)

7. HALF MOON POSE
(page 176)

8. STANDING PIGEON POSE
(page 201)

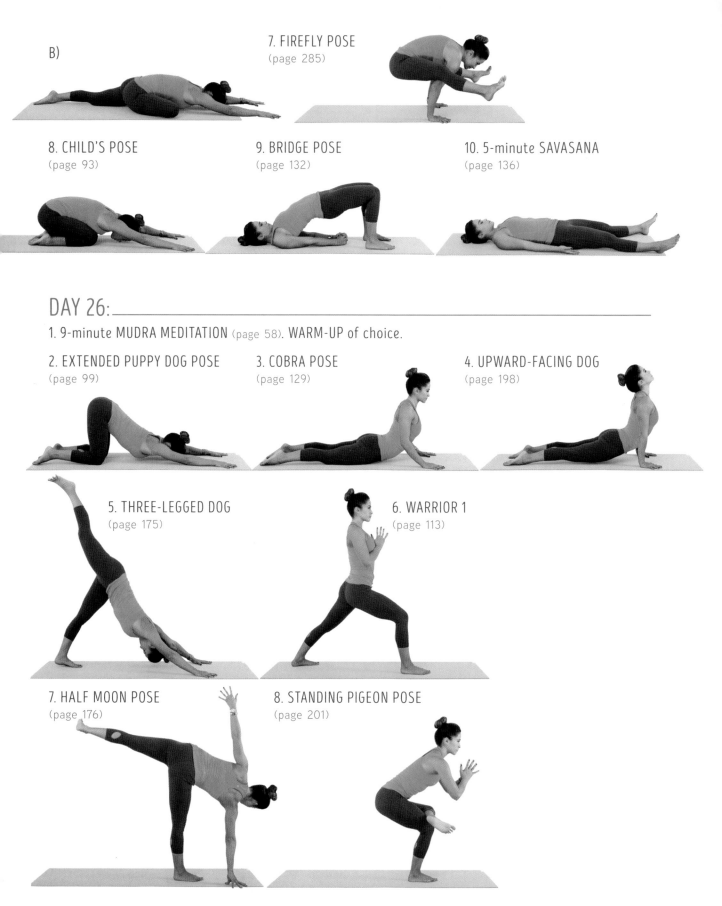

9. BABY FLYING PIGEON POSE (page 228)

A)

B)

10. FLYING PIGEON POSE (page 277)

11. HALF VINYASA

REPEAT OTHER SIDE

12. GORILLA POSE (page 128)

13. COBBLER'S POSE (page 88)

14. RECLINED BOUND ANGLE POSE (page 135)

15. 5-minute SAVASANA (page 136)

DAY 27: REST

DAY 28:

1. 10-minute MEDITATION of choice (page 61).

5-minute PRANAYAMA of choice (page 73).

WARM-UP of choice.

2. EASY POSE (page 90)

3. REVOLVED EASY POSE (page 92)

4. STAFF POSE (page 98)

5. THREE LIMBS FACING INTENSE WEST STRETCH (page 163)

REPEAT OTHER SIDE

6. SAGE TWIST (each side) (page 265)

A)

B)

7. HALF SPINAL TWIST (each side) (page 172)

8. CORPSE POSE with knees in and feet wide (page 136)

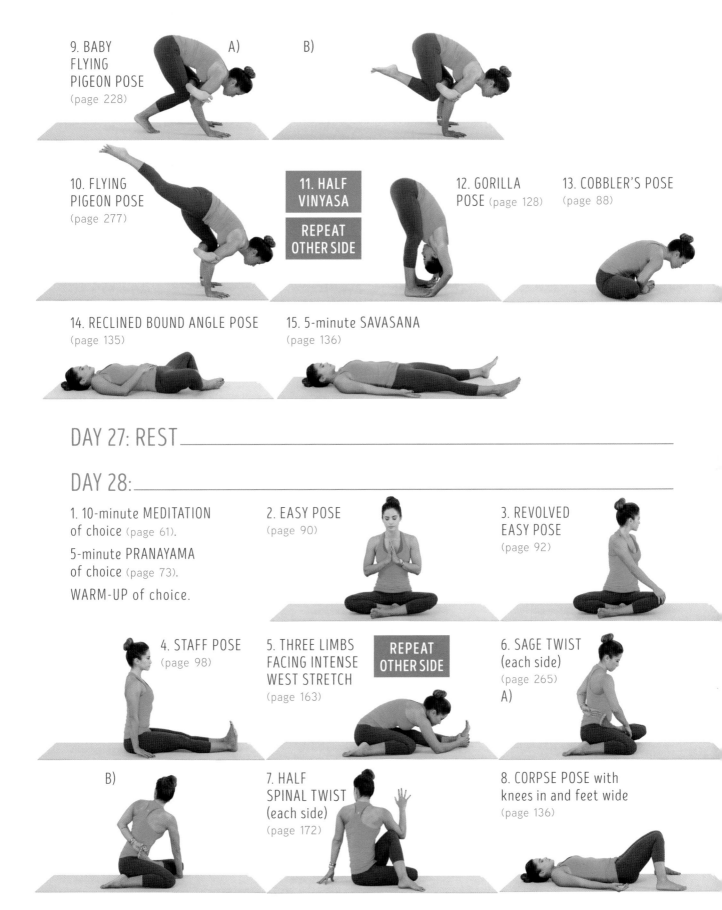

DAY 29:

1. 10-minute **MEDITATION** of choice (page 61).

5-minute **PRANAYAMA** of choice (page 73).

WARM-UP of choice.

RESTORATIVE FLOW (5 minutes in each pose):

2. SUPPORTED BRIDGE POSE (page 310)

3. LEGS ON A CHAIR POSE (page 322)

4. SUPPORTED SUPINE SPINAL TWIST (each side) (page 317)

5. SUPPORTED CORPSE POSE (page 324)

DAY 30:

1. 10-minute **MEDITATION** of choice (page 61).

5-minute **PRANAYAMA** of choice (page 73).

WARM-UP of choice.

2. MOUNTAIN POSE (page 106)

3. TREE POSE (page 105)

4. STANDING PIGEON POSE (page 201)

5. RAG DOLL POSE (page 124)

REPEAT OTHER SIDE

6. VINYASA

7. HIGH LUNGE variation (page 112)

8. HALF VINYASA

REPEAT OTHER SIDE

9. PLANK with lifted leg (each side) (page 109)

10. EXTENDED PUPPY DOG POSE (page 99)

11. BOW POSE (page 271)

12. CHILD'S POSE (page 93)

13. 5-minute SAVASANA (page 136)

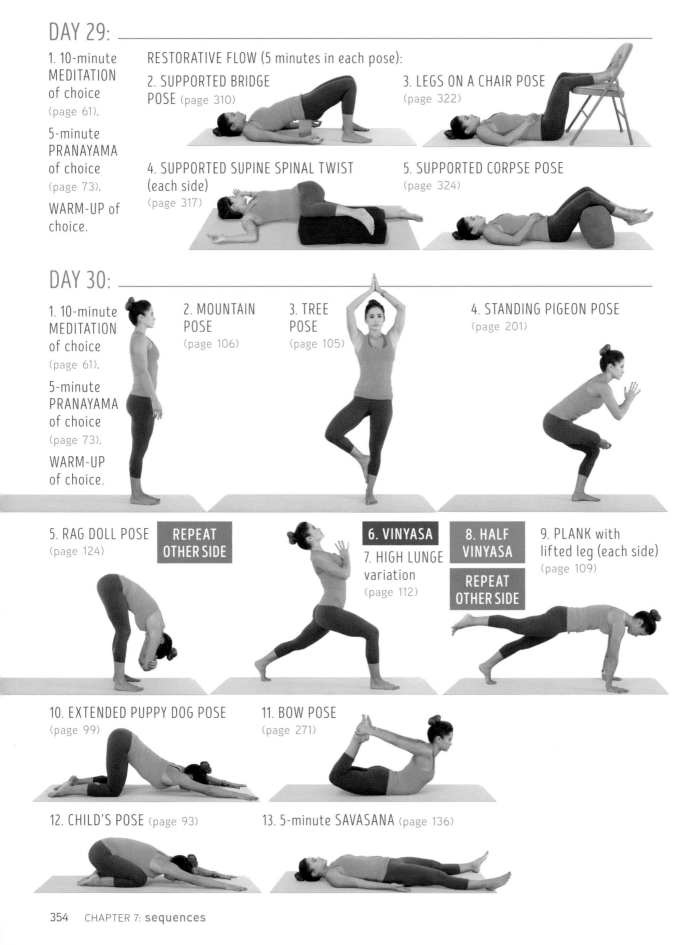

thirty-day core strengthening program

One of the most valuable lessons yoga has taught me is that everything is connected. In a physical sense, this is something to remember when you feel aches and pains. For example, low-back pain is often caused by a weak core and/or tight hamstrings. Working on one or both of those things can help bring relief. I designed this core strengthening program because so many of us could benefit from a more stable core. A strong core can not only relieve minor back pain, but also help improve posture and prevent injuries. Feel free to tailor the program to meet your needs. The sequences are intentionally short so that they'll fit into busy lives, but if you have more time available to practice, add in some of your favorite poses or breathe longer in each suggested pose. Remember to move with intention and mindfulness and always stay within a pain-free range.

Begin each day of this program with a five-minute meditation (see page 61) and a five-minute pranayama of your choice (see page 73), along with the warm-up of your choice except on restorative flow days.

DAY 1:

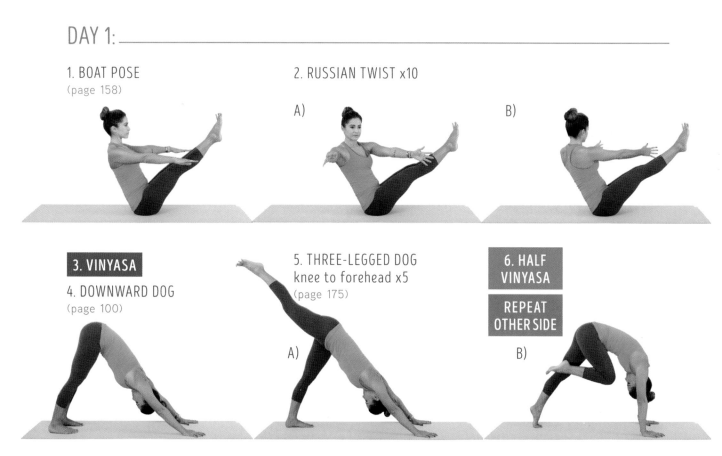

1. BOAT POSE
(page 158)

2. RUSSIAN TWIST x10

A)

B)

3. VINYASA

4. DOWNWARD DOG
(page 100)

5. THREE-LEGGED DOG
knee to forehead x5
(page 175)

A)

6. HALF VINYASA

REPEAT OTHER SIDE

B)

7. HALF VINYASA

REPEAT OTHER SIDE

8. CRUNCH with block x10

A)

B)

C)

D)

9. SUPINE SPINAL TWIST (each side) (page 213)

10. CORPSE POSE (page 136)

DAY 2:

1. VINYASA 2. PLANK (page 109)

3. SIDE PLANK variation (each side) (page 192)

A)

B)

4. VINYASA 5. FOREARM PLANK with leg lift (each side) (page 109)

A)

B)

6. VINYASA TO SEATED 7. BRIDGE POSE (page 132)

8. CORPSE POSE (page 136)

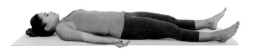

DAY 3: _____

1. CHAIR POSE
(page 125)

2. STANDING FORWARD FOLD
(page 107)

3. VINYASA

4. WARRIOR 2
(page 114)

5. HALF MOON POSE
(page 176)

6. SUGARCANE POSE
(page 178)

7. VINYASA

8. STANDING SPLIT
(page 210)

9. VINYASA TO STANDING

REPEAT OTHER SIDE

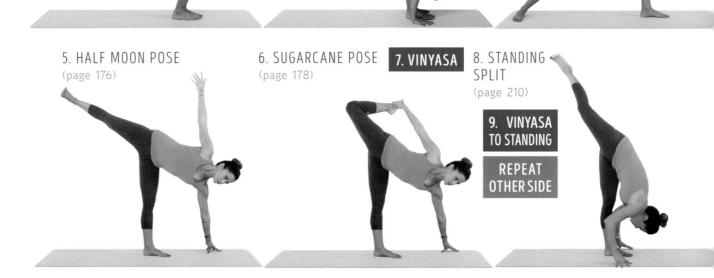

10. VINYASA TO STANDING

11. GARLAND POSE
(page 182)

12. CROW POSE
(page 222)

13. HALF SPINAL TWIST (each side)
(page 172)

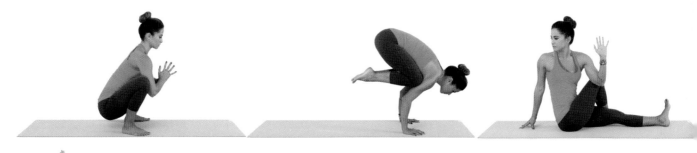

14. SUPPORTED SHOULDER STAND
(page 218)

15. PLOW POSE
(page 235)

16. CORPSE POSE
(page 136)

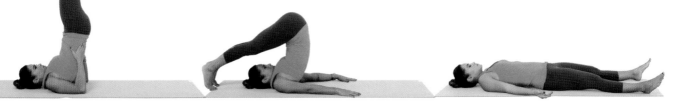

DAY 4:

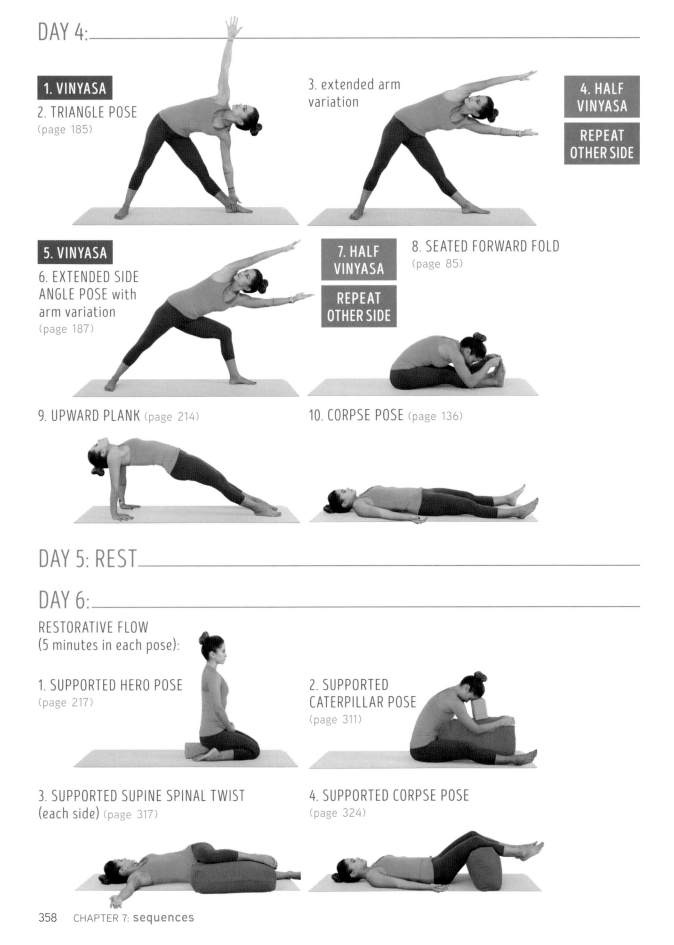

1. VINYASA

2. TRIANGLE POSE
(page 185)

3. extended arm variation

4. HALF VINYASA

REPEAT OTHER SIDE

5. VINYASA

6. EXTENDED SIDE ANGLE POSE with arm variation
(page 187)

7. HALF VINYASA

REPEAT OTHER SIDE

8. SEATED FORWARD FOLD
(page 85)

9. UPWARD PLANK (page 214)

10. CORPSE POSE (page 136)

DAY 5: REST

DAY 6:

RESTORATIVE FLOW
(5 minutes in each pose):

1. SUPPORTED HERO POSE
(page 217)

2. SUPPORTED CATERPILLAR POSE
(page 311)

3. SUPPORTED SUPINE SPINAL TWIST
(each side) (page 317)

4. SUPPORTED CORPSE POSE
(page 324)

DAY 7:

1. CHAIR POSE
(page 125)

2. CHAIR POSE
with leg lift

3. VINYASA **4. LIZARD POSE**
(page 191)

5. ONE-LEGGED SAGE POSE
(page 284)

A)

B)

6. HALF VINYASA

REPEAT OTHER SIDE

7. COBBLER'S POSE
(page 88)

8. HEAD-TO-KNEE POSE
(page 162)

9. CORPSE POSE
(page 136)

DAY 8:

1. FOREARM PLANK (hold for 3 breaths) (page 109)

2. DOLPHIN POSE (hold for 3 breaths)
(page 197)

3. DOWNWARD DOG
(page 100)

4. THREE-LEGGED DOG
(page 175)

5. WARRIOR 3
(page 194)

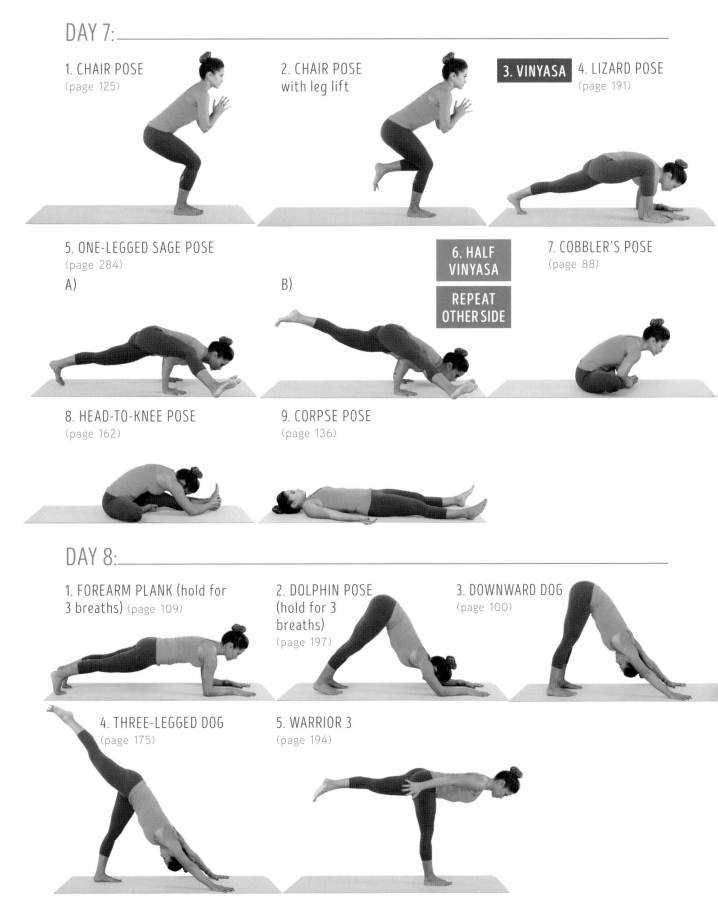

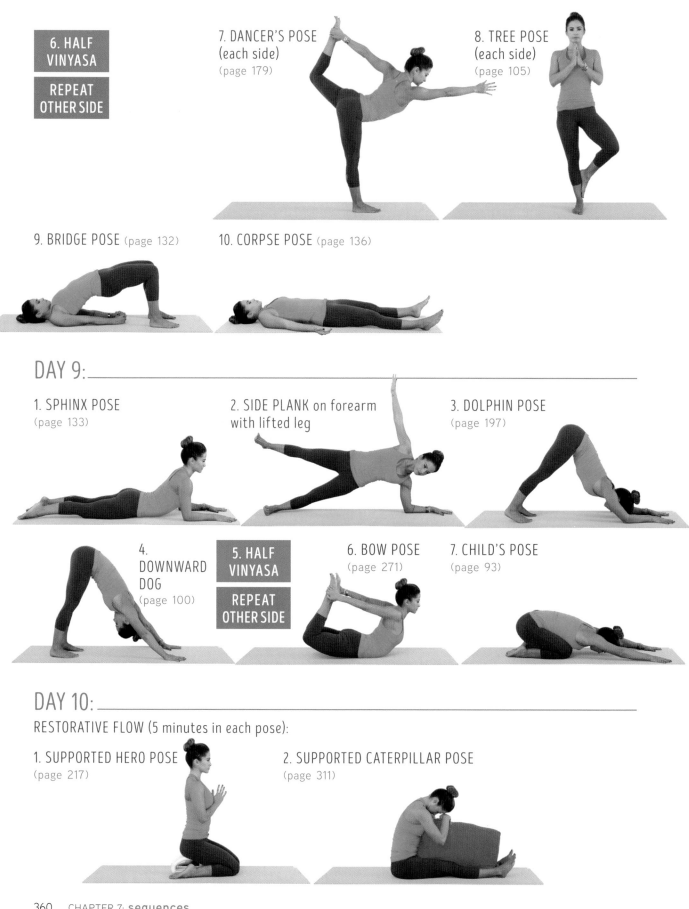

6. HALF VINYASA

REPEAT OTHER SIDE

7. DANCER'S POSE (each side)
(page 179)

8. TREE POSE (each side)
(page 105)

9. BRIDGE POSE (page 132)

10. CORPSE POSE (page 136)

DAY 9:

1. SPHINX POSE
(page 133)

2. SIDE PLANK on forearm with lifted leg

3. DOLPHIN POSE
(page 197)

4. DOWNWARD DOG
(page 100)

5. HALF VINYASA

REPEAT OTHER SIDE

6. BOW POSE
(page 271)

7. CHILD'S POSE
(page 93)

DAY 10:

RESTORATIVE FLOW (5 minutes in each pose):

1. SUPPORTED HERO POSE
(page 217)

2. SUPPORTED CATERPILLAR POSE
(page 311)

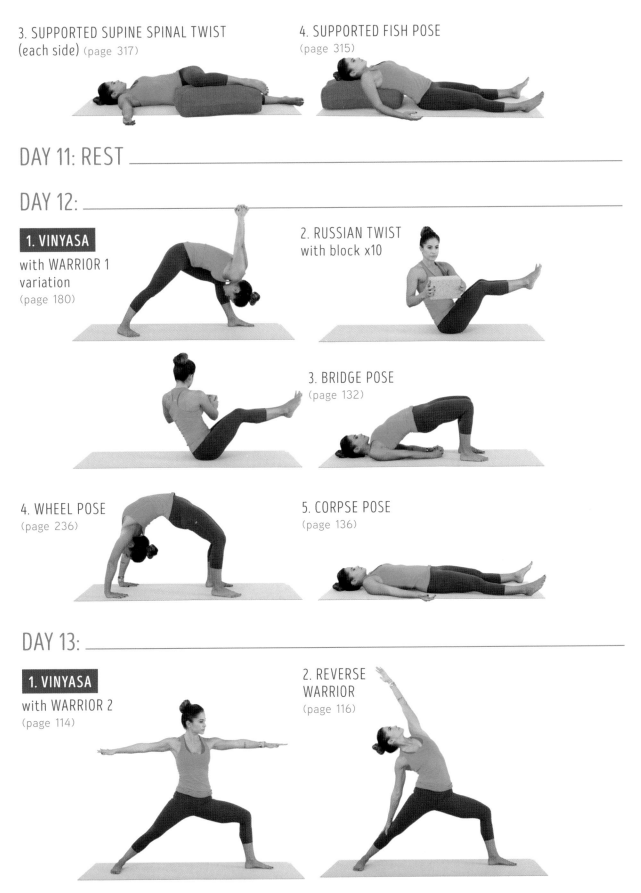

3. SUPPORTED SUPINE SPINAL TWIST
(each side) (page 317)

4. SUPPORTED FISH POSE
(page 315)

DAY 11: REST

DAY 12:

1. VINYASA

with WARRIOR 1
variation
(page 180)

2. RUSSIAN TWIST
with block x10

3. BRIDGE POSE
(page 132)

4. WHEEL POSE
(page 236)

5. CORPSE POSE
(page 136)

DAY 13:

1. VINYASA

with WARRIOR 2
(page 114)

2. REVERSE
WARRIOR
(page 116)

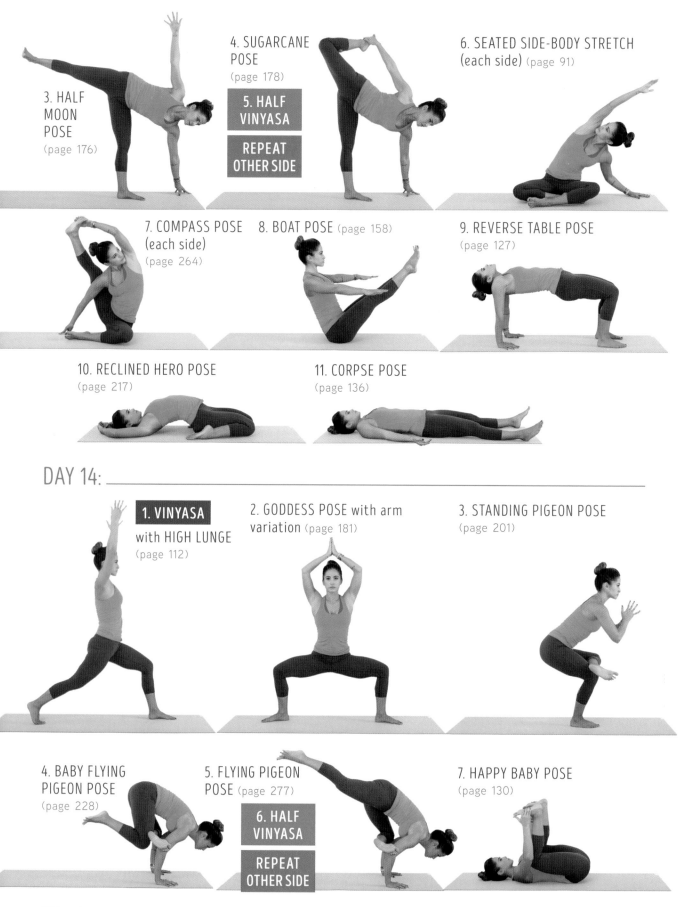

3. HALF MOON POSE (page 176)

4. SUGARCANE POSE (page 178)

5. HALF VINYASA

REPEAT OTHER SIDE

6. SEATED SIDE-BODY STRETCH (each side) (page 91)

7. COMPASS POSE (each side) (page 264)

8. BOAT POSE (page 158)

9. REVERSE TABLE POSE (page 127)

10. RECLINED HERO POSE (page 217)

11. CORPSE POSE (page 136)

DAY 14:

1. VINYASA with HIGH LUNGE (page 112)

2. GODDESS POSE with arm variation (page 181)

3. STANDING PIGEON POSE (page 201)

4. BABY FLYING PIGEON POSE (page 228)

5. FLYING PIGEON POSE (page 277)

6. HALF VINYASA

REPEAT OTHER SIDE

7. HAPPY BABY POSE (page 130)

8. SUPINE SPINAL TWIST with eagle legs (each side) (page 213)

9. CORPSE POSE (page 136)

DAY 15:

1. CHAIR POSE
(page 125)

2. CROW POSE
(page 222)

3. jump back to LOW PLANK
(page 110)

4. VINYASA

5. DOLPHIN POSE
(page 197)

6. SUPPORTED HEADSTAND
(page 229)

A)

B)

C)

7. pike leg reverse crunch in SUPPORTED HEADSTAND x10

A)

B)

C)

D)

E)

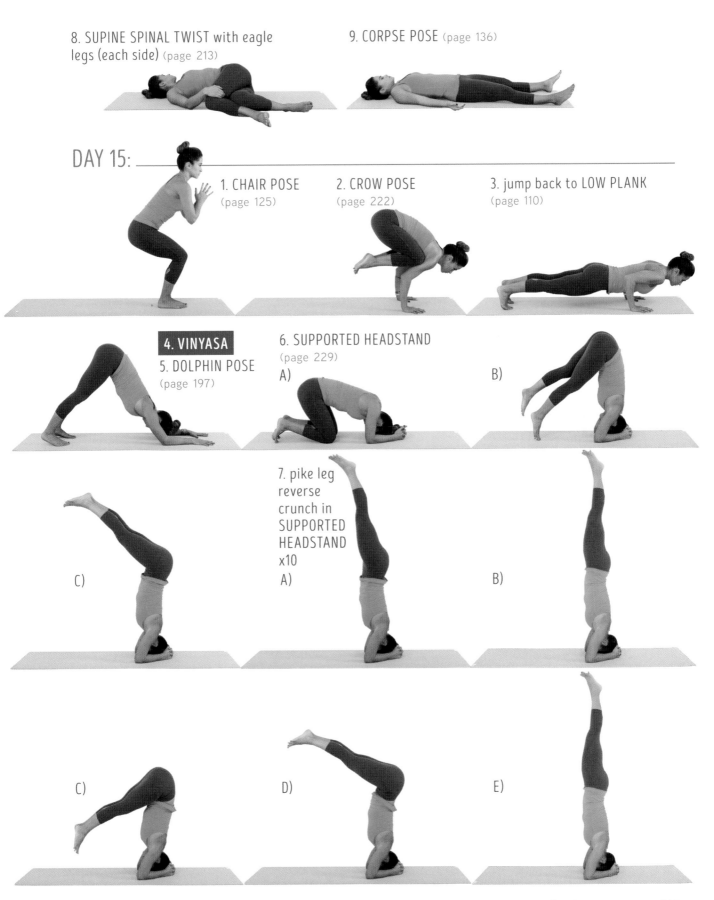

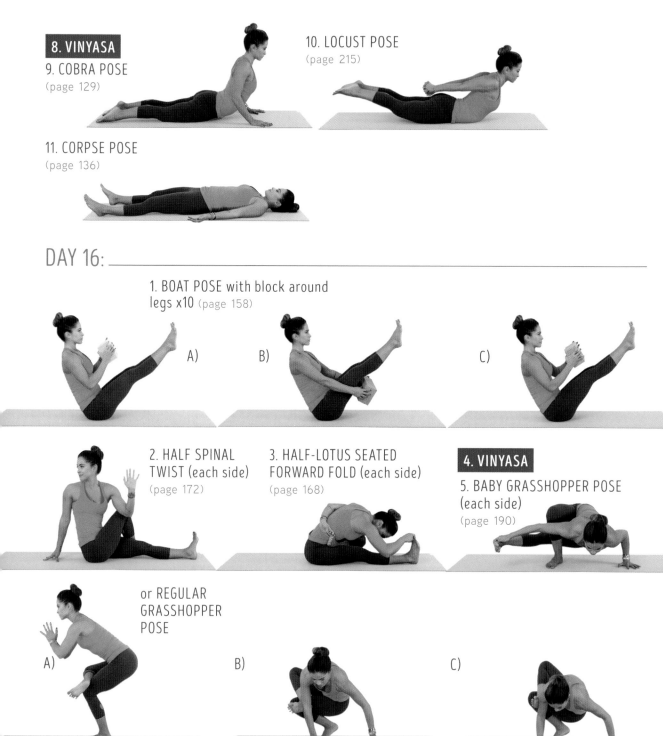

8. VINYASA

9. COBRA POSE
(page 129)

10. LOCUST POSE
(page 215)

11. CORPSE POSE
(page 136)

DAY 16:

1. BOAT POSE with block around legs x10 (page 158)

A)

B)

C)

2. HALF SPINAL TWIST (each side)
(page 172)

3. HALF-LOTUS SEATED FORWARD FOLD (each side)
(page 168)

4. VINYASA

5. BABY GRASSHOPPER POSE (each side)
(page 190)

or REGULAR GRASSHOPPER POSE

A)

B)

C)

D)

E)

F)

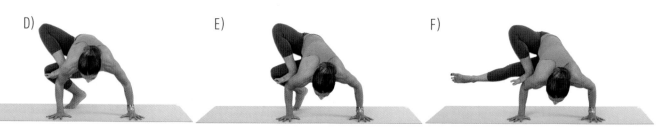

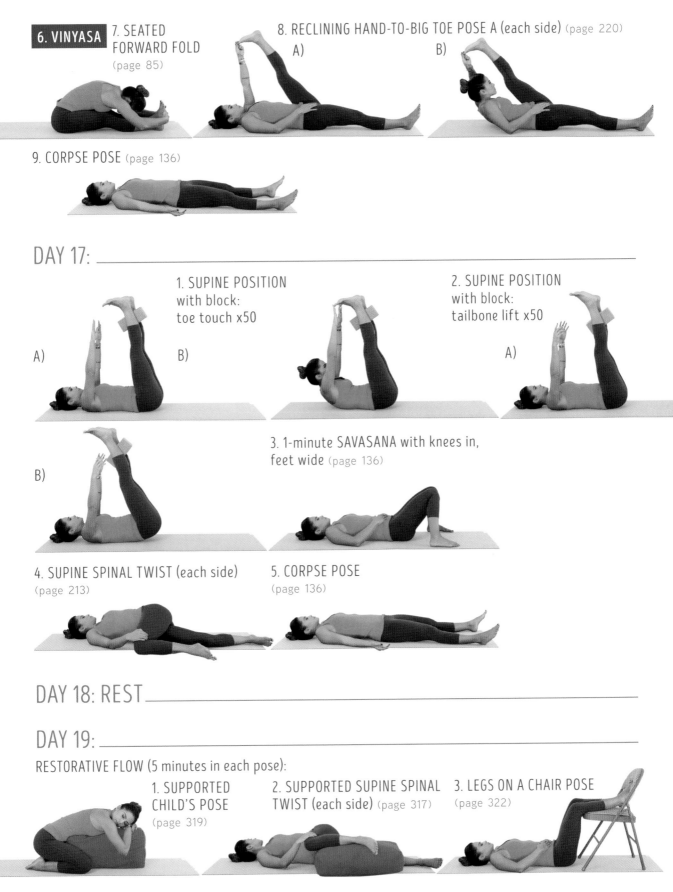

6. VINYASA

7. SEATED FORWARD FOLD (page 85)

8. RECLINING HAND-TO-BIG TOE POSE A (each side) (page 220)

A)

B)

9. CORPSE POSE (page 136)

DAY 17:

1. SUPINE POSITION with block: toe touch x50

A)

B)

2. SUPINE POSITION with block: tailbone lift x50

A)

B)

3. 1-minute SAVASANA with knees in, feet wide (page 136)

4. SUPINE SPINAL TWIST (each side) (page 213)

5. CORPSE POSE (page 136)

DAY 18: REST

DAY 19:

RESTORATIVE FLOW (5 minutes in each pose):

1. SUPPORTED CHILD'S POSE (page 319)

2. SUPPORTED SUPINE SPINAL TWIST (each side) (page 317)

3. LEGS ON A CHAIR POSE (page 322)

DAY 20:

1. BOAT POSE (30 seconds)
(page 158)

2. HALF VINYASA

3. to DOLPHIN POSE (page 197)

4. THREE-LEGGED DOLPHIN (each side) (page 197)

5. VINYASA TO SEATED

6. 20-second RUSSIAN TWIST HOLD with block (each side)

7. HALF VINYASA

8. to DOLPHIN POSE

9. FOREARM STAND
(page 273)

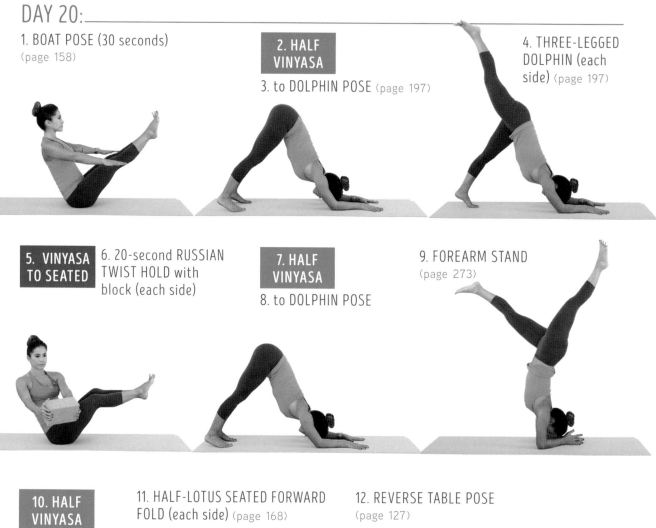

10. HALF VINYASA

11. HALF-LOTUS SEATED FORWARD FOLD (each side) (page 168)

12. REVERSE TABLE POSE
(page 127)

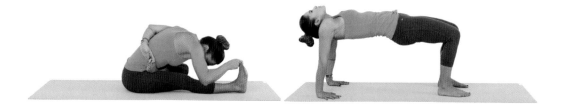

13. CORPSE POSE (page 136)

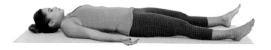

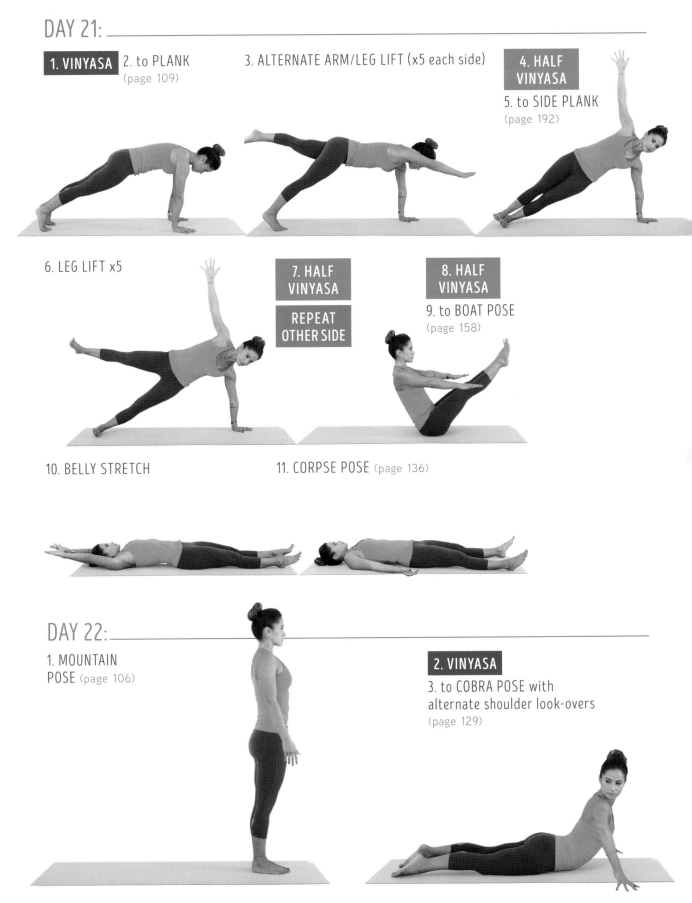

DAY 21:

1. VINYASA 2. to PLANK
(page 109)

3. ALTERNATE ARM/LEG LIFT (x5 each side)

4. HALF VINYASA

5. to SIDE PLANK
(page 192)

6. LEG LIFT x5

7. HALF VINYASA

REPEAT OTHER SIDE

8. HALF VINYASA

9. to BOAT POSE
(page 158)

10. BELLY STRETCH

11. CORPSE POSE (page 136)

DAY 22:

1. MOUNTAIN POSE (page 106)

2. VINYASA

3. to COBRA POSE with alternate shoulder look-overs
(page 129)

4. CAMEL prep

5. CAMEL POSE
(page 258)

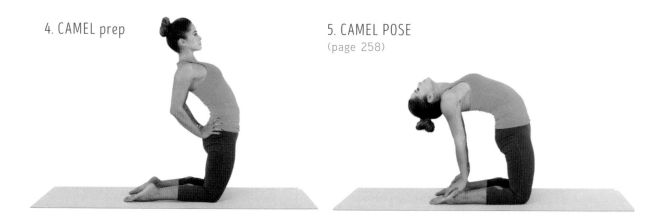

6. RABBIT POSE (page 165)

7. CORPSE POSE (page 136)

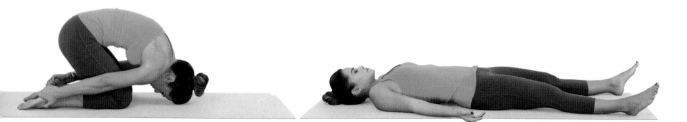

DAY 23:

1. VINYASA 2. to STANDING HAND-TO-BIG-TOE POSE A & B
(page 188)

3. SIDE PLANK variation
(page 192)

A)

B)

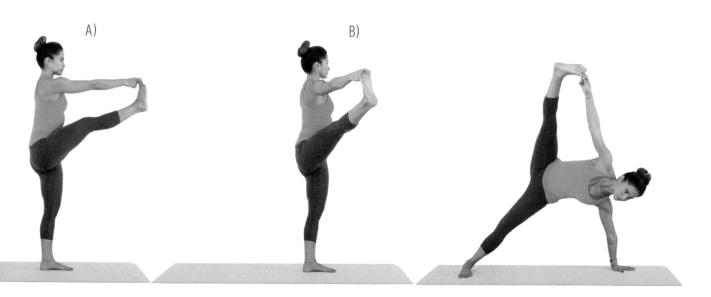

4. WILD THING
(page 208)

REPEAT OTHER SIDE

5. VINYASA

6. to DANCER'S POSE (each side) (page 179)

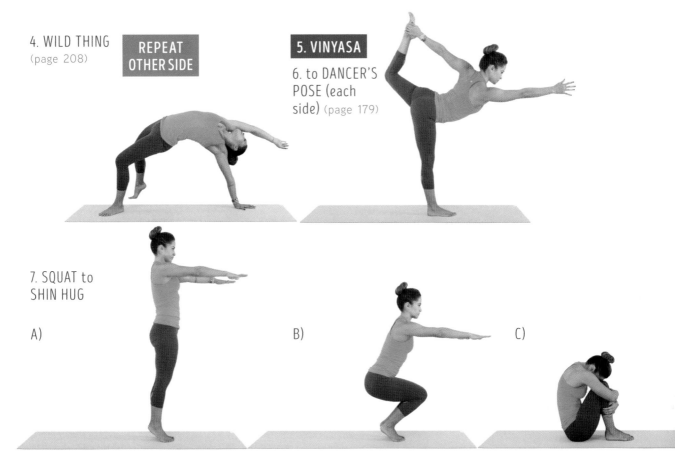

7. SQUAT to SHIN HUG

A)

B)

C)

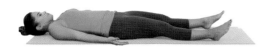

8. CORPSE POSE (page 136)

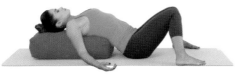

DAY 24: REST _____

DAY 25: _____

RESTORATIVE FLOW
(5 minutes in each pose):

1. LEGS ON A CHAIR POSE
(page 322)

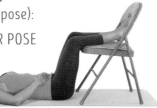

2. SUPPORTED FISH POSE with reclined bound angle pose legs (page 315)

3. SUPPORTED FISH POSE with leg variation

4. SUPPORTED CORPSE POSE
(page 324)

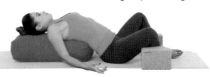

DAY 26: _____

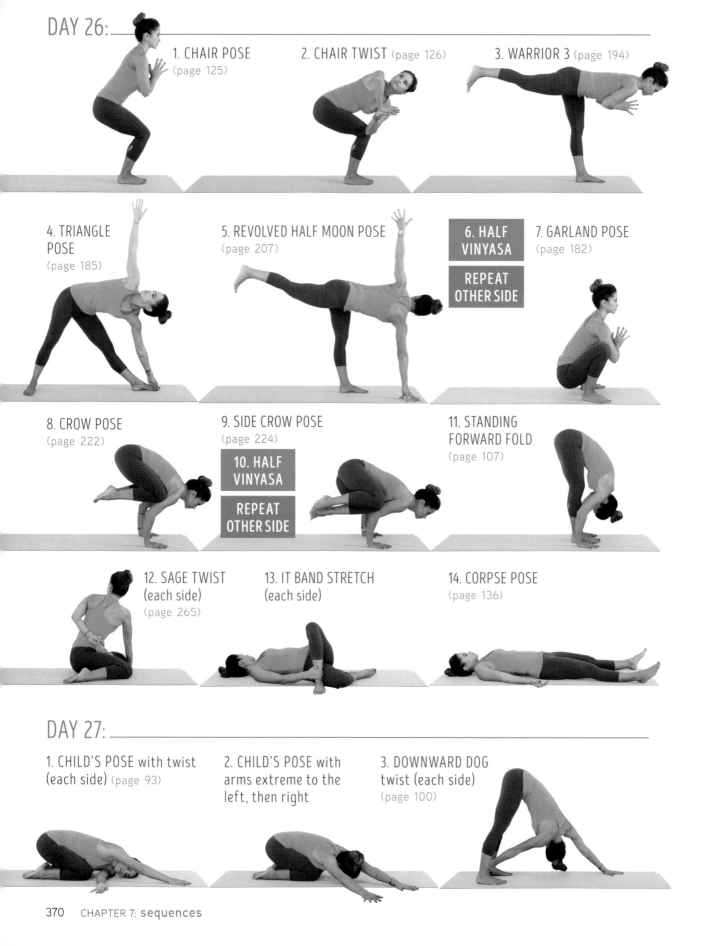

1. CHAIR POSE (page 125)

2. CHAIR TWIST (page 126)

3. WARRIOR 3 (page 194)

4. TRIANGLE POSE (page 185)

5. REVOLVED HALF MOON POSE (page 207)

6. HALF VINYASA

REPEAT OTHER SIDE

7. GARLAND POSE (page 182)

8. CROW POSE (page 222)

9. SIDE CROW POSE (page 224)

10. HALF VINYASA

REPEAT OTHER SIDE

11. STANDING FORWARD FOLD (page 107)

12. SAGE TWIST (each side) (page 265)

13. IT BAND STRETCH (each side)

14. CORPSE POSE (page 136)

DAY 27: _____

1. CHILD'S POSE with twist (each side) (page 93)

2. CHILD'S POSE with arms extreme to the left, then right

3. DOWNWARD DOG twist (each side) (page 100)

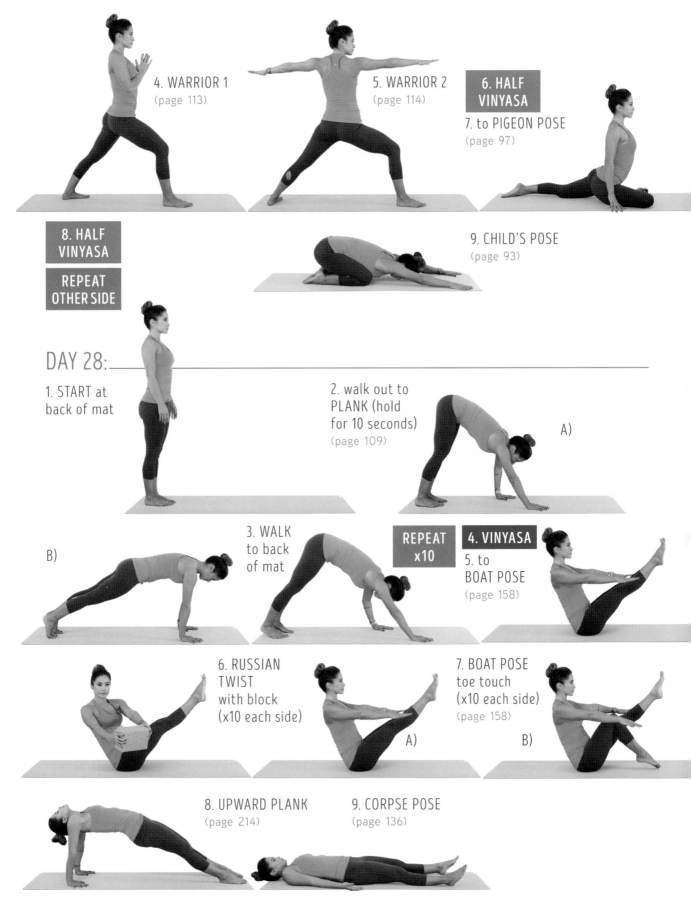

4. WARRIOR 1
(page 113)

5. WARRIOR 2
(page 114)

6. HALF VINYASA

7. to PIGEON POSE
(page 97)

8. HALF VINYASA

REPEAT OTHER SIDE

9. CHILD'S POSE
(page 93)

DAY 28:

1. START at back of mat

2. walk out to PLANK (hold for 10 seconds)
(page 109)

A)

B)

3. WALK to back of mat

REPEAT x10

4. VINYASA

5. to BOAT POSE
(page 158)

6. RUSSIAN TWIST with block
(x10 each side)

A)

7. BOAT POSE toe touch (x10 each side)
(page 158)

B)

8. UPWARD PLANK
(page 214)

9. CORPSE POSE
(page 136)

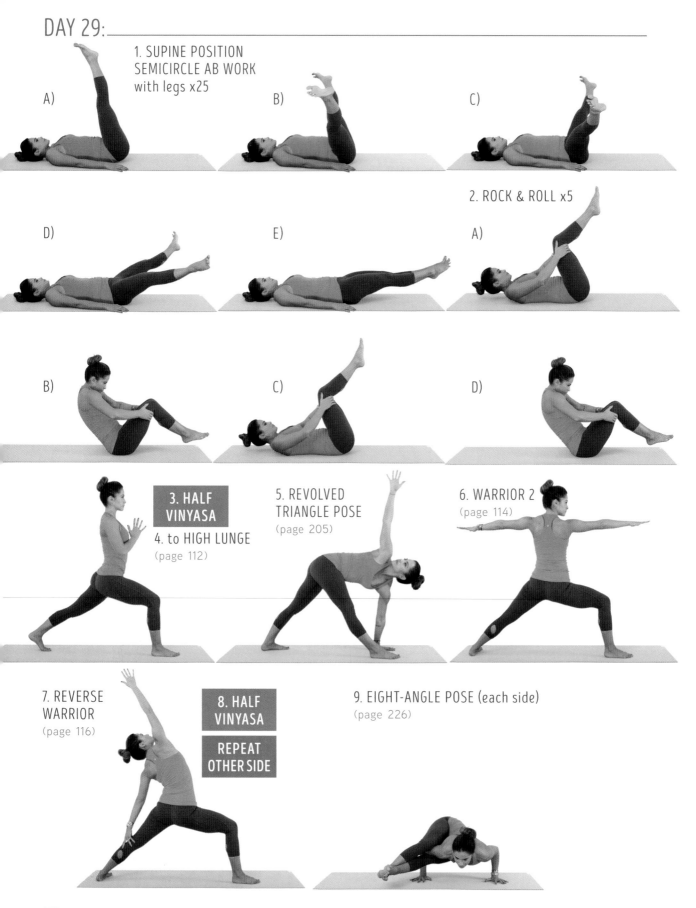

1. SUPINE POSITION SEMICIRCLE AB WORK with legs x25

A)

B)

C)

D)

E)

2. ROCK & ROLL x5

A)

B)

C)

D)

3. HALF VINYASA

4. to HIGH LUNGE (page 112)

5. REVOLVED TRIANGLE POSE (page 205)

6. WARRIOR 2 (page 114)

7. REVERSE WARRIOR (page 116)

8. HALF VINYASA

REPEAT OTHER SIDE

9. EIGHT-ANGLE POSE (each side) (page 226)

10. SUPINE SPINAL TWIST
(page 213)

11. CORPSE POSE
(page 136)

DAY 30:

1. BLOCK EXCHANGE CRUNCH x50

A)

B)

C)

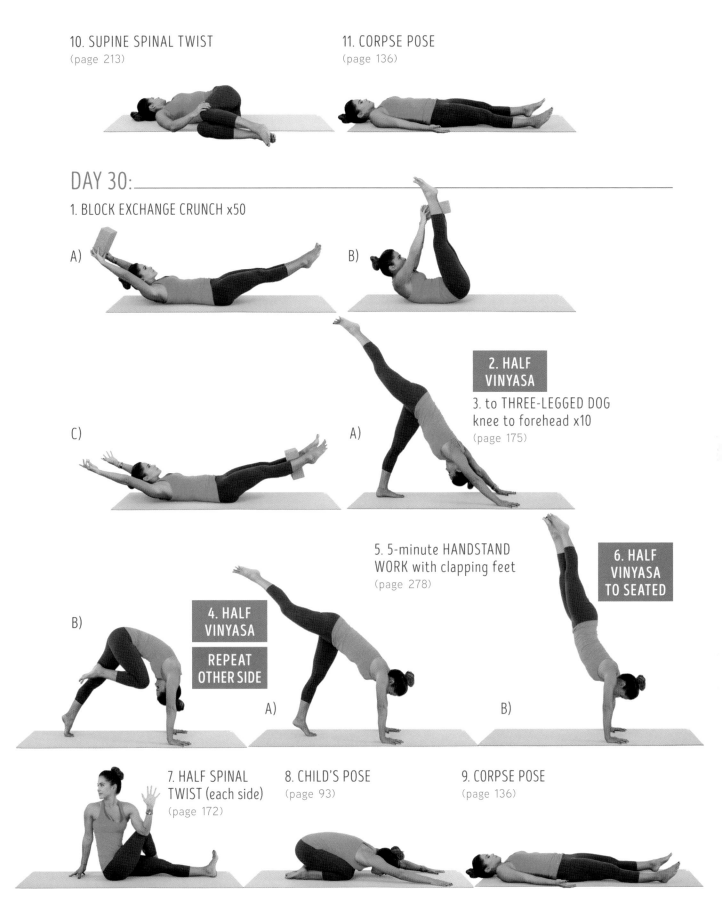

2. HALF VINYASA

3. to THREE-LEGGED DOG knee to forehead x10
(page 175)

A)

5. 5-minute HANDSTAND WORK with clapping feet
(page 278)

6. HALF VINYASA TO SEATED

B)

4. HALF VINYASA

REPEAT OTHER SIDE

A)

B)

7. HALF SPINAL TWIST (each side)
(page 172)

8. CHILD'S POSE
(page 93)

9. CORPSE POSE
(page 136)

thirty-day program for back pain and chest opening

This thirty-day yoga program focuses on back pain and chest opening. The program is suitable for people with tight hips, a tight chest, and mild back pain. The thing to remember about yoga is that everything is connected. What I mean is that while you might experience mild upper-back pain, the root cause could be a tight chest and/or tight shoulders. Everything in the body is connected, which is why this program covers the entire body with the aim of alleviating tension in the back and chest. Make this program work for you. Modify it to fit your lifestyle and schedule. If you need to skip a day, skip a day. If you need to shorten a practice or feel like lengthening a practice, do so. There is no right or wrong way to do this. As long as you loosely follow the program and maintain a consistent practice, you should see a noticeable difference by the end of the thirty days. You may notice core strengthening, improved posture, and reduced back pain.

Begin each day's practice with a five-minute meditation (from chapter 1) and a five-minute pranayama (from chapter 2).

DAY 1:

RESTORATIVE FLOW (5 minutes in each pose):

1. SUPPORTED FISH POSE
(page 314)

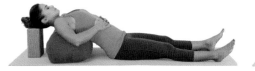

2. SUPPORTED FISH POSE with leg variation
(page 315)

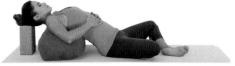

3. SUPPORTED FISH POSE

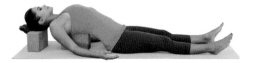

4. SUPPORTED RECLINED BOUND ANGLE POSE
(page 312)

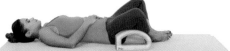

5. SUPPORTED CORPSE POSE
(page 324)

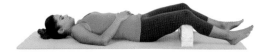

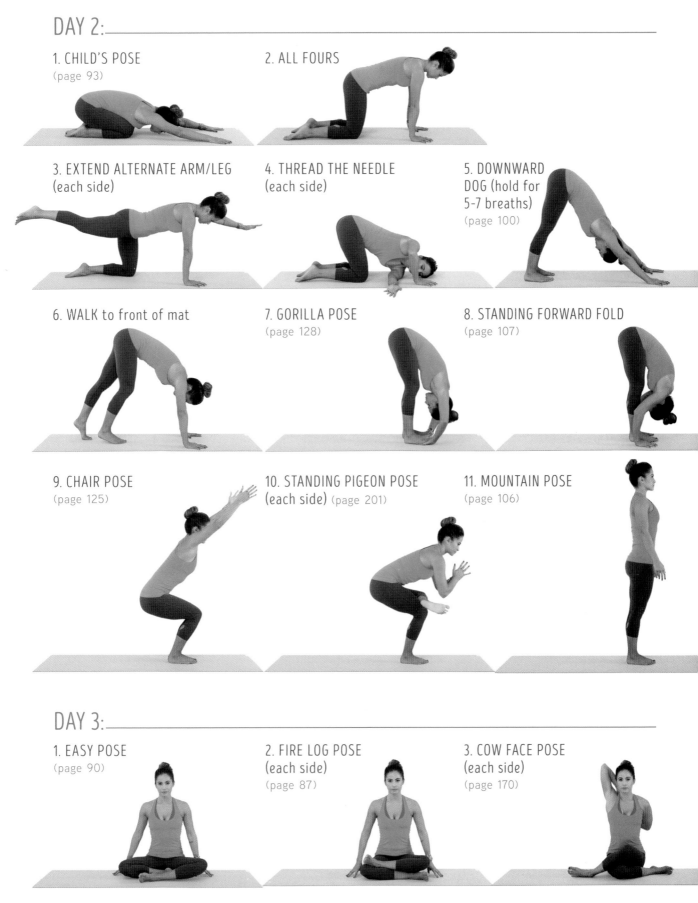

DAY 2:

1. CHILD'S POSE
(page 93)

2. ALL FOURS

3. EXTEND ALTERNATE ARM/LEG
(each side)

4. THREAD THE NEEDLE
(each side)

5. DOWNWARD DOG (hold for 5-7 breaths)
(page 100)

6. WALK to front of mat

7. GORILLA POSE
(page 128)

8. STANDING FORWARD FOLD
(page 107)

9. CHAIR POSE
(page 125)

10. STANDING PIGEON POSE
(each side) (page 201)

11. MOUNTAIN POSE
(page 106)

DAY 3:

1. EASY POSE
(page 90)

2. FIRE LOG POSE
(each side)
(page 87)

3. COW FACE POSE
(each side)
(page 170)

thirty-day program for back pain and chest opening 375

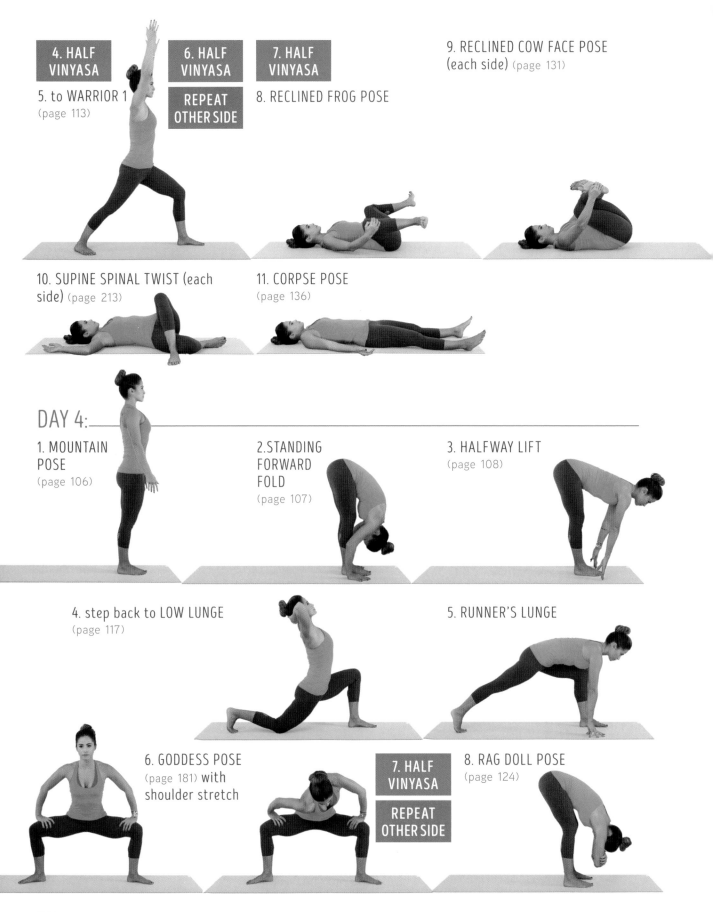

4. HALF VINYASA

5. to WARRIOR 1 (page 113)

6. HALF VINYASA

REPEAT OTHER SIDE

7. HALF VINYASA

8. RECLINED FROG POSE

9. RECLINED COW FACE POSE (each side) (page 131)

10. SUPINE SPINAL TWIST (each side) (page 213)

11. CORPSE POSE (page 136)

DAY 4:

1. MOUNTAIN POSE (page 106)

2. STANDING FORWARD FOLD (page 107)

3. HALFWAY LIFT (page 108)

4. step back to LOW LUNGE (page 117)

5. RUNNER'S LUNGE

6. GODDESS POSE (page 181) with shoulder stretch

7. HALF VINYASA

REPEAT OTHER SIDE

8. RAG DOLL POSE (page 124)

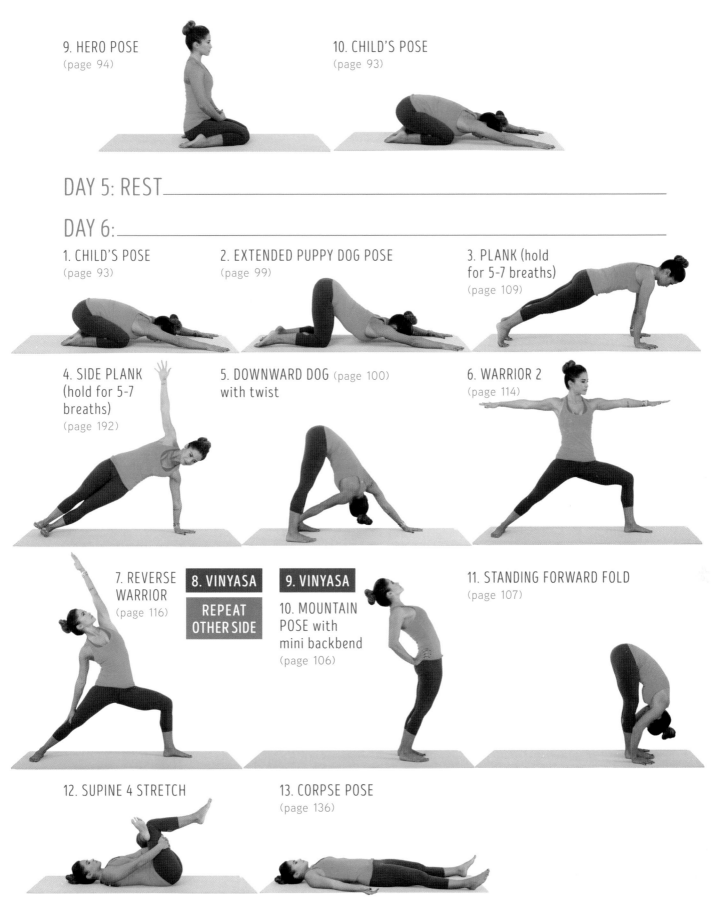

9. HERO POSE
(page 94)

10. CHILD'S POSE
(page 93)

DAY 5: REST_____

DAY 6:_____

1. CHILD'S POSE
(page 93)

2. EXTENDED PUPPY DOG POSE
(page 99)

3. PLANK (hold for 5-7 breaths)
(page 109)

4. SIDE PLANK (hold for 5-7 breaths)
(page 192)

5. DOWNWARD DOG (page 100) with twist

6. WARRIOR 2
(page 114)

7. REVERSE WARRIOR
(page 116)

8. VINYASA

REPEAT OTHER SIDE

9. VINYASA

10. MOUNTAIN POSE with mini backbend
(page 106)

11. STANDING FORWARD FOLD
(page 107)

12. SUPINE 4 STRETCH

13. CORPSE POSE
(page 136)

DAY 7:

1. START at back of mat

2. walk to PLANK POSE
(page 109)

A)

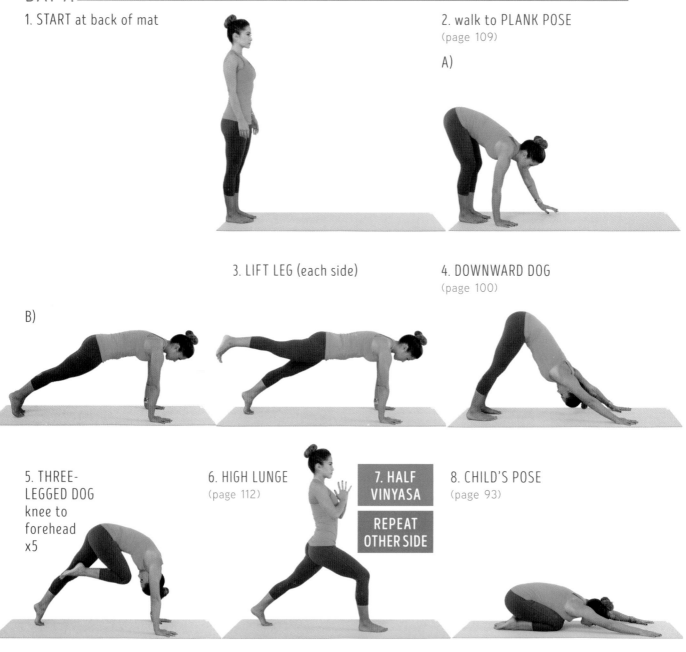

3. LIFT LEG (each side)

4. DOWNWARD DOG
(page 100)

B)

5. THREE-LEGGED DOG
knee to forehead
x5

6. HIGH LUNGE
(page 112)

7. HALF VINYASA

REPEAT OTHER SIDE

8. CHILD'S POSE
(page 93)

DAY 8:

1. SEATED FORWARD FOLD
(page 85)

2. SEATED FORWARD FOLD
with legs mat width

3. HIP-OPENING WIDE-LEG SEATED FORWARD FOLD

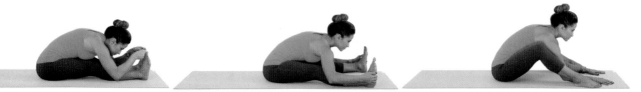

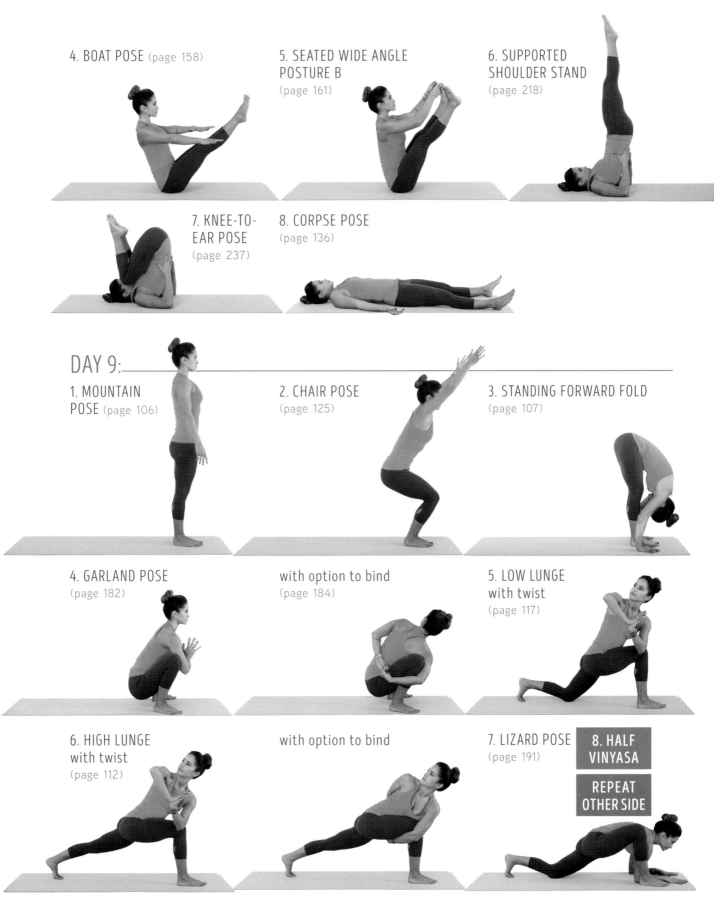

4. BOAT POSE (page 158)

5. SEATED WIDE ANGLE POSTURE B (page 161)

6. SUPPORTED SHOULDER STAND (page 218)

7. KNEE-TO-EAR POSE (page 237)

8. CORPSE POSE (page 136)

DAY 9:

1. MOUNTAIN POSE (page 106)

2. CHAIR POSE (page 125)

3. STANDING FORWARD FOLD (page 107)

4. GARLAND POSE (page 182)

with option to bind (page 184)

5. LOW LUNGE with twist (page 117)

6. HIGH LUNGE with twist (page 112)

with option to bind

7. LIZARD POSE (page 191)

8. HALF VINYASA

REPEAT OTHER SIDE

9. BABY GRASSHOPPER (each side) (page 190) **or REGULAR GRASSHOPPER** (each side)

10. HAPPY BABY POSE (page 130)

11. RECLINING HAND-TO-BIG TOE POSE A (each side) (page 220)

A)

B)

12. CORPSE POSE (page 136)

DAY 10: REST_____

DAY 11: _____

1. STANDING HAND-TO-BIG-TOE POSE (each side) (page 118)

A)

B)

2. HALF VINYASA

3. SEATED WIDE ANGLE POSTURE A (page 160)

4. SEATED WIDE ANGLE POSTURE A side-body stretch (each side)

5. SUPPORTED HEADSTAND with twist (each side) (page 229)

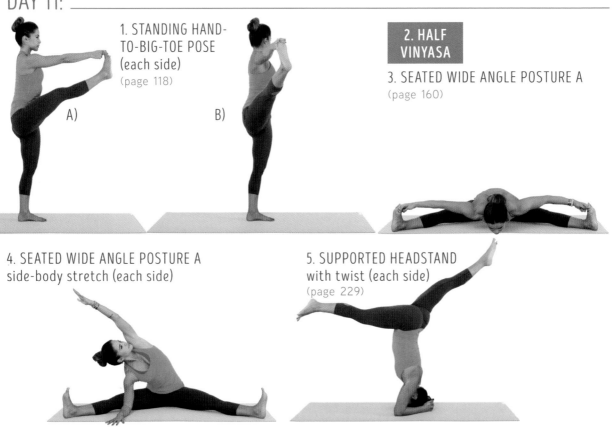
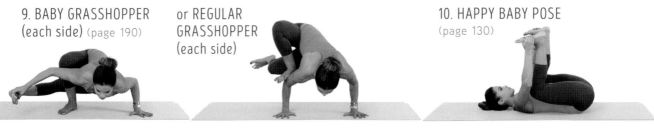
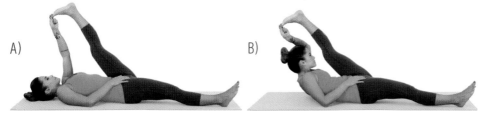
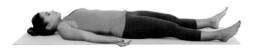

6. CRUNCH x25

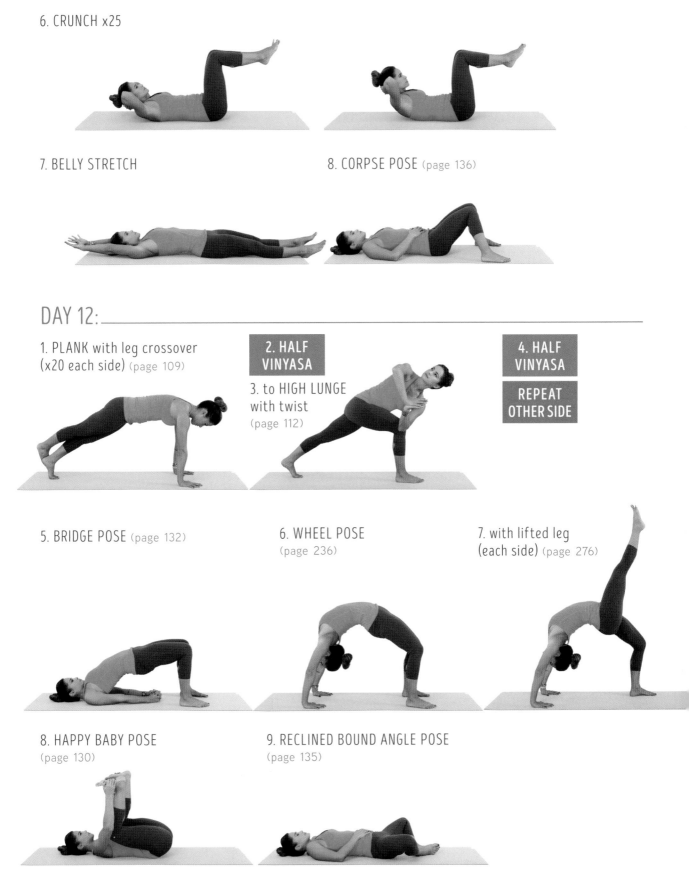

7. BELLY STRETCH

8. CORPSE POSE (page 136)

DAY 12:

1. PLANK with leg crossover
(x20 each side) (page 109)

2. HALF VINYASA

3. to HIGH LUNGE with twist
(page 112)

4. HALF VINYASA

REPEAT OTHER SIDE

5. BRIDGE POSE (page 132)

6. WHEEL POSE
(page 236)

7. with lifted leg
(each side) (page 276)

8. HAPPY BABY POSE
(page 130)

9. RECLINED BOUND ANGLE POSE
(page 135)

DAY 13:

1. VINYASA

2. to INTENSE STRETCH
(page 206)

3. LOW LUNGE
(page 117)

4. RUNNER'S LUNGE

5. HALF VINYASA

REPEAT OTHER SIDE

6. PIGEON POSE
(each side)
(page 97)

A)

B)

7. L-SHAPE LEG STRETCH (each side)

8. MONKEY POSE
(each side)
(page 260)

9. COBBLER'S POSE
(page 88)

10. SUPINE SPINAL TWIST
(each side) (page 213)

11. CORPSE POSE (page 136)

DAY 14:

1. VINYASA with WARRIOR 1 variation
(page 180)

2. SIDE PLANK tree pose variation
(page 192)

3. HALF-BOUND LOTUS TREE POSE (page 199)

4. RECLINED BOUND ANGLE POSE
(page 135)

5. SUPPORTED CORPSE POSE
(page 324)

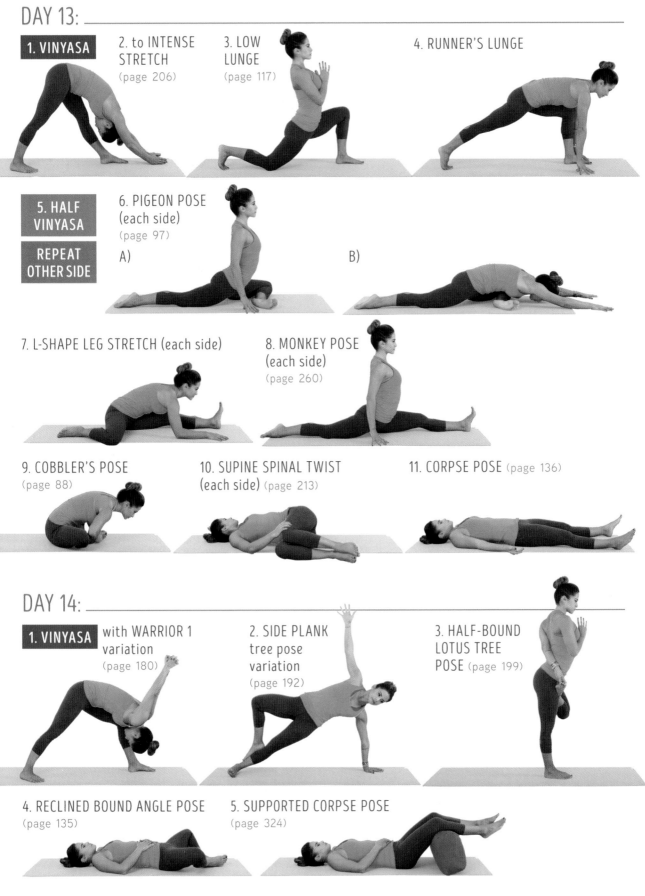

DAY 15:

1. VINYASA

2. to EXTENDED SIDE ANGLE POSE (each side) (page 187)

with option to bind

3. GARLAND POSE (page 182)

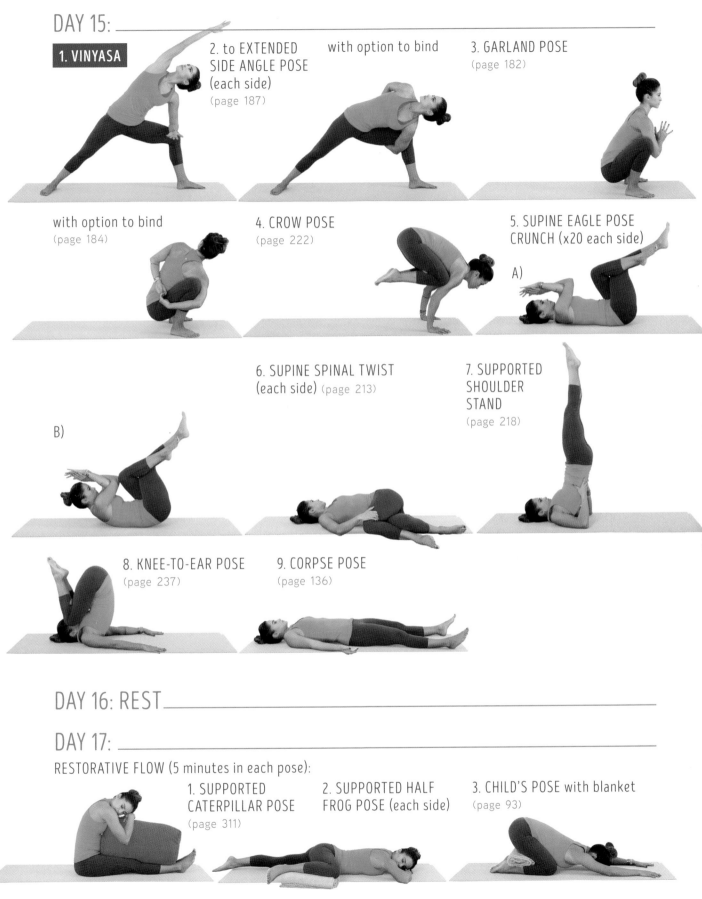

with option to bind (page 184)

4. CROW POSE (page 222)

5. SUPINE EAGLE POSE CRUNCH (x20 each side)

A)

6. SUPINE SPINAL TWIST (each side) (page 213)

7. SUPPORTED SHOULDER STAND (page 218)

B)

8. KNEE-TO-EAR POSE (page 237)

9. CORPSE POSE (page 136)

DAY 16: REST

DAY 17:

RESTORATIVE FLOW (5 minutes in each pose):

1. SUPPORTED CATERPILLAR POSE (page 311)

2. SUPPORTED HALF FROG POSE (each side)

3. CHILD'S POSE with blanket (page 93)

DAY 18:

1. VINYASA 2. to WARRIOR 2
(page 114)

3. REVERSE WARRIOR
(page 116)

4. HALF MOON POSE
(page 176)

5. HALF VINYASA

REPEAT OTHER SIDE

6. HALF VINYASA

7. to BRIDGE POSE
(page 132)

8. CORPSE POSE
(page 136)

DAY 19:

1. MOUNTAIN POSE with hands clasped behind back
(page 106)

2. TOPPLING TREE POSE (each side)

3. LOW LUNGE with cow face arms (page 117)

4. HALF VINYASA

5. to CAMEL prep

6. CAMEL POSE (page 258)

7. CHILD'S POSE (page 93)

8. SUPINE SPINAL TWIST (each side)
(page 213)

9. CORPSE POSE (page 136)

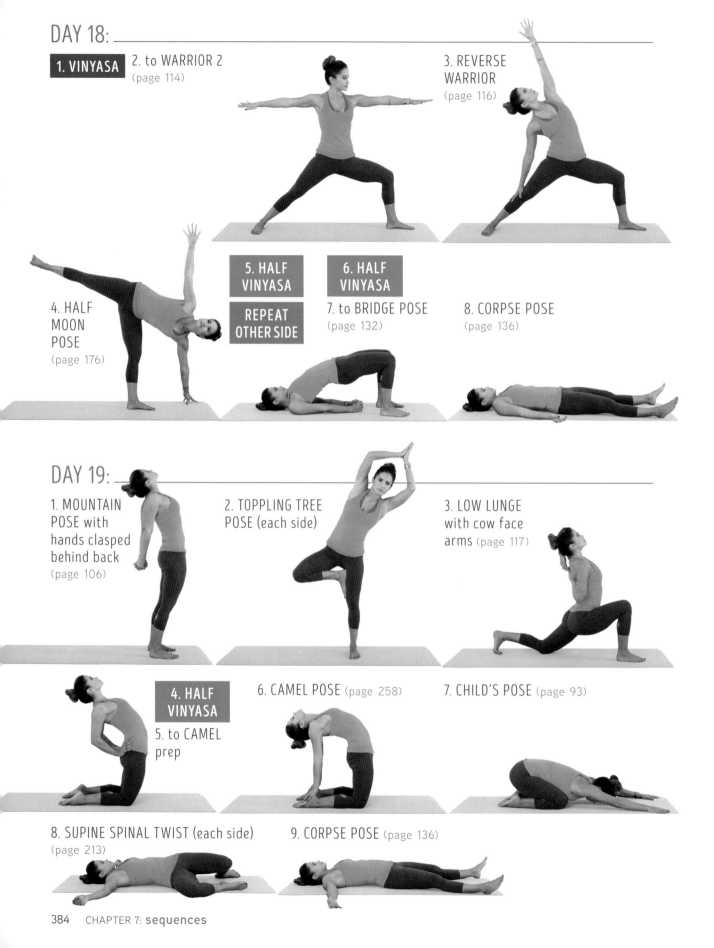

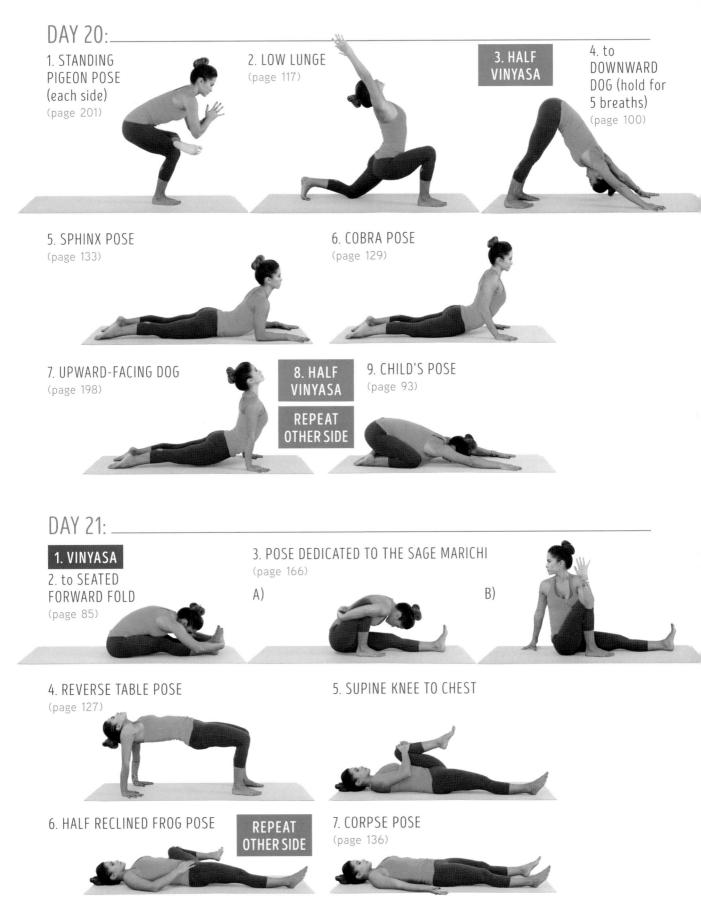

DAY 20:

1. STANDING PIGEON POSE (each side)
(page 201)

2. LOW LUNGE
(page 117)

3. HALF VINYASA

4. to DOWNWARD DOG (hold for 5 breaths)
(page 100)

5. SPHINX POSE
(page 133)

6. COBRA POSE
(page 129)

7. UPWARD-FACING DOG
(page 198)

8. HALF VINYASA

REPEAT OTHER SIDE

9. CHILD'S POSE
(page 93)

DAY 21:

1. VINYASA

2. to SEATED FORWARD FOLD
(page 85)

3. POSE DEDICATED TO THE SAGE MARICHI
(page 166)

A)

B)

4. REVERSE TABLE POSE
(page 127)

5. SUPINE KNEE TO CHEST

6. HALF RECLINED FROG POSE

REPEAT OTHER SIDE

7. CORPSE POSE
(page 136)

DAY 23:

1. BOAT POSE ROCK & ROLL x5 (page 158)

A)

B)

C)

2. BOAT POSE ALTERNATING TOE TOUCH x20

A)

B)

3. SUPINE WINDSHIELD WASHER LEGS x10

4. SUPINE KNEE CIRCLE x10

A)

B)

C)

D)

5. SUPINE HALF-CIRCLE x10

A)

B)

C)

D)

E)

6. ROCK & ROLL to

7. HALF VINYASA

8. BELLY STRETCH

9. CHILD'S POSE
(page 93)

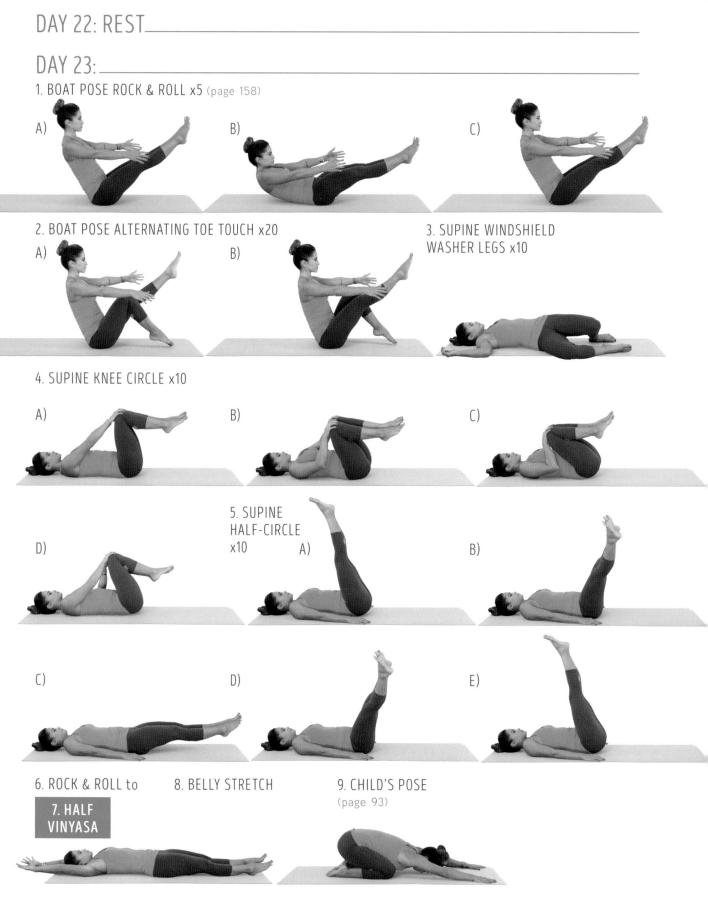

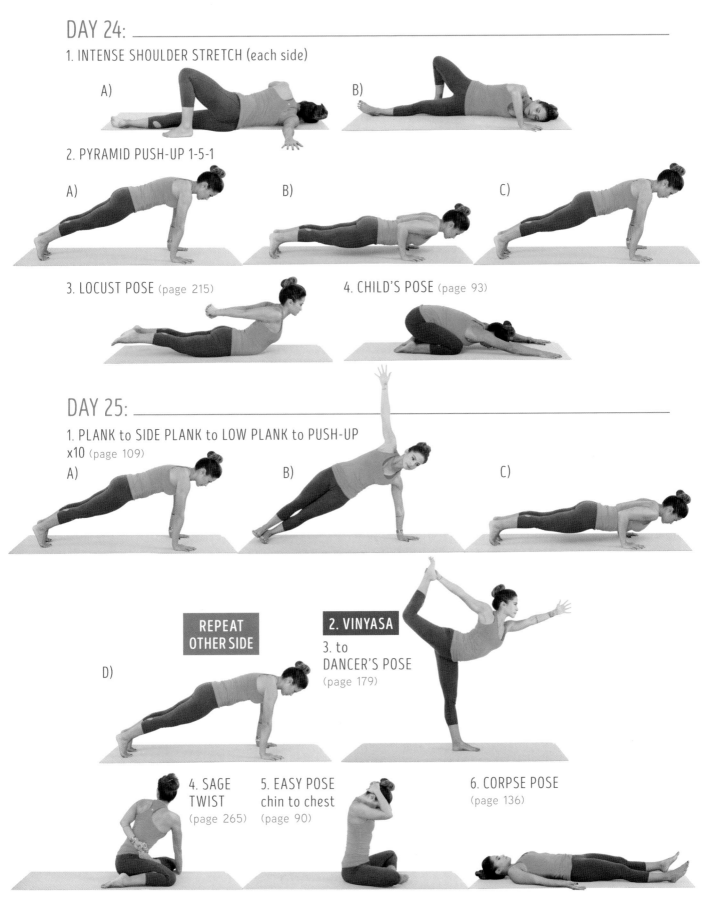

DAY 24:

1. INTENSE SHOULDER STRETCH (each side)

A)

B)

2. PYRAMID PUSH-UP 1-5-1

A)

B)

C)

3. LOCUST POSE (page 215)

4. CHILD'S POSE (page 93)

DAY 25:

1. PLANK to SIDE PLANK to LOW PLANK to PUSH-UP x10 (page 109)

A)

B)

C)

REPEAT OTHER SIDE

D)

2. VINYASA

3. to DANCER'S POSE (page 179)

4. SAGE TWIST (page 265)

5. EASY POSE chin to chest (page 90)

6. CORPSE POSE (page 136)

DAY 26: _____

RESTORATIVE FLOW (5 minutes in each pose):

1. LEGS ON A CHAIR POSE
(page 322)

2. SIDE-LYING CORPSE POSE (each side)
(page 323)

3. SUPPORTED HERO POSE
(page 217)

4. SUPPORTED RECLINING HERO POSE (page 325)

5. SUPPORTED FISH POSE
with two bolsters (page 315)

DAY 27: REST _____

DAY 28: _____

1. TREE POSE
(page 105)

2. BALANCING STICK POSE

3. WARRIOR 3
(page 194)

4. HALF VINYASA

TO OTHER SIDE

5. VINYASA TO SEATED

6. COBBLER'S POSE
(page 88)

7. WIDE LEGS with arms threaded under knees

8. HALF SPINAL TWIST (each side)
(page 172)

9. CORPSE POSE
(page 136)

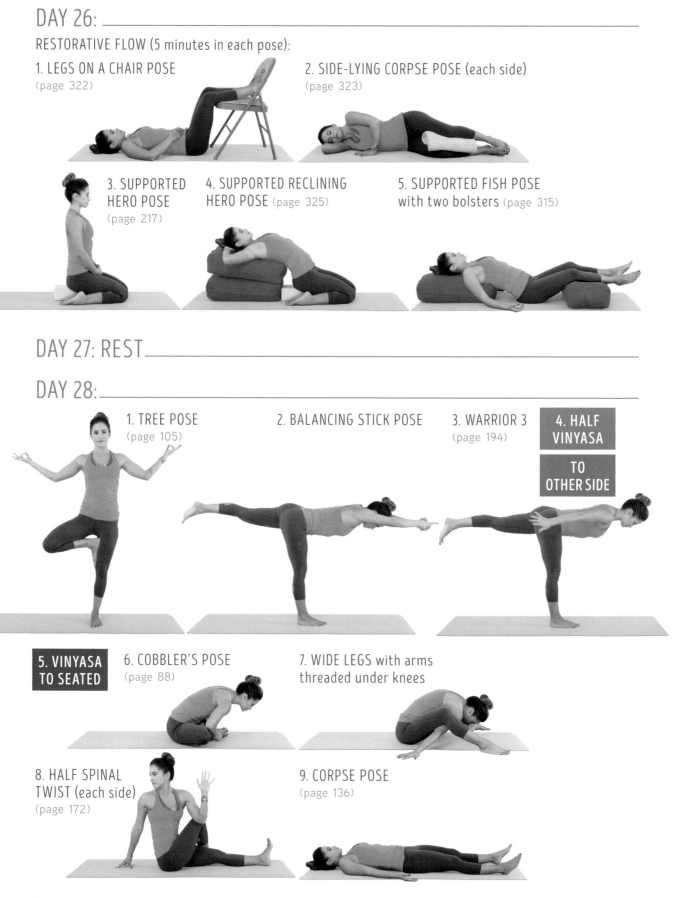

DAY 29:

1. CHAIR POSE
(page 125)

2. CHAIR TWIST
(page 126)

3. STANDING FORWARD FOLD
(page 107)

4. LOW LUNGE
with hands
behind head
(page 117)

5. LOW LUNGE
with prayer
hands

6. LOW LUNGE
with twist

7. HIGH LUNGE with twist
(page 112)

8. LIZARD POSE
(page 191)

9. HALF VINYASA

TO OTHER SIDE

10. TRIANGLE POSE
(each side) (page 185)

with option
to bind
(page 186)

11. FROG POSE
(page 212)

12. BABY GRASSHOPPER (each side)
(page 190)

or REGULAR
GRASSHOPPER
(each side)

13. IT BAND STRETCH
(each side)

14. BRIDGE POSE
(page 132)

15. CORPSE POSE
(page 136)

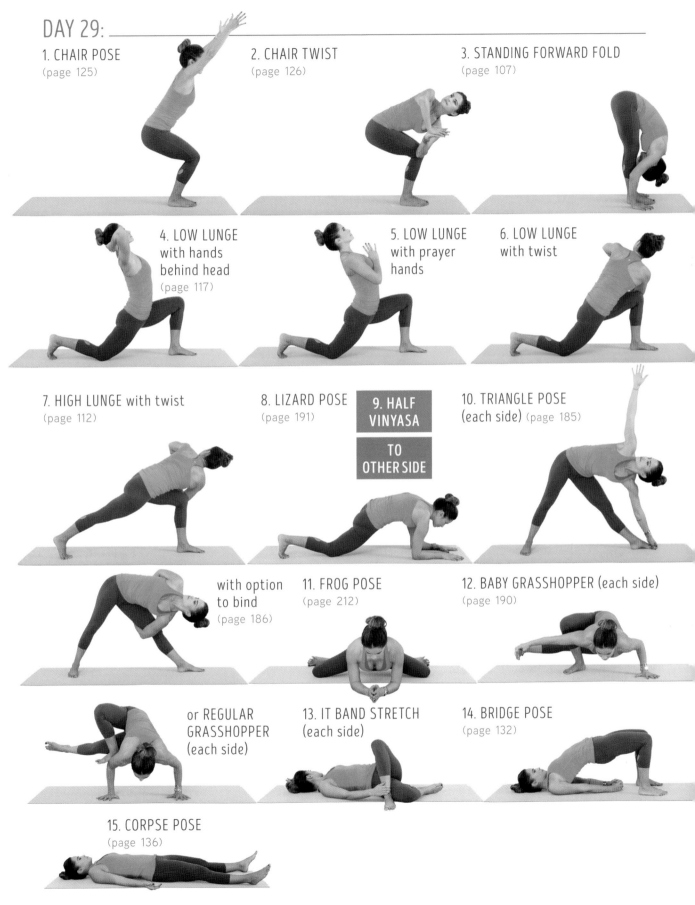

DAY 30: _____

1. BLOCK EXCHANGE CRUNCH x25

A)

B)

C)

2. TAILBONE LIFT x25

A)

B)

3. BOAT POSE TOE TOUCH x10

A)

B)

C)

4. VINYASA

5. to WARRIOR 1 (page 113)

6. WARRIOR 2 (page 114)

7. HALF MOON POSE (page 176)

8. HALF VINYASA   **9. VINYASA TO SEATED**

REPEAT OTHER SIDE

10. COBBLER'S POSE (page 88)

11. SEATED FORWARD FOLD (page 85)

12. RECLINED COW FACE POSE (each side) (page 131)

13. CORPSE POSE (page 136)

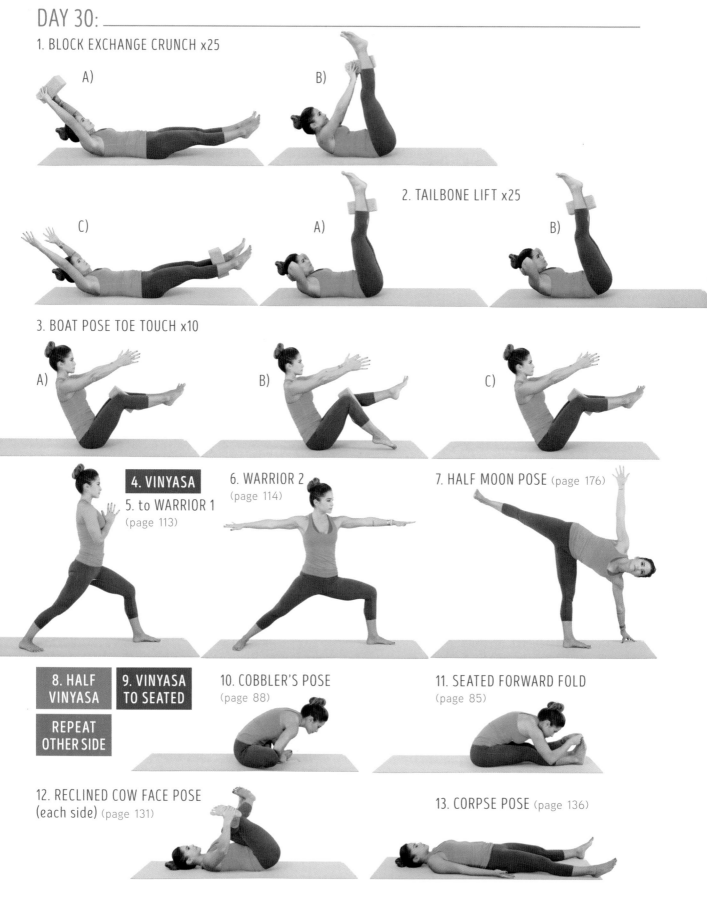

complementary practices

These complementary practices offer quick and effective doses of yoga asana that can easily be implemented into your life. The chair yoga sequence is wonderful for anyone with a desk job, while the gym and pre- and post-run yoga sequences make for excellent warm-ups and cool-downs when you're active. Lastly, the insomnia sequences work well not only when you're having trouble sleeping, but also when you're feeling exhausted or under the weather. Make the sequences work for you and your lifestyle and schedule. If you stumble across a pose that doesn't feel great for your body, just swap it out for one that does work for you. Do what feels best and stay consistent in your practice to reap the most benefits.

chair yoga at the office

You can easily incorporate these five-minute sequences into your workday. Take five breaths in each pose before moving on.

HIPS SEQUENCE: _____

1. LEGS ON A CHAIR POSE (page 322)

2. SUPINE 4 STRETCH (each side)

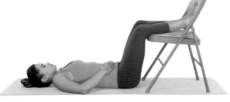

3. RECLINING HAND-TO-BIG TOE POSE A (each side) (page 220)

A)   B)

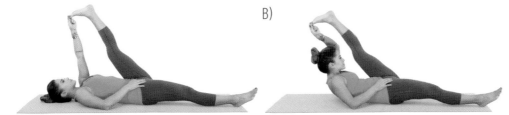

CHEST SEQUENCE:

1. SEATED CHEST STRETCH

2. SEATED CHEST STRETCH with hands interlaced behind back

3. SEATED FORWARD FOLD with arm variation (page 107)

4. SEATED TWIST (each side)

BACK PAIN SEQUENCE:

1. SEATED PIGEON POSE (each side) (page 97)

2. EAGLE POSE in chair (each side) (page 204)

3. UPWARD PLANK in chair (page 214)

4. LOW LUNGE (each side) (page 117)

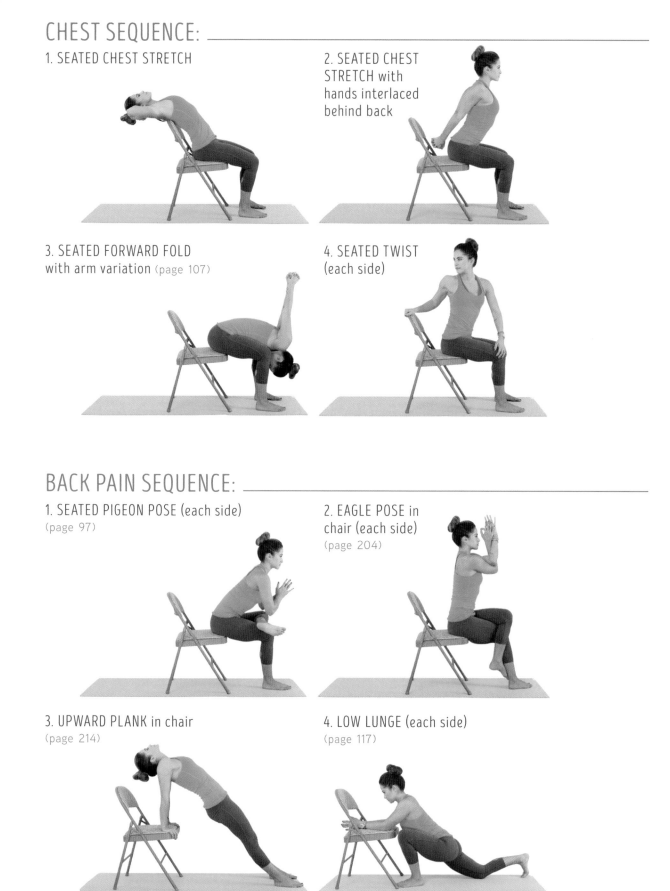

NECK AND SHOULDERS SEQUENCE

1. SEATED EAR TO SHOULDER (each side)   **2. LOOK LEFT, THEN RIGHT**   **3. CHIN TO CHEST**

4. TRICEPS STRETCH (each side)   **5. SHOULDER ROLLS**

A)

B)

C)

6. COW FACE ARMS
(each side)
(page 170)

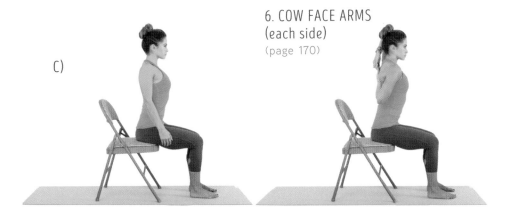

CHEST SEQUENCE:

1. WARRIOR 1 with chair
(page 113)

2. TRIANGLE POSE with chair
(page 185)

3. WARRIOR 3 with chair
(page 194)

**4. REVOLVED
TRIANGLE POSE
with chair**
(page 205)

**REPEAT
OTHER SIDE**

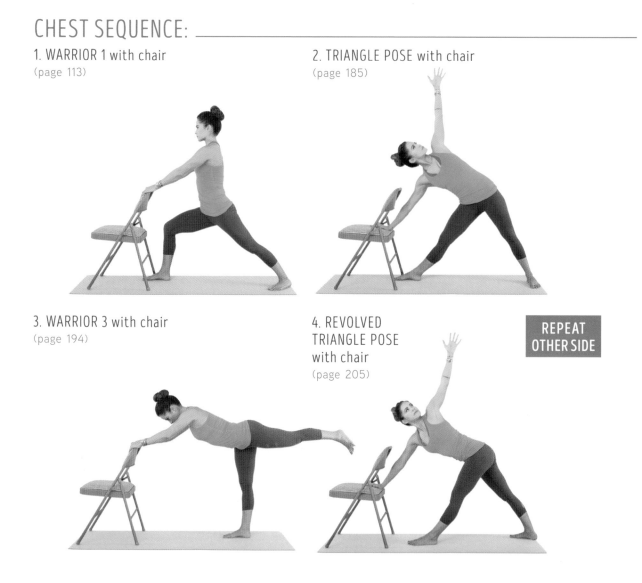

yoga for the gym

These quick sequences are designed to help warm up the body prior to a workout. Take three to five deep breaths in each pose before moving on.

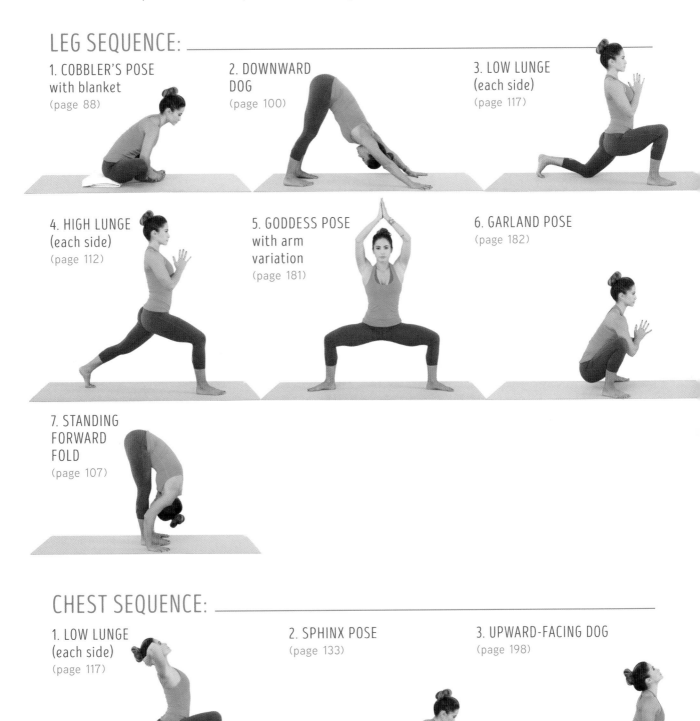

LEG SEQUENCE:

1. COBBLER'S POSE
with blanket
(page 88)

2. DOWNWARD DOG
(page 100)

3. LOW LUNGE
(each side)
(page 117)

4. HIGH LUNGE
(each side)
(page 112)

5. GODDESS POSE
with arm variation
(page 181)

6. GARLAND POSE
(page 182)

7. STANDING FORWARD FOLD
(page 107)

CHEST SEQUENCE:

1. LOW LUNGE
(each side)
(page 117)

2. SPHINX POSE
(page 133)

3. UPWARD-FACING DOG
(page 198)

4. HIGH LUNGE
variation (each side)
(page 112)

5. WIDE-LEG FORWARD FOLD C
(page 122)

6. UPWARD PLANK
(page 214)

7. CAMEL prep

8. CAMEL POSE (page 258)

9. CHILD'S POSE (page 93)

BACK SEQUENCE:

1. RAG DOLL POSE
(page 124)

2. SQUAT with rag doll arms overhead

3. DOWNWARD DOG (page 100)

4. CAT/COW POSE (page 83)

A)

B)

5. GATE POSE
(each side)
(page 84)

6. HALF SPINAL TWIST
(each side) (page 172)

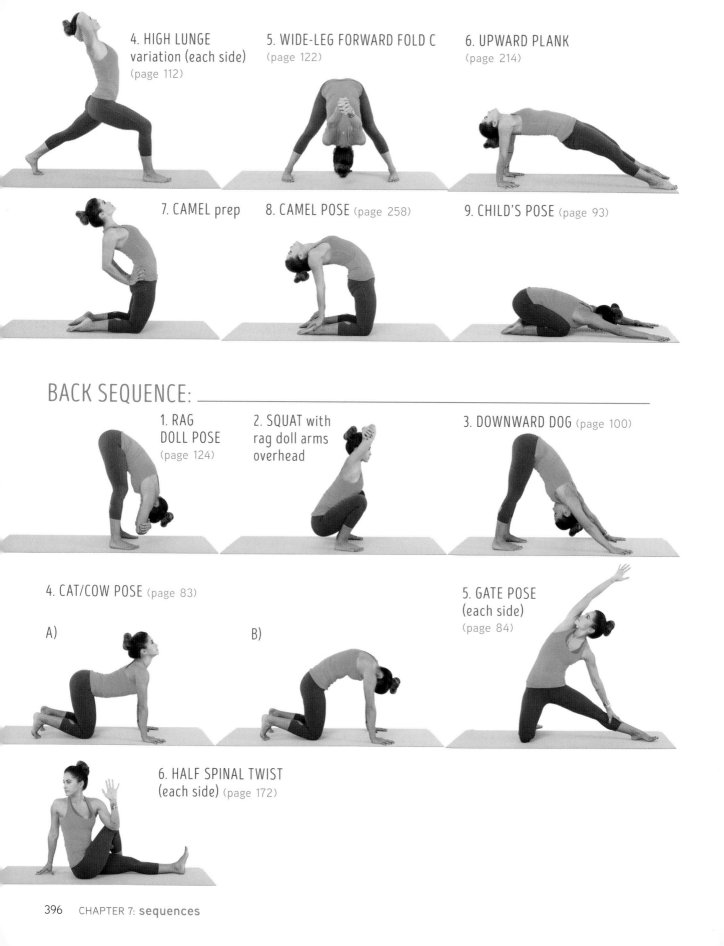

ARMS SEQUENCE:

1. THREAD THE NEEDLE (each side)

2. COW FACE ARMS (each side)
(page 170)

3. TRICEPS AND NECK STRETCH

A)

B)

C)

4. INTENSE SHOULDER STRETCH (each side)

A)

B)

5. DOWNWARD DOG
(page 100)

6. DOLPHIN POSE
(page 197)

7. CHILD'S POSE
(page 93)

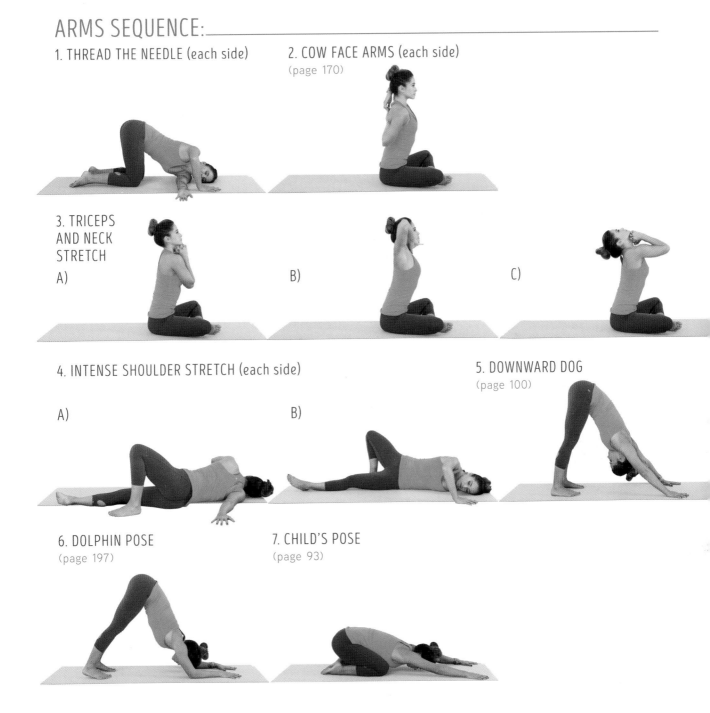

pre-run yoga

These sequences are designed to help stretch the entire body prior to a run. Aim for three to five deep breaths in each pose before lacing up and being on your way.

PRE-RUN SEQUENCE 1:

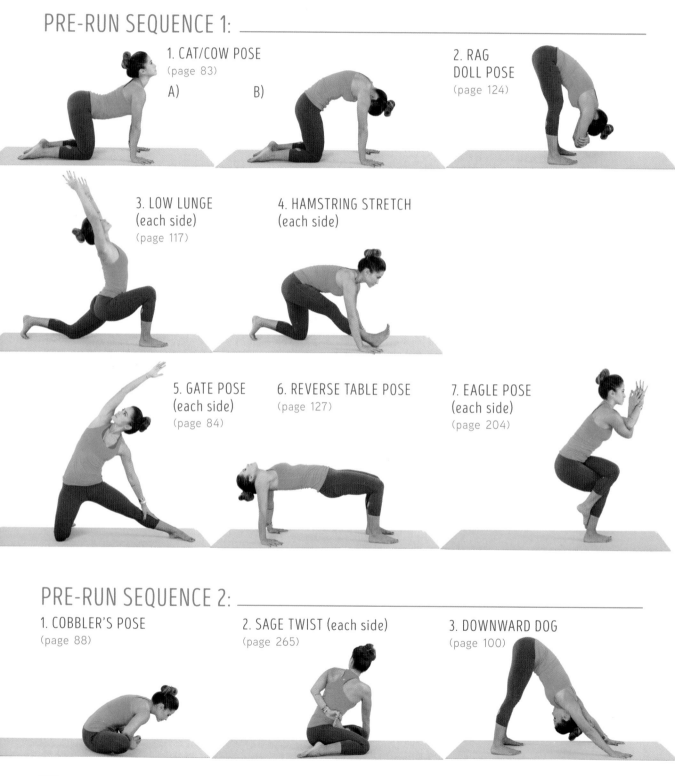

1. CAT/COW POSE
(page 83)

A)

B)

2. RAG DOLL POSE
(page 124)

3. LOW LUNGE
(each side)
(page 117)

4. HAMSTRING STRETCH
(each side)

5. GATE POSE
(each side)
(page 84)

6. REVERSE TABLE POSE
(page 127)

7. EAGLE POSE
(each side)
(page 204)

PRE-RUN SEQUENCE 2:

1. COBBLER'S POSE
(page 88)

2. SAGE TWIST (each side)
(page 265)

3. DOWNWARD DOG
(page 100)

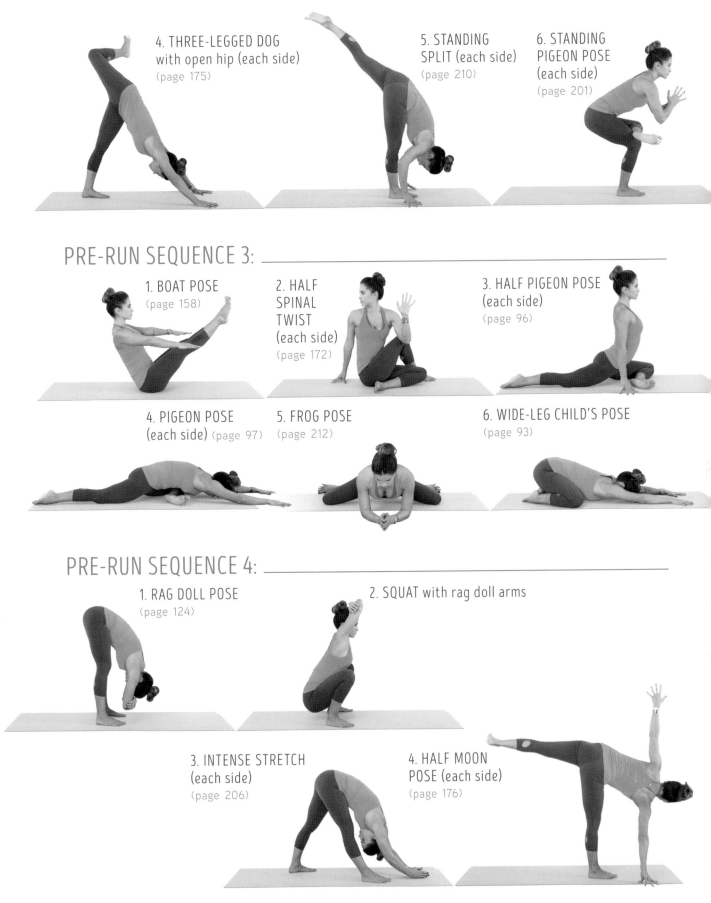

4. THREE-LEGGED DOG
with open hip (each side)
(page 175)

5. STANDING SPLIT (each side)
(page 210)

6. STANDING PIGEON POSE (each side)
(page 201)

PRE-RUN SEQUENCE 3:

1. BOAT POSE
(page 158)

2. HALF SPINAL TWIST (each side)
(page 172)

3. HALF PIGEON POSE (each side)
(page 96)

4. PIGEON POSE (each side) (page 97)

5. FROG POSE (page 212)

6. WIDE-LEG CHILD'S POSE (page 93)

PRE-RUN SEQUENCE 4:

1. RAG DOLL POSE
(page 124)

2. SQUAT with rag doll arms

3. INTENSE STRETCH (each side)
(page 206)

4. HALF MOON POSE (each side)
(page 176)

PRE-RUN SEQUENCE 5: _____

1. SUPINE 4 STRETCH
(each side)

2. roll up to BOAT POSE
(page 158)

A)

B) C) D)

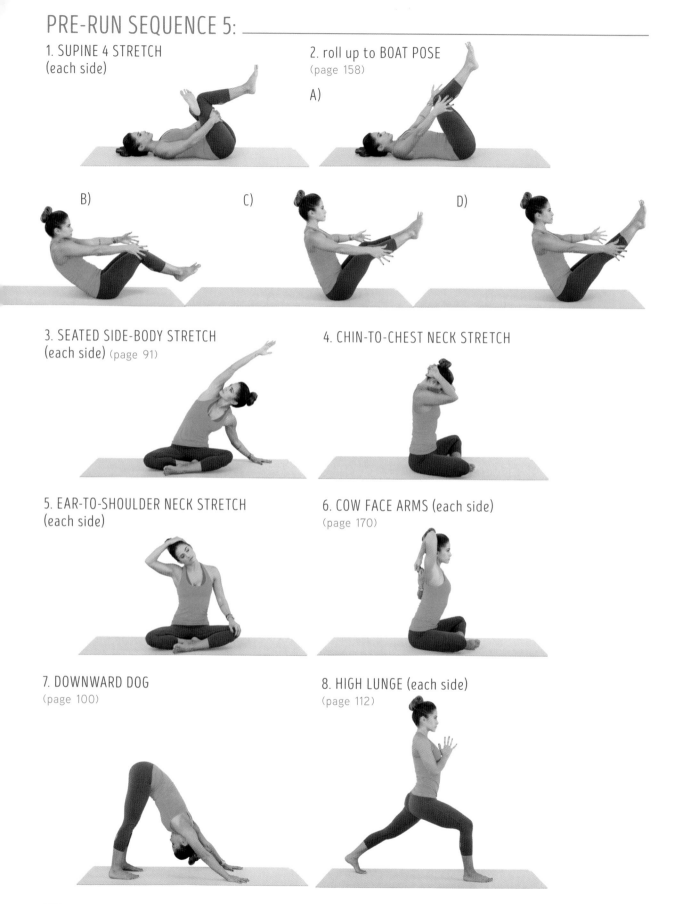

3. SEATED SIDE-BODY STRETCH
(each side) (page 91)

4. CHIN-TO-CHEST NECK STRETCH

5. EAR-TO-SHOULDER NECK STRETCH
(each side)

6. COW FACE ARMS (each side)
(page 170)

7. DOWNWARD DOG
(page 100)

8. HIGH LUNGE (each side)
(page 112)

post-run yoga

These quick sequences are designed to cool down the body after a run. Take three to five deep breaths (or more if you like) in each pose before moving on.

POST-RUN SEQUENCE 1:

1. FIRE LOG POSE (each side) (page 87)

2. COW FACE POSE (each side) (page 170)

A)

B)

3. SUPPORTED BRIDGE POSE (page 310)

4. HERON POSE (each side) (page 174)

5. HERO POSE (page 94)

6. RECLINED HERO POSE (page 217)

7. RECLINED BOUND ANGLE POSE (page 135)

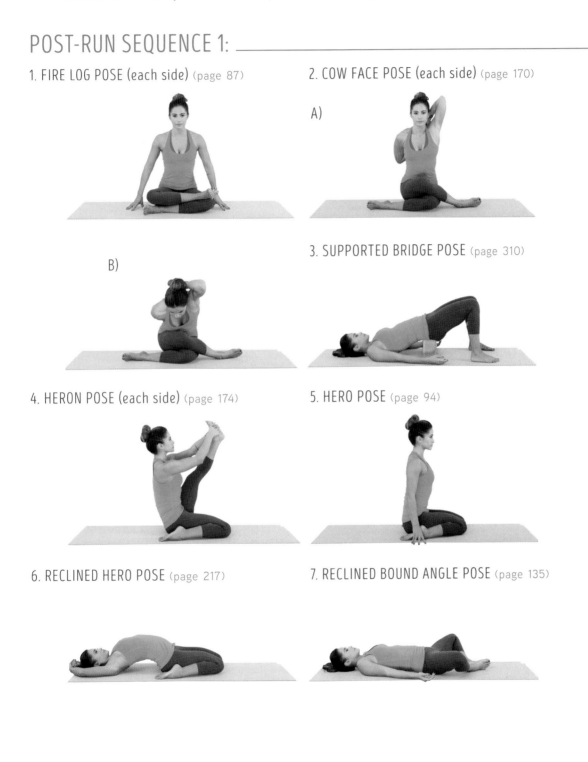

POST-RUN SEQUENCE 2:

1. GARLAND POSE (page 182)

with option to bind (each side) (page 184)

2. SEATED PIRIFORMIS STRETCH

A)

B)

alternate view

with option to take arms under

3. HAPPY BABY POSE (page 130)

4. RECLINED FROG POSE

5. SUPINE SPINAL TWIST (each side) (page 213)

POST-RUN SEQUENCE 3:

1. EASY POSE forward fold (each side) (page 90)

2. STANDING HAND-TO-BIG-TOE POSE A (each side) (page 188)

3. TRIANGLE POSE (each side) (page 185)

4. LOCUST POSE A (page 215)

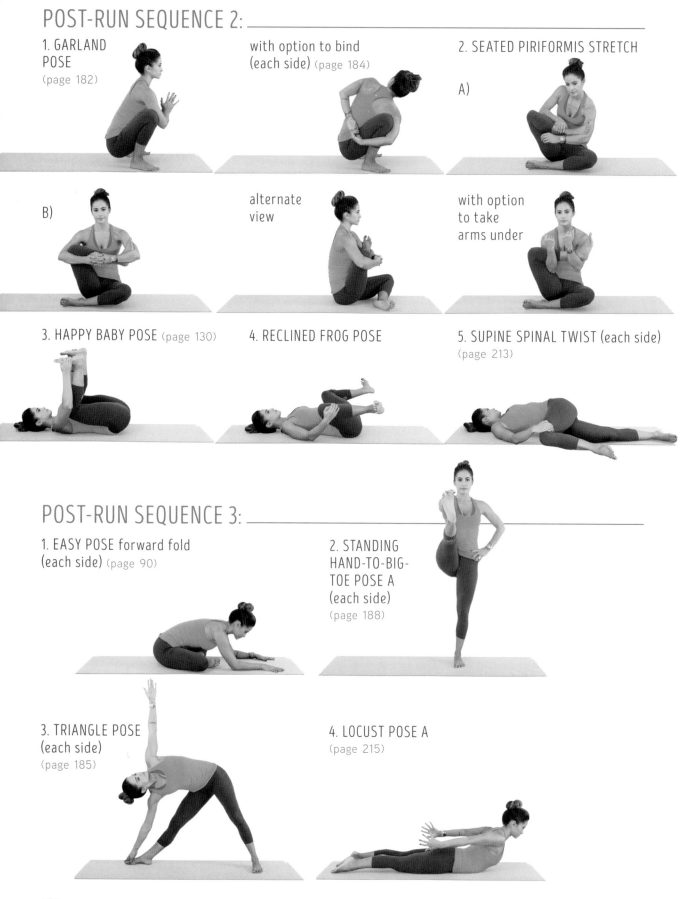

POST-RUN SEQUENCE 4:

1. SEATED FORWARD FOLD with feet mat width (page 85)

2. SEATED FORWARD FOLD hip-opening variation

3. HALF-LOTUS SEATED FORWARD FOLD (each side) (page 168)

4. HALF HAPPY BABY POSE (each side) (page 130)

5. SUPINE SPINAL TWIST with eagle legs (each side) (page 213)

6. HALF RECLINED FROG POSE (each side)

POST-RUN SEQUENCE 5:

1. GATE POSE (each side) (page 84)

2. CAT/COW POSE (page 83)

A)

B)

3. EXTENDED PUPPY DOG POSE (page 99)

4. INTENSE SHOULDER STRETCH (each side)

5. CHILD'S POSE with twist (each side) (page 93)

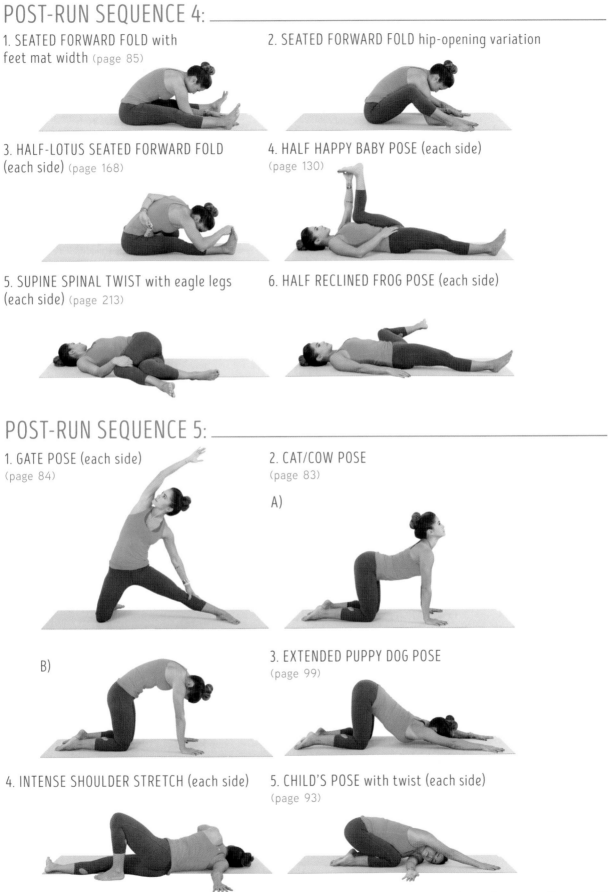

yoga for insomnia

These sequences are designed to be relaxing and calming to help ensure a solid night's sleep. Take three to five deep breaths in each pose (or more if you like) before moving on.

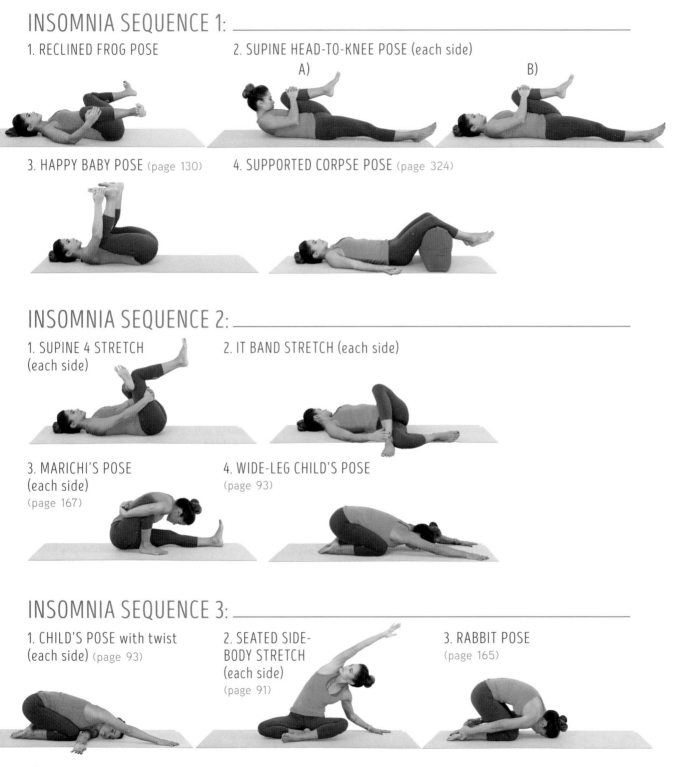

INSOMNIA SEQUENCE 1:

1. RECLINED FROG POSE

2. SUPINE HEAD-TO-KNEE POSE (each side)
   A)
   B)

3. HAPPY BABY POSE (page 130)

4. SUPPORTED CORPSE POSE (page 324)

INSOMNIA SEQUENCE 2:

1. SUPINE 4 STRETCH (each side)

2. IT BAND STRETCH (each side)

3. MARICHI'S POSE (each side) (page 167)

4. WIDE-LEG CHILD'S POSE (page 93)

INSOMNIA SEQUENCE 3:

1. CHILD'S POSE with twist (each side) (page 93)

2. SEATED SIDE-BODY STRETCH (each side) (page 91)

3. RABBIT POSE (page 165)

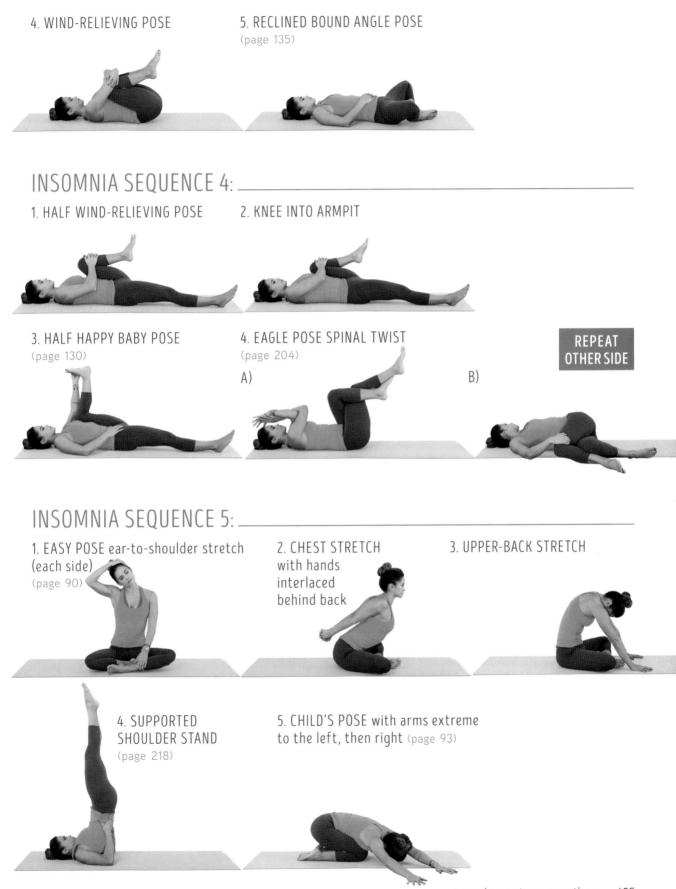

4. WIND-RELIEVING POSE

5. RECLINED BOUND ANGLE POSE
(page 135)

INSOMNIA SEQUENCE 4:

1. HALF WIND-RELIEVING POSE

2. KNEE INTO ARMPIT

3. HALF HAPPY BABY POSE
(page 130)

4. EAGLE POSE SPINAL TWIST
(page 204)

A)

B)

REPEAT OTHER SIDE

INSOMNIA SEQUENCE 5:

1. EASY POSE ear-to-shoulder stretch
(each side)
(page 90)

2. CHEST STRETCH
with hands
interlaced
behind back

3. UPPER-BACK STRETCH

4. SUPPORTED SHOULDER STAND
(page 218)

5. CHILD'S POSE with arms extreme
to the left, then right (page 93)

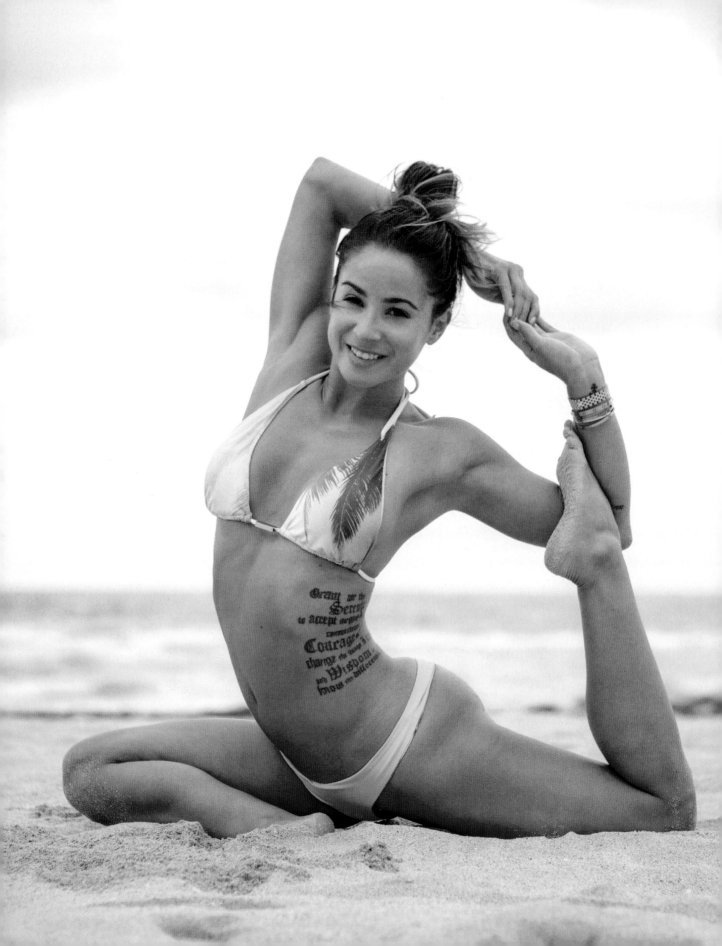

afterword:
Namaslay

Admittedly, I'm only in my early thirties, so I don't have ~~anything~~ it all figured out, but I'm on a good path. These days, I feel so good. I feel unstoppable. I wake up every day and jump out of bed, psyched to get the day started.

Sometimes I wonder how long this sense of wonder will last—the way I look at the world around me in awe, with gratitude for all the simple things. Like the sunrise I catch as I drink my morning tea. And the fact that there are, like, seven billion of us roaming around on this spinning planet that revolves perfectly around the sun next to a moon that controls the oceans. You know, the little things.

But seriously.

No, seriously.

It's pretty incredible to feel this way, but yeah, I worry that maybe it's not real. Maybe this light that drives my days will burn out. Maybe this is a fleeting, temporary joy.

When I travel to New York, I sometimes find myself on edge, and I understand where the angry New Yorker stereotype came from. When I fail to seal a deal for work, I get irritable, annoyed, and frustrated. When I am lacking quality sleep, my days don't look as bright. Some days I'm not a Hell Yeah person. Sometimes I fall into the victim mentality. I still get a case of the Poor Me's now and then.

But I'll tell you something: it never lasts very long. Because living in that way isn't enjoyable. It's stressful.

I've come to realize that life goes on. Whatever is going to happen will happen, regardless of whether I'm hating the world for all its ugliness or I'm seeking its beauty. So why not live with eyes wide open and a heart that's full?

Why not smile more? Offer a kind word? Manifest gratitude? Celebrate my strength? Go after what I want without considering what might go wrong? Why not allow myself to dream big, listen to my heart, and give it what it needs?

It feels good to do this, but it's work. It takes effort, especially at first, to look on the bright side. To commit to believing in myself. To manifest gratitude. To get out of my comfort zone. To act kinder than I feel. To take the time to do the little things.

But when I do?

Oh man, when I do, it's like living a dream—a dream in which I am able to get through anything. In which the people around me are good and kind and lift me up. In which I am strong, confident, and able to do whatever it is I put my mind to and work toward. In the dream, the world around me is vibrant and buzzing, and everything is so alive. It's the most incredible dream I could dream up. And the best part? It's my reality.

So when I encounter people who don't feel the same way, who feel tired, angry, defeated, and defensive, I want to simultaneously give them a hug and shake them and tell them, "Wake up! You don't have to feel this way!"

Are you one of those people?

If you are, I feel for you. That defensive place where you wear armor to protect yourself, where you feel the world is out to get you, is a tough place to be. It is a constant battle. It's exhausting. I've been there. I do not want to return.

It's like you've built a wall to keep out the pain, and I understand putting up that barrier to protect yourself. If you've been dealt a shitty hand time and again, I understand wanting to retreat to that place. I'd even argue that for a hot second, it's a good place to stop, catch your breath, and regroup. But don't hang out there for long. The same wall you built up to keep out the pain will also keep out the good—all the too-big smiles, all the throw-your-head-back laughs, all the things that make life so mind-blowingly beautiful.

The thing I've come to realize is that every moment is an opportunity to learn. If you approach the things that have brought you pain with eyes and heart wide open, then they become lessons. Don't run away from the hard stuff—from the fear and the unknown. Instead, carve out a little space to sit in the discomfort and breathe it all in. And then make your decision. Will you lie down and give in to the discomfort, or will you get up and soldier on?

I encourage you to get up, no matter how many times you're knocked down. Strain to hear the little voice inside you that lets you know you are bigger than any obstacle you may encounter. Ask yourself how you can grow from each experience. Cultivate a willingness to soften despite the things that may have hardened you.

The yoga practice is the perfect vehicle to do this. The beautiful thing about yoga is that what happens on the mat is often reflective of what's going on in our lives. So when you're on your mat, check in with yourself. Notice where you are tense. Notice the poses that you avoid. Notice when you're fidgety and irritable and how that translates into your practice. Use the yoga practice to get to know yourself, and then approach these facets of your practice bravely and confidently. Sift through the stuff you're carrying with you and discard anything you're holding onto that's not helping you progress in your practice and in your life. It won't be easy. You may face demons. You may have to weed through layers upon layers of hard exterior that you've put up to protect yourself. But it will feel freeing, and it will be worth it.

Make the commitment to press pause on your busy life and take time to get to know yourself. Ask yourself what is it that you need. What is it that you want? And is what you are doing, being, and experiencing expanding and adding vibrancy to your life? If the answer is no, it's time to make a change.

Don't focus on the destination because real life is not a destination. Real life beats to a pulse of constant change. So allow yourself to march, dance, and soar through life with an open heart, knowing that you have the opportunity to learn from every situation, and that in every moment you have the privilege of experiencing and growing. Be unapologetic in the evolution of your life and own every moment, knowing that you are meant to be there. When you get knocked down, remember that our brightest moments are often born from our darkest struggles. Keep fighting. Run and leap over your perceived limits. Tap into your inherent greatness. Keep working on the phenomenal masterpiece of your life, making it as beautiful as you can. And don't take any shit.

Namaslay.

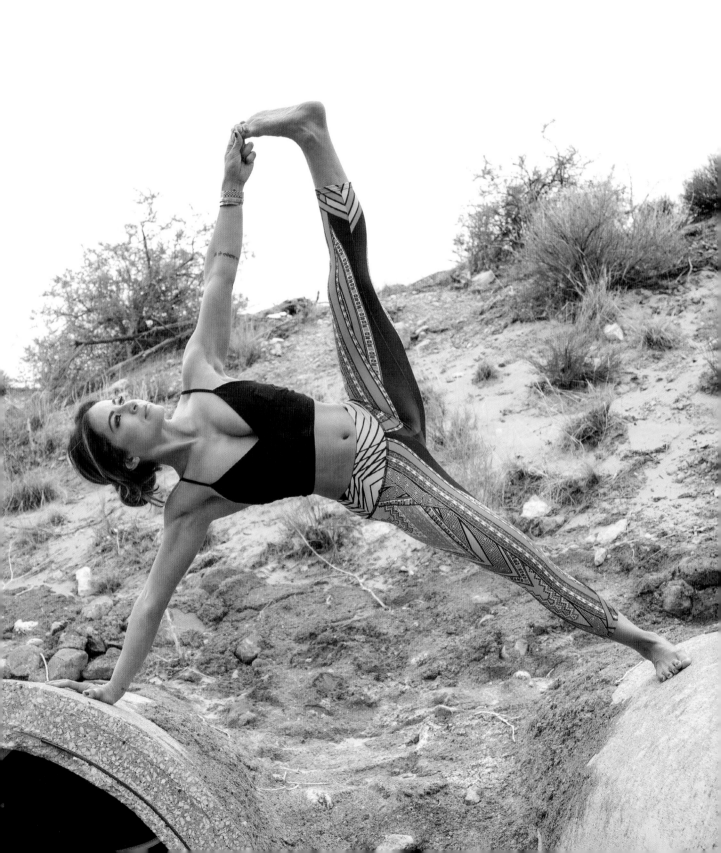

acknowledgments

First and foremost, thank you to the YBC Community. You have made the world feel like a small town. I wouldn't be where I am today without you, and I thank each and every one of you from the bottom of my heart for your support.

This book would not be possible without the support of those around me. Biggest thanks to my right-hand woman and marketing director, Lauren Wotherspoon, for your determination, hard work, yes-I-can attitude, and dedication to YBC. Thank you to Madison Mundy for your attention to detail and feedback.

Thank you to Hayley Mason for your support from the very beginning and for introducing me to Victory Belt.

Thank you to the entire Victory Belt family—you have literally helped make a dream come true and were a joy to work with throughout this entire process. Special thanks to Glen Cordoza, who shot with us for thirteen hours straight, for your hell-yeah attitude and for being down with the old-school hip hop playlist. Thanks to Jaqueline Shepherd and Whitney VanOsdel for bringing such contagious great energy to the photo shoot and for making me look as beautiful on the outside as I felt on the inside. Thanks to Coach Bryan Zobre for getting me in the best shape of my life—I still hear you saying, "And drive!" A huge thank you to Coach James Keeler for keeping me in the best shape of my life, for the constant encouragement, and for being such a huge inspiration in my continued pursuit of health and fitness.

My deepest gratitude goes to all my incredible yoga instructors over the years, including the lovely teachers at Kripalu and the brilliant duo of Raquel Salvador and Mark Ansari. Your teachings have helped shape me into the instructor and person I am today.

As a former (Spanish) teacher, I want to be sure to take time to thank my own teachers. Teachers have one of the toughest jobs out there, and it's often a thankless one. Please know that whether you're a kindergarten teacher or a college professor, what you say and how you teach matter. The following people have had a huge impact on my personal development as well as my writing. I feel tremendously thankful to have had the privilege of being a student of some of the best educators in the world. To Janet Neary and Margaret Ruotolo—thank you for helping to instill self-confidence from an early age. To Joan Wingard—thank you for your collaborative teaching style, which fueled my passion to teach. To Paula Rogers—thank you for teaching me that cookies and cakes are done and people are finished, and for teaching with a sense of humor and joy; you made middle school a place I wanted to be. To Don Looney—thank you for teaching me to watch out for "staccato" writing, for your wry sense of humor, and for being unapologetically yourself. To Denise Feikema—I use what you've taught me on a daily basis and cannot thank you enough for the fact that you put so much time and energy into helping me write with confidence. To all teachers everywhere, thank you for what you're doing.

To my dear friends Spencer, Kent, Zach, Julius, Geoff, Sean, and my gang of Cool Girls: Kat, Meredith, Maryann, Misty, Jenna, and Carley. They say you're the sum of the people around you, and I am so thankful you are all in my life. Thank you for always giving it to me straight, having my back, your constant encouragement, and your brilliant sense of humor. I love you guys.

index

A huge thank you to my in-laws, Jan and Moe, for their constant support and willingness to drop everything and help. I appreciate you both so much. To my dad and brother for their unconditional love and support. And to my biggest cheerleader, my mom, the original Cool Girl, I love you to the moon and back and thank you from the bottom of my heart for being the most wonderful mother.

And last but definitely not least, thank you to my husband, Greg, for for shooting such incredible images for the blog and this book and for being the best human I know. Your quiet determination, calm nature, and tireless pursuit of your dreams have always been such inspirations to me.